English for Paramedics

English for Paramedics

Case Studies

Angličtina pro záchranáře: Kazuistiky

IRENA BAUMRUKOVÁ

To order additional copies of this book, contact:
Xlibris LLC
0-800-056-3182
www.xlibrispublishing.co.uk
Orders@xlibrispublishing.co.uk
521019

CONTENTS

VOLUME 2

Angličtina pro záchranáře je určena **studentům středních a vyšších zdravotnických škol a studentům medicíny**, kteří se chtějí zdokonalit v angličtině a současně si zajímavou formou procvičit odborné učivo.

V prvním díle učebnice se případy týkají **dýchacích cest, dýchání a oběhového systému** (zhodnocení a intervence u pacientů s dýchacími obtížemi, dodávání kyslíku, podpory ventilace, anatomie a fyziologie dýchacího systému, základního ošetření dýchacích cest, základní kardiopulmonární resuscitace).

Jiné kazuistiky popisují naléhavé stavy v **oblasti neurologie, endokrinologie, gastroenterologie, urologie, toxikologie** a obtíže spojené s **vlivy prostředí.** Další případy se týkají **problémů chování**, či radí jak **posoudit a ošetřit úrazy.**

Samostatná kapitola je věnována **gynekologii, porodnictví a pediatrii.** Poslední část se zabývá obecnými **zásadami při zásahu** (základní fyziologie a posouzení stavu pacienta, bezpečnost místa, manipulace s vozidly, operace na místě nehody, ochrana před infekcí, právní zřetele, komunikace, dokumentace, hromadné nehody, nebezpečné materiály).

Druhý díl je rozdělen do **24 jednotek**, z nichž každá obsahuje kolem 20 případů. Texty obsahově pokrývají veškerou problematiku, nejsou však rozřazeny do tematických skupin, což umožňuje opakovat a **doplňovat učivo** prvního dílu novým a objevným způsobem.

Kazuistiky byly převzaty z materiálů určených k **samostatnému testování znalostí** studentů, **budoucích záchranářů**. Při výběru byly zohledněny jazykové potřeby **středně pokročilých** studentů a u každé lekce jsou uvedena obsažená slovíčka. Podrobný anglicko český slovník na konci publikace obsahuje i nejzákladnější výrazy a proto rovněž **motivovaní začátečníci** mohou snadno postupovat při studiu pomalejším tempem.

Texty jsou krátké, přehledné, psané aktuálním jazykem a vždy **obsahují i správnou odpověď** (ta je označena hvězdičkou). **Metoda**

doplňování vhodných výrazů je zábavná a obzvláště účinná při nenásilném osvojování nových slov v kontextu známých faktů.

Učitelé jistě najdou **inspiraci pro další využití** kazuistik, např. jako doplnění teoretických lekcí, pro vytváření modelových situací, procvičování dialogů ap.

Autorka přeje studentům hodně úspěchů a radosti z učení.

Praha 2013

Case studies

Check your professional knowledge. Practise your language skills. Fill in suitable words. Translate into Czech.

Kazuistiky

Ověřte si své odborné znalosti. Procvičujte jazykové dovednosti. Doplňte vhodné výrazy. Přeložte do češtiny.

VOLUME I

Part I
Airway and breathing

Airway and breathing assessment; proper interventions for patients with respiratory compromise; oxygen delivery systems; ventilatory support; respiratory anatomy and physiology; basic airway management; basic cardiopulmonary resuscitation; advanced interventions

Unit I
1
The absence of carbon dioxide in _____ ___ indicates the endotracheal tube has been placed in the oesophagus.*
The _____ __ carbon dioxide likely indicates that the _____ ____ has been placed in the oesophagus.
_____ correct endotracheal tube placement is absolutely essential.
Your next action is to remove the endotracheal tube and provide several ventilations prior to attempting intubation again.*
The endotracheal tube is likely placed in the _____. Your next action is to _____ the endotracheal tube and provide _____ _____ with

supplemental oxygen _____ __ attempting another intubation.

remove, prior to, several ventilations, oesophagus, Verifying, absence of, endotracheal tube, exhaled air

2
The ____ used to describe normal breath sounds heard over most of the _____ ____ is:
- _____
- _____
- vesicular*
- bronchovesicular

chest wall, term, bronchial, adventitious

3
Breath sounds such as _____ ___ _____ that are not normally heard are _____ __:
- bronchial
- adventitious*
- vesicular
- bronchovesicular

crackles and rhonchi, defined as

4
The following correctly describes the flow of air from outside the body into the trachea: nose, _____ _____, nasopharynx, oropharynx, _____, larynx, _____.*

nasal cavities, trachea,
laryngopharynx

5

You are called for an unresponsive 29-year-old man. Bystanders report he has been drinking heavily all day. Assessment reveals the patient to be responsive only to painful stimuli. His breathing is shallow at a rate of 4 times per minute.

How would you manage this patient? Bag-valve device with a reservoir at 10-15 LPM.*

Breathing must be supported with a ___-_____ _____ with _____ high-flow oxygen. This patient's breathing is too ____ and too _____ to receive enough oxygen for proper ___ _____ to take place.

slow, gas exchange, bag-valve
device, shallow, supplemental

6

The area where the trachea _____ into the right and left main stem _____ is known as the:

- pleura
- xiphoid process
- carina*
- _____ angle

divides, bronchi, sternal

7

The administration of which of the following may result in a decrease in the respiratory rate? Morphine sulphate.*

_____ is an opiate that can cause _____ _____ _____ depression. Administration may result in a _____ in the respiratory rate. Patients receiving morphine must be monitored closely for _____ _____.

respiratory depression, central
nervous system, Morphine,
decrease

8

The _____ _____ between the base of the _____ and the _____ into which the tip of the curved blade (Macintosh blade) is placed during _____ intubation is the:

- carina
- vallecula*
- glottis
- oesophagus

tongue, orotracheal, anatomical
structure, epiglottis

9

When blood levels of carbon dioxide or hydrogen ions _____ above normal, the respiratory centre of the brain responds by increasing the rate and depth of respiration.*

_____ ___ _____ of respiration are increased to _____ excess CO_2 and therefore decrease hydrogen ion concentrations. This is a normal _____ _____ of the body.

compensatory mechanism, increase, Rate and depth, eliminate

10

The blood component _____ for transporting oxygen from the _____ to the ____ _____ and transporting _____ _____ from the body tissues to the lungs is the:

- plasma
- platelets
- leukocytes
- erythrocytes*

responsible, carbon dioxide, lungs, body tissues

11

What is the _____ of the laryngeal mask airway (___)? It is blindly inserted.*
LMA insertion does not require _____.

LMA, laryngoscopy, advantage

12

What is often a ____ _____ in patients with respiratory distress? Cyanosis.

_____ is a late finding and may not __ _____ even when the patient is severely _____.

Cyanosis, hypoxic, be present, late finding

13

You have a female patient with a long history of COPD who complains of worsening shortness of breath. She is on continuous 2 LMP of home oxygen.
You are concerned that increasing the oxygen flow may eliminate the hypoxic drive to breathe because the hypoxic rate is regulated by low PaO_2.*

_____ _____ to breathe is common in patients with COPD or other _____ respiratory disorders. Hypoxic drive is regulated by a low PaO_2 (_____ __ _____). Delivering an _____ _____ of oxygen may increase the PaO_2 and therefore eliminate the drive to breathe.

increased concentration, degenerative, Hypoxic drive, partial pressure of oxygen

14

You arrive on the scene of a patient who is receiving bag-valve mask ventilation. The abdomen is extremely distended. After intubation, you have resistance while _____ the patient.
Lung sounds are diminished _____, and the trachea is midline.
What should you do? Insert a naso/oral gastric tube.*
When _____ _____ interferes with _____, insertion of a naso/oral gastric tube into the stomach __ _____.

> ventilations, is indicated, gastric distension, bagging, bilaterally

15

The simplest airway management _____ in a patient without suspected _____ _____ injury is the head-tilt/chin-lift _____.

> manoeuvre,* cervical spine, technique

16

The proper size of the _____ airway is determined __ _____ from the corner of the mouth to the tip of the earlobe at the angle of the jaw.*
It is essential that the OPA be sized appropriately because improper sizing can lead to _____ _____.

> airway obstruction, by measuring, oropharyngeal

17

The maximum water pressure recommended for _____ _____ ventilation should not exceed 30 cm.*
The valve opening at the cardiac sphincter (opening into the _____) is approximately 30 cm/H_2O. Not exceeding 30 cm/H_2O will reduce (not eliminate) the occurrence of _____ _____.

> positive pressure, stomach, gastric distension

18

Manual manoeuvres used __ _____ a patient's airway include the head tilt/chin lift and jaw thrust.*
The ____-____/____-____ and ___-_____ manoeuvres are both very effective in initial management of the airway.

> head-tilt/chin-lift, jaw-thrust, to open

19

Advantages of the Oesophageal Tracheal Combitube include all of the following:

- _____ is rapid and easy.*
- It can be used on _____ patients.*
- It can provide ventilation when _____ in the oesophagus.*

It is not indicated for _____ patients due to its large diameter and the risk of _____ of the oesophagus.

> insertion, paediatric, perforation, trauma, placed

20

Causes for decreased ETCO₂ readings include:

- nonperfusing patient*
- presence of severe _____*
- presence of _____ emboli*

All the conditions listed will result in a decreased ETCO₂ reading. Other _____ include shock, bronchospasm, and incomplete airway obstruction (such as _____ plugging).

> causes, mucus, acidosis, pulmonary

21

You are caring for a male patient with ventricular tachycardia. He is lethargic, diaphoretic, and pale and has vomited once. His vital signs are as follows: BP, 74/P; pulse, 184; respirations, 14. You are assigned to manage the airway.

_____ _____ should include _____ the airway for vomitus.*

Remember the basics! You must first open the airway and suction it _____ any other airway management.

Your patient becomes unresponsive and apnoeic. Further airway management should include endotracheal _____.*

> intubation, Initial management, before, suctioning

22

Succinylcholine is contraindicated in patients with crush injures because of risk of hyperkalaemia. Succinylcholine should not be used on _____ trauma, _____, or _____ injuries because these conditions can result in _____.

> crush, hyperkalaemia, blunt, burns

Vocabulary I

abdomen /ˈæb.də.mən/ břicho

acidosis /ˌæs.ɪˈdəʊ.sɪs/ acidóza, porucha acidobazické rovnováhy ve prospěch kyselin, zvýšení kyselé reakce tělesných tekutin, zvýšení aktivity vodíkových iontů

administration /ədˌmɪn.ɪˈstreɪ.ʃən/ podávání léků

advanced /ədˈvɑːnt st/ pokročilý

advantage /ədˈvɑːn.tɪdʒ/ výhoda, přednost

adventitious /ˌæd.vənˈtɪʃ.əs/ nahodilý, vyskytující se na nesprávném místě

airway /ˈeə.weɪ/ dýchací cesty

angle /ˈæŋɡəl/ úhel, hrana, šikmý, nasměrovat, natočit do jistého úhlu

apnoeic /æpˈniː.ɪk/ apnoický, bez dechu

appropriately /əˈprəʊ.pri.ət.li/ vhodně, náležitě, přiměřeně

assessment /əˈses.mənt/ hodnocení, ohodnocení, posudek

assign /əˈsaɪn/ zadat, přidělit

attempt /əˈtemp t/ pokus, pokoušet se, snažit

bag /bæɡ/ pytel, dát do pytle

bag /bæɡ/ **valve** /vælv/ dýchací vak, ruční zařízení, poskytnutí ventilace pozitivním tlakem pacientovi, který nedýchá, nebo dýchá nedostatečně

bag-valve mask /mɑːsk/ dýchací maska

base /beɪs/ spodina, základ, základna

basic /ˈbeɪ.sɪk/ základ, základní

bilaterally /ˌbaɪˈlæt.ər.ə.li/ bilaterálně, dvoustranně

blade /bleɪd/ čepel

blindly /ˈblaɪnd.li/ slepě, naslepo

blunt / blʌnt/ tupý, oblý, přímý

brain /breɪn/ mozek

bronchospasm /ˌbrɒŋ.kəʊ.ˈspæz.əm/ bronchospasmus, křeč průdušek

bronchus /ˈbrɒŋ.kəs/ pl bronchi /-kaɪ/ průduška

burn /bɜːn/ popálenina, hořet

bystander /ˈbaɪˌstæn.dər/ náhodný divák, přihlížející, svědek

carbon /ˈkɑː.bən/ **dioxide** /daɪˈɒk.saɪd/ oxid uhličitý

care / keə/ **for** / fɔː/ starat se, mít zájem, ošetřovat

carina /kəˈraɪn.ə/ člunek, výběžek

cavity /ˈkæv.ɪ.ti/ dutina

chest /tʃest/ **wall** /wɔːl/ hrudní stěna

chin-lift /tʃɪn/, /lɪft/ zvednutí brady

Combi tube /komˈbi.tju:b/ trubice s dvěma průsvity k ventilaci průdušnice při vložení naslepo

common /ˈkɒmən/ běžný, obvyklý

compensatory /ˌkɒm.pənˈseɪt.ə ri/ kompenzační

complain /kəmˈpleɪn/ stěžovat si, naříkat si

component /kəmˈpəʊnənt/ složka, součást

compromise /ˈkɒmprəˌmaɪz/ zhoršení

concern /kənˈsɜːn/ zájem, starost, obavy, znepokojení

continuous /kənˈtɪn.ju.əs/ nepřetržitý, neustálý

contraindicate /ˌkɒn.trəˈɪn.dɪ.keɪt/ kontraindikovat

corner /ˈkɔː.nər/ koutek

correct /kəˈrekt/ správný, přesný, napravit

crackle /ˈkræk.|/ praskot, praskání, šustění

crush /krʌʃ/ drtit, rozdrtit, rozmačkat, rozmáčknout

curved /kɜːvd/ zahnutý, zakřivený

cyanosis /ˌsaɪəˈnəʊ.sɪs/ cyanóza

decrease /dɪˈkriːs/ snížit se, zmenšit, pokles

degenerative /dɪˈdʒen.ər.ə.tɪv/ degenerativní

delivery /dɪˈlɪv.ər.i/ dodání

depression /dɪˈpreʃ.ən/ pokles, krize, deprese, stlačení

depth /depθ/ hloubka, intenzita

device /dɪˈvaɪs/ zařízení, prostředek, vybavení, přístroj

diameter /daɪˈæm.ɪ.tər/ průměr (kružnice)

diaphoretic /ˌdaɪ.ə.fəˈret.ɪk/ diaforetický, opocený

diminish /dɪˈmɪnɪʃ/ zmenšit se, slábnout, ubývat

disorder /dɪˈsɔː.dər/ porucha, choroba, potíže

distend /dɪˈstend/ roztáhnout se, zduřet

distension /dɪˈsten.tʃən/ distenze, roztažení, rozepětí, rozšíření

divide /dɪˈvaɪd/ rozdělit, dělit se

drive /draɪv/ úsilí, snaha

due /djuː/ **to** /tʊ/ kvůli, následkem, v důsledku, díky

earlobe /ˈɪə.ləʊb/ ušní lalůček

eliminate /ɪˈlɪm.ɪ.neɪt/ eliminovat, odstranit

endotracheal /en.dɒ.trəˈkiː.əl/ **tube** /tjuːb/ (**ET tube**) endotracheální trubice, trubice do průdušnice

epiglottis /ˌep.ɪˈglɒt.ɪs/ příklopka hrtanová

erythrocyte /ɪˈrɪθ.rəʊ.saɪt/ erytrocyt, červená krvinka

essential /ɪˈsen.tʃəl/ základní, důležitý, hlavní

excess /ekˈses/ nadměrný, přebytečný

exchange /ɪksˈtʃeɪndʒ/ výměna

extremely /ɪkˈstriːm.li/ extrémně, nesmírně, neobyčejně

flow /fləʊ/ tok, proud, příliv, téci, proudit

gastric /ˈgæs.trɪk/ gastrický, žaludeční

gastric /ˈgæs.trɪk/ **tube** /tjuːb/ žaludeční sonda

glottis /ˈglɒt.ɪs/ pl glotides glotis, hlasivková štěrbina, nejužší část hrtanu

hydrogen /ˈhaɪ.drɪ.dʒən/ vodík

hyperkalaemia /ˌhaɪ.pə.kæˈliː.mi.ə/ hyperkalemie, nadbytek draslíku v krvi

hypoxic /haɪˈpɒk.sɪk/ **drive** /draɪv/ stimulace dýchání nízkým stavem PaO$_2$ (parciální tlak kyslíku v tepenné arteriální krvi)

improper /ɪmˈprɒp.ər/ nevhodný, nesprávný

incomplete /ˌɪn.kəmˈpliːt/ neúplný, nedokončený

initial /ɪˈnɪʃəl/ počáteční, výchozí

insert /ɪnˈsɜːt/ vložit, vsunout

insertion /ɪnˈsɜː.ʃən/ zasazení, aplikace (vložka)

interfere /ˌɪn.təˈfɪər/ interferovat, narušovat, vadit, obtěžovat

intervention /ˌɪn.təˈven.ʃən/
intervence, zákrok
intubation /ˌɪn.tjuːˈbeɪ.ʃən/
intubace, zavedení rourky do
průdušnice
ion /ˈaɪ.ɒn/ iont
jaw /dʒɔː/ čelist
jaw /dʒɔː/ thrust /θrʌst/ zajištění
otevřených dýchacích cest,
předsunutí spodní čelisti
laryngeal /ləˈrɪn.dʒi.əl/ laringeální,
hrtanový
laryngoscopy /ˌlærɪŋˈgɒ.skə.pi/
laryngoskopie, zrakové vyšetření
hrtanu pomocí laryngoskopu
larynx /ˈlær.ɪŋks/ (pl. larynges)
larynx, hrtan
lead /liːd/ zavést, řídit, vedení,
vést, být v čele
lethargic /ləˈθɑːˌdʒɪk/ letargický,
otupělý, netečný
leukocyte /ˈljuː.kə.saɪt/ leukocyt,
bílá krvinka
likely /ˈlaɪklɪ/ pravděpodobný,
vhodný
LPM, Liter /ˈliːtə/ Per /pə/ Minute /
ˈmɪnɪt/ litrů za minutu
lung /lʌŋ/ plíce
mainstem /meɪn.stəm/ bronchus /
ˈbrɒŋ.kəs/ hlavní průduška
manage /ˈmæn.ɪdʒ/ řídit, vést,
organizovat, zvládnout, dokázat
management /ˈmænɪdʒmənt/
řízení, ošetření, léčba
manoeuvre /məˈnuː.və/ manévr,
manipulace, řídit, vést
manual /ˈmæn.ju.əl/ ruční, návod,
pokyny
measure /ˈmeʒ.ər/ měřit

midline /ˈmɪd.laɪn/ střednice
morphine /ˈmɔː.fiːn/ sulphate /ˈsʌl.
feɪt/ morfin sulfát
mouth /maʊθ/ ústa, hrdlo, otvor
mucus /ˈmjuː.kəs/ mukus, hlen, sliz
nasal /ˈneɪ.zəl/ nosní
nasopharynx /ˌneɪ.zəˈfær.ɪŋks/
nosohltan
obstruction /əbˈstrʌk.ʃən/
překážka, ucpání
occurrence /əˈkʌr.ənt s/ případ
výskytu
oesophagus /ɪˈsɒf.ə.gəs/ ezofagus,
jícen
OPA, Oropharyngeal /ˈɔː.rə .fəˈrɪn.
dʒi.əl/ Airway /ˈeə.weɪ/ zařízení
používané k udržení otevřených
horních dýchacích cest
opiate /ˈəʊ.pi.ət/ opiát, lék
obsahující opium nebo jeho
alkaloidy
paediatric /ˌpiː.diˈæt.rɪk/
pediatrický
painful /ˈpeɪn.fəl/ bolestivý,
působící bolest
pale /peɪl/ bledý
partial /ˈpɑː.ʃəl/ pressure /ˈpreʃ.ər/
parciální tlak
perforation /ˌpɜː.fərˈeɪ.ʃən/
perforace, proniknutí, propíchnutí
placement /ˈpleɪs.mənt/ umístění,
rozmístění
plasma /ˈplæz.mə/ plazma
platelet /ˈpleɪt.lət/ krevní destička
pleura /ˈplʊə.rə/ pleura,
pohrudnice
plug /plʌg/ čípek, zátka, zásuvka,
ucpat, uzavřít
pressure /ˈpreʃ.ə/ tlak, stisk, napětí

prior /'praɪə/ **to** /tʊ/ před, přede
proper /'prɒpə/ vhodný
provide /prə'vaɪd/ poskytnout, dodat, zajistit
pulmonary /'pʊl.mə.nə.ri/ pulmonální, plicní
rate /reɪt/ tempo, rychlost, frekvence, míra
recommended /ˌrekə'mendɪd/ doporučený
remove / rɪ'muːv/ odstranit, vyjmout, svléknout si
report /rɪ'pɔːt/ oznámit, podat zprávu, hlášení
require /rɪ'kwaɪər/ nutně potřebovat, požadovat
reservoir /'rez.ə.vwɑːr/ ložisko, rezervoár, nádrž
resistance /rɪ'zɪs.tənt s/ rezistence, odpor, odolnost
respond /rɪ'spɒnd/ odpovědět, reagovat
responsible /rɪ'spɒnt.sɪ.b̩l/ odpovědný, zodpovídat se
responsive /rɪ'spɒnt.sɪv/ vnímavý, reagující, citlivý na co
reveal /rɪ'viːl/ odhalit, prozradit, objevit
rhonchus /rong'kəs/ pl. -chi chrapot
shallow /'ʃæl.əʊ/ mělký
shortness /'ʃɔːt.nəs/ nedostatečnost
shortness /'ʃɔːt.nəs/ **of breath** / breθ/ dyspnoe, dušnost
size /saɪz/ velikost, rozměry
sound /saʊnd/ zvuk, znít
sphincter /'sfɪŋk.tər/ svěrač

sternal /'stɔː.nəl/ sternální, týkající se hrudní kosti
stimulus /'stɪm.jʊ.ləs/ pl stimuli podnět, popud
suction /'sʌk.ʃən/ odsávání, odsávat
supplemental /ˌsʌp.lɪ'men.təl/ doplňkový, dodatečný
support /'sə.pɔːt/ podpora
tachycardia /ˌtæk.ɪ'kɑː.di.ə/ tachykardie
therefore /'ðeə.fɔːr/ proto, toho důvodu
tilt /tɪlt/ naklonit, sklon, sklopit
tip /tɪp/ špička, hrot
tissue /'tɪʃ.uː/, /'tɪs.juː/ tkáň
tongue /tʌŋ/ jazyk, špice
trachea /trə'kiː.ə/ trachea, průdušnice
trauma /'trɔː.mə/ trauma, zranění
unresponsive /ˌʌn.rɪ'spɒnt .sɪv/ bez reakce, nereagující, netečný
vallecula /və'lek.jʊl.ə/ valekula, jamka, žlábek
ventilation /ˌven.tɪ'leɪ.ʃən/ ventilace, dýchání, výměna plynů
ventilatory /'ventɪˌleɪtə.rɪ/ ventilační, dechový
ventricular /ven'trɪk.jə.lər/ ventrikulární, komorový
verify /'ver.ɪ.faɪ/ verifikovat, ověřit si, potvrdit
vomitus /'vɒm.ɪ.təs/ vomitus, zvratky
xiphoid /zi.foid/ **process** /'proʊ.ses/ měčovitý výběžek

Unit 2

I

What effects does hyperventilation have on cerebral circulation and intracranial pressure? More pronounced decrease in circulation than decrease in intracranial pressure.*
CO_2 is a very potent _____. When a patient is hyperventilating, CO_2 is removed, and the _____ will become constricted. This vasoconstriction leads to decreased _____ _____ by _____ cerebral blood flow.

> decreasing, vessels, vasodilator, cerebral pressure

2

A respiratory pattern characterized by an _____ _____, rate, and volume with _____ periods of apnoea is called Biot's (ataxic) respiration.*
This pattern is seen in patients with increased _____ _____.

> intermittent, intracranial pressure, irregular pattern

3

A _____ _____ characterized by deep, rapid _____ is called central neurogenic hyperventilation.*

This breathing pattern is usually seen as a loss of normal _____ of ventilatory control.

> regulation, respiratory pattern, respirations

4

A respiratory pattern characterized by ____, shallow, irregular respirations is called bradypnoea.*
This breathing pattern can be associated with _____ or several other _____ _____ disorders.

> nervous system, stroke, slow

5

All of the following can affect the accuracy reading of a pulse oximeter:
- hypoperfusion*
- anaemia*
- carbon monoxide poisoning*

Other circumstances that can affect the _____ include exposure to nail polish or acrylic nails, dark pigmentation or _____, and high bilirubin concentration. Hyperthermia (fever) should not affect the accuracy of a pulse oximeter _____.

> bruising, reading, accuracy

6

Complications of endotracheal intubation include all of the following:
- _____ to the teeth*
- oesophageal intubation*
- laryngospasm*

Gastric distension usually occurs with bag-valve mask ventilations _____ intubation. A correctly placed endotracheal tube should not contribute to _____ _____.

> gastric distension, prior to, trauma

7

Confirmation of _____ ____ placement should be evaluated:
- _____ after insertion*
- each time the patient is moved*
- by __ ____ two methods*

> immediately, at least, endotracheal tube

8

You are using an end-tidal carbon dioxide detector as a tool to assist in proper endotracheal intubation placement. The absence of carbon dioxide in exhaled air indicates that the endotracheal tube has been:

- placed in the right main stem bronchus
- correctly placed in the trachea
- placed in the oesophagus*
- placed in the left main stem bronchus

The use of end-tidal _____ _____ (ETCO$_2$) detection is one tool to assess for proper _____ ____ placement. The _____ of carbon dioxide likely indicates that the endotracheal tube has been placed in the _____. Verifying correct endotracheal tube placement is absolutely _____. ETCO$_2$ detection is only one method to assist in the verification of proper placement.

> endotracheal tube, absence, essential, carbon dioxide, oesophagus

9

The minimum-size bag-valve mask device used for neonates, infants, and children should be 450 ml. Although it is likely that the ___-_____ ____ will not deliver 450 ml of volume, it is important to have a device _____ __ delivering excessive volumes because, as the bag __ _____, there is dead space from which air cannot be _____ expelled.

> is compressed, fully, bag-valve mask, capable of

10

A high-pitched noise associated with upper-airway _____ is known as:
- wheezing
- rhonchi
- stridor*
- rales

This can be __ _____ of pending complete airway obstruction when associated with _____ such as anaphylactic shock.

> conditions, an indication, constriction

11

The next five questions are basic life-support questions:
- Before providing _____ _____ to an unresponsive victim, you must _____ ___ breathing. You do this by looking, listening, and feeling _____ through the victim's nose or mouth.*
- You are performing rescue breathing on an adult. How many _____ do you give? One breath every 5 seconds.*

- Where would you place your hands on the chest of an adult victim when you are performing _____ _____? On the lower half of the sternum, at the nipple line.*
- What is the ratio of compressions to _____ when performing one-person CPR on an adult? 30 compressions to 2 ventilations.*
- What is the correct rate you should use to perform chest compressions for an adult victim of _____ _____? 100 times per minute.*

> airflow, check for, ventilations, chest compressions, rescue breathing, breaths, cardiac arrest

12

You are _____ rescue breathing with a ___-____ device for an apnoeic child. How often should you provide rescue breaths?____ _____ 3 seconds.*

> performing, once every, bag-mask

13

In a patient in _____ _____, the development of which sign/symptom would lead you __ _____ the patient is significantly _____? Cyanosis.*

---
decompensating, respiratory
distress, to believe

14
You respond to a cafeteria for a 16-year-old patient who is choking. Your patient is conscious and coughing forcefully. She appears anxious and is difficult to communicate with due to the coughing but is able to _____ _____. Assessment reveals a respiratory rate of 28, _____, diminished breath sounds on the right side, and a SpO$_2$ reading of 96%. Based on the history and _____ _____, you suspect aspiration of food into the right main stem bronchus causing obstruction.*
Based on the history of the patient _____, a constant cough (from bronchospasm), and diminished breath sounds (obstruction) on the right should lead you to suspect _____ of food.

---
shallow, choking, assessment
findings, follow commands,
aspiration

15
Nasotracheal intubation is _____ in a patient with a suspected basilar skull fracture.*

A suspected basilar _____ _____ is a contraindication for nasotracheal intubation because the _____ ___ of the endotracheal tube could enter the _____ _____ through the fracture site.

---
skull fracture, cranial cavity,
contraindicated, distal tip

16
Blind nasotracheal intubation should be attempted on a patient with spontaneous respirations.* _____ nasotracheal intubation requires the patient to have _____ respirations because the endotracheal tube __ _____ as the patient inhales.

---
spontaneous, is inserted, Blind

17
You arrive on the scene of a 40-year-old male with a _____ __ palpitations and dizziness. _____ are as follows: BP, 102/78; pulse, 128 and slightly irregular; and respirations of 26. A pulse oximeter reading of 86% is obtained. He has __ ____ medical problems. With this information, you suspect:
- hyperventilation syndrome
- hypoxaemia*
- congestive heart failure
- pending respiratory arrest

A patient with a pulse oximeter reading of 86% with no significant past medical history of _____ _____ is considered hypoxic.

> no past, pulmonary disorders, complaint of, Vitals

18
The presence of rhonchi in a patient _____ ____ pneumonia indicates:
- narrowing of the airways
- normal finding in a pneumonia patient
- onset of bronchitis
- mucus in the airways*

Rhonchi are abnormal ____ _____ heard on auscultation of airway that is obstructed by thick _____.

> lung sounds, secretions, diagnosed with

19
When using a bulb syringe device to assist in the verification of proper endotracheal tube placement, all of the following are true:
- If the ____ _____ easily inflates, the endotracheal tube is correctly placed in the trachea.*
- If the bulb syringe does not _____, the endotracheal

tube is placed in the oesophagus.*
- The ____ on the endotracheal tube should not be inflated prior to using a bulb syringe device.*

If the endotracheal tube has been placed in the _____, inflating the cuff on the endotracheal tube will hold the oesophagus ____ and allow the bulb syringe to inflate. It is important to not inflate the endotracheal tube cuff prior to using any bulb syringe device.

> inflate, bulb syringe, oesophagus, cuff, open

20
You respond to a 17-year-old male because his father was unable to wake him. The father states that his son was at a party last night and has a history of _____ ____ ___. He is unconscious and unresponsive. BP is not obtainable, pulse 42 and weak, and respirations of 4. You have orally intubated the patient. Auscultation of lung sounds post-intubation _____ breath sounds heard over the right chest and an absence of breath sounds over the left chest. Your ____ _____ would be to deflate the endotracheal tube cuff, withdraw the tube by 2 cm and

reevaluate breath sounds, and
reinflate the cuff.*
This patient was ____ _____
intubated in the right main
stem bronchus. Deflating
the endotracheal tube cuff,
withdrawing the tube slightly,
_____ the cuff, and
_____ breath sounds is
the proper procedure when a right
main stem bronchus intubation is
suspected.

> reveal, most likely, recreational
> drug use, reinflating, next action,
> reevaluating

21
All of the following are reasons for
a pulse oximeter to read 'Error':
- low capillary blood ____*
- _____
  vasoconstriction*
- extremity _____*

> flow, movement, peripheral

22
Field extubation is indicated if
the patient is awake and able to
maintain his or her own airway.*
Field extubation is ___ _____. If
it must be _____, the patient
must clearly be able to
_____ ___ _____ his or her
own airway and have _____
spontaneous respirations.

> maintain and protect, adequate,
> performed, not common

Vocabulary 2
accuracy /ˈæk.jʊ.rə.si/ přesnost,
správnost
acrylic /əˈkrɪl.ɪk/ akryl, akrylový
adequate /ˈæd.ə.kwət/ dostatečný,
přiměřený
adult /ˈæd.ʌlt/,/əˈdʌlt/ dospělý,
zletilý
affect /əˈfekt/ ovlivnit, působit,
postihnout, zasáhnout
airflow /ˈeə.fləʊ/ proud vzduchu
anaemia /əˈniːmɪə/ anémie,
chudokrevnost
anxious /ˈæŋk.ʃəs/ úzkostlivý,
zneklidněný
apnoea /ˈæp.ni.ə/ apnoe, zástava
dechu
apnoeic /æpˈniː.ɪk/ apnoický, bez
dechu
appear /əˈpɪər/ zdát se, jevit se,
vypadat, objevit se
arrest /əˈrest/ zástava
aspiration /ˌæspɪˈreɪʃən/ aspirace,
dýchání
associated /əˈsəʊ.si.eɪ.tɪd/
spojený, související
at /ət/ **least** /liːst/ při nejmenším,
alespoň
ataxic /əˈtæk.sɪk/ ataktický,
nesouladný, nekoordinovaný
pohyb
attempt /əˈtemp t/ pokus,
pokoušet se, snažit
auscultation /ˌɔː.skəlˈteɪ.ʃən/
auskultace, vyšetření poslechem

awake /ə'weɪk/ probudit se, probrat se, být vzhůru, bdělý
based /beɪst/ založený, vycházející z, působící
basilar /'bæz.ɪ.lər/ basilární, základnový
bilirubin /ˌbɪl.ɪ'ru:.bɪn/ bilirubin, žlučové barvivo
blind /blaɪnd/ slepý
bradypnoea /ˌbræd.ɪ.'pni.ə/ bradypnoe, zpomalené dýchání
breath /breθ/ dech, dýchání
bronchitis /brɒŋ'kaɪ.tɪs/ bronchitida, zánět průdušek
bruising /'bru:.zɪŋ/ pohmožděniny, podlitiny
bulb /bʌlb/ baňka
cafeteria /ˌkæf.ə'tɪə.ri.ə/ jídelna, restaurace
capillary /kə'pɪl.ər.i/ kapilára, vlásečnice, kapilární
carbon monoxide /ˌkɑ:.bən.mə'nɒk.saɪd/ oxid uhelnatý
cardiac arrest /'kɑr.di.ˌæk ə'rest/ zástava srdce
central /'sen.trəl/ centrální, středový
cerebral /'ser.ɪ.brəl/ mozkový
check /tʃek/ kontrolovat, zkontrolovat, kontrola
choke /tʃəʊk/ dusit se
circulation /ˌsɜ:.kjʊ'leɪ.ʃən/ cirkulace, oběh
circumstance /'sɜ:.kəm.stɑ:nt s/ okolnost, poměry
command /kə'mɑ:nd/ příkaz, ovládnutí, kontrola, velení

communicate /kə'mju:.nɪ.keɪt/ komunikovat
complaint /kəm'pleɪnt/ stížnost, nemoc, neduh, potíž
complete /kəm'pli:t/ úplný
compression /kəm'preʃən/ komprese, stlačení, stisknutí, slisování
condition /kən'dɪʃ.ən/ stav, fyzická kondice, potíže, podmínka
confirmation /ˌkɒn.fə'meɪ.ʃən/ potvrzení, schválení
congestive /kən'dʒes.tɪv/ **heart** / hɑ:t/ **failure** /'feɪ.ljər/ městnavé srdeční selhání, k městnavému srdečnímu selhání dochází, když srdce selže jako pumpa a krev se hromadí před pravou komorou v pravé síni a žilním systému nebo před levou komorou v levé síni a plicním oběhu
conscious /'kɒn.tʃəs/ při vědomí, vědomý si
constant /'kɒn.stənt/ neustálý, nepřetržitý
constricted /kən'strɪkt.ɪd/ zúžený, stáhnutý
constriction /kən'strɪk.ʃən/ stažení, zúžení
contraindication /ˌkɒn.trə.ˌɪn.dɪ'keɪ.ʃən/ kontraindikace, příčiny vylučující užití určitých léků nebo léčebných postupů
contribute /kən'trɪb.ju:t/ přispět, přispívat, darovat, podílet
cough /kɒf/ kašel, kašlat
cranial /'kreɪ.ni.əl/ kraniální, lebeční

cuff /kʌf/ manžeta, záložka
decompensation /di:ˌkɒm.penˈseɪ.
ʃən/ dekompenzace, selhání
kompenzačních mechanismů,
udržujících určitou chorobu
v přijatelných mezích, vzniká
postupem nemoci, následkem
přidružení jiné choroby nebo
nedodržením léčby
deflate /dɪˈfleɪt/ vyfouknout,
splasknout
detector /dɪˈtek.tər/ detektor, čidlo
device /dɪˈvaɪs/ zařízení, vybavení,
přístroj
diagnose /ˈdaɪəgˌnəʊz/ stanovit
diagnózu
distal /dɪ.stəl/ distální, vzdálený
od centra, periferní
dizziness /ˈdɪz.ɪ.nəs/ závrať, točení
hlavy, mrákotný stav
effect /ɪˈfekt/ efekt, účinek, dopad
error /ˈer.ər / omyl, chyba
exposure /ɪkˈspəʊ.ʒə/ obnažení,
vystavení
extremity /ɪkˈstrem.ɪ.ti/ končetina
extubation /ˌeks.tjʊˈbeɪ.ʃən/
extubace
feeling /ˈfiː.lɪŋ/ pocit, mínění
fever /ˈfiː.vər/ horečka
field /fiːld/ terén
finding /ˈfaɪndɪŋ/ závěr, zjištění,
nález
fracture /ˈfræk.tʃə/ zlomenina
high-pitched /ˌhaɪˈpɪtʃt/ vysoký,
ostrý, pronikavý zvuk
history /ˈhɪs.tər.i/ anamnéza
hyperthermia /ˌhaɪ.pəˈθɜ:.mɪ.ə/
hypertermie, přehřátí

hyperventilation /ˌhaɪ.pəˌven.tɪˈleɪ.
ʃən/ hyperventilace, chorobně
zvýšená plicní ventilace
hypoperfusion /ˌhaɪ.pəʊ.pəˈfju:.
ʒən/ nedokrvení, snížená perfuze,
nedostatečné zásobování orgánů
tekutinou
hypoxaemia /ˌhai.pɒkˈsi:.mi.ə/
hypoxemie, snížené množství
kyslíku v krvi
immediately /ɪˈmi:.di.ət.li/
okamžitě, ihned
indication /ˌɪn.dɪˈkeɪ.ʃən/ indikace,
údaj, označení, léčebný příkaz
inflate /ɪnˈfleɪt/ nafouknout
inhale /ɪnˈheɪl/ nadechovat
intermittent /ˌɪn.təˈmɪt.ənt/
občasný, přerušovaný
intracranial /ɪn.trəˈkreɪ.ni.əl/
intrakraniální, nitrolebeční
irregular /ɪˈreg.jə.lər/ nepravidelný
laryngospasm /læˈrɪŋ.gə.spæz.əm/
křeč hrtanu
life support /ˈlaɪf.səˌpɔ:t/ podpora
života
listening /ˈlɪs.ən.ɪŋ / poslech,
naslouchání
looking /lʊk.ɪŋ/ vzhled, vypadající
loss /lɒs/ ztráta, úbytek
maintain /meɪnˈteɪn/ udržovat,
uchovat, zachovat
move /mu:v/ pohnout, hnout
movement /ˈmu:v.mənt/ pohyb
nail /neɪl/ **polish** /ˈpɒl.ɪʃ/ lak na
nehty
narrow /ˈnær.əʊ/ úzký, těsný,
omezený

27

nasotracheal /ˌneɪ.zə.trəˈkiː.əl/ nazotracheální, týkající se nosu a průdušnice

neurogenic /ˌnjʊə.rəˈdʒen.ɪk/ neurogenní, nervového původu, vznikající v nervovém systému

niple /ˈnɪpͺl/ prsní bradavka

noise /nɔɪz/ hluk, rámus

obstruct /əbˈstrʌkt/ zablokovat, ucpat

onset /ˈɒnˌset/ propuknutí, začátek

palpitations /ˌpæl.pɪˈteɪ.ʃənz/ palpitace, zrychlené bušení srdce

pattern /ˈpæt.ən/ model, schéma, systém, obrazec, struktura

pending /ˈpen.dɪŋ/ brzký, bezprostředně hrozící

perform /pəˈfɔːm/ vykonat, provést, udělat, fungovat

period /ˈpɪə.ri.əd/ doba, lhůta

pigmentation /ˌpɪg.mənˈteɪ.ʃən/ pigmentace

pneumonia /njuːˈməʊ.ni.ə/ zápal plic

poisoning /ˈpɔɪ.zən.ɪŋ/ otrava

potent /ˈpəʊ.tənt/ silný, účinný

procedure /prəˈsiːdʒə/ postup, procedura

pronounced /prəˈnaʊnst/ vyslovovaný, zřetelný, výrazný

pulse /pʌls/ **oximetry** /ˈɒk.sɪ.m.ə.tri/ pulzní oxymetrie, neinvazivně měří saturaci hemoglobinu kyslíkem v arteriální části krevního řečiště (pulzatilní tok), místem umístění detektoru jsou prsty končetin nebo ušní lalůčky

rale /raːl/ šelest, šelesty

ratio /ˈreɪ.ʃi.əʊ/ podíl, vzájemný poměr, vztah

reading /ˈriː.dɪŋ/ odečet

reevaluate /ˌriː.ɪˈvæljueɪt/ znovu zhodnotit, přehodnotit

regulation /ˌreg.jʊˈleɪ.ʃən/ regulace, řízení, usměrňování

reinflate /ˌriː.ɪnˈfleɪt/ znovu nafouknout

rescue /ˈreskjuː/ zachránit, pomoc, vysvobodit

secretion /sɪˈkriː.ʃən/ sekrece, vylučování, výměšky

shallow /ˈʃæl.əʊ/ mělký

significant /sɪgˈnɪf.ɪ.kənt/ důležitý, význačný, významný

skull /skʌl/ lebka

slightly /ˈslaɪt.li/ trochu, nepatrně

spontaneous /spɒnˈteɪ.ni.əs/ spontánní, samovolný

sternum /ˈstɜː.nəm/ sternum, hrudní kost

stridor /straɪd.ər/ stridor, pískavý zvuk při ztíženém dýchaní

stroke /strəʊk/ mozková mrtvice, úder, bití pulsu

suspect /səˈspekt/ mít podezření, domnívat se

syringe /sɪˈrɪndʒ/ injekční stříkačka

thick /θɪk/ hustý

times /taɪmz/ krát, opakovaně

tool /tuːl/ nástroj, pomůcka, prostředek

upper /ˈʌp.ər/ horní

vasoconstriction /ˌveɪ.zə.kənˈstrɪk.ʃən/ vazokonstrikce, zúžení cév

vasodilator /ˌveɪ.zə.daɪˈleɪ.tər/ vazodilátor, vyvolávající rozšíření cévy

verification /ˌver.ɪ.fɪˈkeɪ.ʃən/ verifikace, ověření, potvrzení

vessel /ˈves.əl/ céva

victim /ˈvɪk.tɪm/ oběť

vitals /ˈvaɪ.təlz/ známky života, fyziologické funkce

volume /ˈvɒl.juːm/ objem, množství, hlasitost

wheeze /wiːz/ sípat, těžce dýchat, sípání

withdraw /wɪðˈdrɔː/ stáhnout, ustoupit, odejít

Unit 3

1

You have successfully resuscitated a patient who suffered a cardiac arrest. You are __ _____ to the hospital when the patient wakes up and is not tolerating the endotracheal tube. The medical director at the _____ _____ has ordered you to extubate the patient. All of the following should be done:

- removing the endotracheal tube on a cough or respiration*
- deflating the endotracheal tube cuff _____*
- providing _____ oxygen once the tube is removed*

The endotracheal tube must be removed swiftly on a _____ __ _____.

en route, supplemental, cough or expiration, receiving hospital, completely

2

You have orally intubated a patient. While your partner ventilates the patient with a bag-valve device, you assess for proper placement. Auscultation reveals sounds heard over the right chest and an absence of breath sounds over the left chest. Your best course of action would be to deflate the endotracheal tube cuff, withdraw the tube by 2 cm and reevaluate breath sounds, and reinflate the cuff.*
This patient was most likely intubated in the right ____ ____ _____ the endotracheal tube cuff, _____ the tube slightly, reinflating the cuff and _____ breath sounds is the proper procedure.

Deflating, reevaluating, main stem bronchus, withdrawing

3

The Sellick manoeuvre may be used to minimize gastric distension and facilitate the placement of an endotracheal tube into the glottic opening.* Posterior pressure exerted on the _____ _____ (the Sellick manoeuvre) will effectively _____ the oesophagus, minimizing the potential for gastric _____. This manoeuvre will also reposition the _____ _____ for clearer _____ of anatomic structures.

compress, visualization, distension, cricoid cartilage, vocal cords

4

You arrive at the scene of an accident in which a car ___ _____ a telephone pole. You find a 17-year-old female _____ from her vehicle, lying 25 feet from the point of impact.

Which is an _____ method of opening the airway? Jaw thrust.* This is a trauma victim and should be managed utilizing C-spine _____.

> Ejected, precautions, has struck, acceptable

5

Which is NOT considered a ____ __ _____ indicating a tension pneumothorax?
- dyspnoea
- hyperresonance to percussion
- distended jugular veins
- clear lung sounds*

_____ lung sounds do not indicate the presence of a _____ pneumothorax.

> Clear, tension, sign or symptom

6

When confirming an endotracheal tube placement, it is imperative to auscultate:
- at the midaxillary line*
- over the trachea*
- over the epigastrium*

_____ individual lung fields is of great benefit because they help to _____ tube placement. Auscultation of the epigastrium is beneficial because it will help to verify _____ tube placement or problems with the ____ ____ of the tube.

> improper, cuff seal, Auscultating, confirm

7

A respiratory pattern characterized by a gradually increasing rate and tidal volume followed by a gradual _____ with intermittent periods of _____ is called:
- Cheyne-Stokes*
- Biot's (ataxic)
- central neurogenic hyperventilation
- agonal

This breathing pattern is usually seen in patients with _____ _____ or elderly patients with terminal illness.

> brain injury, decrease, apnoea

8

You observe a COPD patient utilizing the pursed-lip breathing technique. It helps maintain pressure within the airways.*

_____-___ breathing technique helps _____ _____ within the airways (even during exhalation) to _____ bronchial walls that have been damaged as a result of _____.

> support, maintain pressure,
> Pursed-lip, disease

9

When intubating an adult patient with a _____ _____ (Macintosh blade), the tip of the blade should __ _____ in the vallecula __ ___ ____ of the tongue.*

> at the base, curved blade, be placed

10

After _____ the chest of the victim with a tension pneumothorax, you determine your _____ was successful by observing for an improvement in the patient's ventilatory and circulatory status.* In a tension pneumothorax, the patient is dealing with _____ _____ and circulation problems. This tension pneumothorax creates an intrathoracic shift, impending _____ ____ return to the heart.

> venous blood, intervention,
> oxygenation problems,
> decompressing

11

During needle decompression, ___ _____ is inserted on the top of the rib for what purpose? To ensure that the vein, artery, and _____ _____ under each rib are not damaged.*
Each _____ _____ contains a vein, artery, and nerve, which lie underneath each rib.

> the needle, intercostal space,
> nerve bundle

12

You have intubated a patient with a long history of chronic bronchitis. During transport you notice that _____ are becoming increasingly difficult. You _____ the chest and hear faint equal breath sounds. What intervention is most likely indicated for this patient? Tracheobronchial suctioning.* In this scenario, suctioning is indicated. A patient with _____ _____ produces copious amounts of _____, which is capable of plugging the larger airways of an __ ____. This would result in difficult ventilation.

> ET tube, mucus, chronic
> bronchitis, ventilations, auscultate

13

A drop in systolic _____ _____ of 10 mmHg or more or the absence of a _____ _____ during inspiration is known as:
- pericardial tamponade
- pulsus paradoxus*
- orthostatic _____

- pulse pressure change

> radial pulse, change, blood
> pressure

14

Suctioning (application of
_____ _____) should be
activated upon extraction of the
suction catheter.*
Prolonged suctioning has been
found __ _____ hypoxia; therefore,
suctioning should __ _____ to
extraction only.

> be limited, to cause, negative
> pressure

15

When using a _____ _____
(Miller blade) to _____ an adult
patient, the tip of the blade should
be placed:

- directly __ __ _____ the
  epiglottis.*
- above the epiglottis
- in the vellecula
- past the epiglottis at the
  vocal cord

> intubate, on or under, straight
> blade

16

Digital intubation may be helpful
when:

- there is suspected spinal
  cord injury*
- the tongue is swollen

- the respiratory rate is 4/
  minute
- upper-airway obstruction
  is suspected

The sniffing position is not
required to perform _____
_____. The head can remain
in a _____ _____; therefore,
digital intubation may be helpful
with _____ spinal cord injury.

> suspected, digital intubation,
> neutral position

17

An infant should not be _____
for more than 5 seconds.*
Suctioning should not _____
10 seconds in a child and 15
seconds in an _____.

> exceed, adult, suctioned

18

A child in respiratory distress may
grunt as the child breathes. This
is a result of creating pressure to
help maintain open airways.*
_____ involves exhaling
against a partially closed glottis.
This creates pressure to help
maintain open _____ _____
similar to pursed-lip breathing
in adults with COPD. This short
low-pitched sound is often
_____ ___ whimpering and
suggests _____ _____.

mistaken for, severe hypoxia,
Grunting, lower airways

19
You are caring for a 77-year-old
male patient who is short of
breath and has a history of
____. He is alert and oriented
to person, place, and time but
is able to speak only in two- to
three-word sentences. What does
the patient's ability to speak in
two- to three-word sentences
indicate? Inadequate tidal volume
is present.*
A patient not being able to
speak in full sentences due to
_____ _____ indicates
that the patient does not have
an adequate tidal volume. This
assessment finding can be
a significant _____ ____ of
pending respiratory failure.

breathing difficulty, warning sign,
COPD

20
One reason the respiratory
system of a geriatric patient
becomes less effective is that
there is decreased chest wall
compliance.*
There is no escaping the fact that
the body becomes ___ _____
with age. Decreased chest wall
compliance, loss of lung elasticity,
___ _____, decreased
_____ of gases, and

_____ of the respiratory
muscles can all contribute to a
less active respiratory system in a
_____ _____.

air trapping, geriatric patient,
hypertrophy, less efficient,
diffusion

21
You respond to a 72-year-old
man with syncope. He is sitting in
the kitchen when you arrive. He
is alert and oriented to _____,
_____, and ____. He complains of
dizziness. Current vitals are as
follows: BP, 108/60; pulse, 96 and
slightly irregular; and respirations
of 28. Pulse oximeter reading is
97%. ECG shows a sinus rhythm
with occasional PVCs. This
patient should receive oxygen by
a nonrebreather mask.*
This patient needs oxygen by a
_____ ____. He has an
increased respiratory rate and
PVCs on the monitor that may
indicate hypoxia. A normal pulse
oximeter of 97% is an excellent
_____, but oxygen should
not be withheld based on this
reading. Always remember __
_____ your patient and not the
pulse oximeter.

nonrebreather mask, to treat,
finding, person, place, time

22
Respiratory acidosis is caused by:
- an excess of _____
- excess carbon dioxide*
- _ ____ __ bicarbonate
- _____ carbon dioxide excretion

excess, bicarbonate, a loss of

23
The nasopharyngeal airway should be measured:
- from the _____ of the mouth to the earlobe
- from the tip of the nose to the earlobe*
- from the ___ __ ___ ____ to the corner of the mouth
- from the tip of the nose to the ____

corner, chin, tip of the nose

Vocabulary 3
above /ə'bʌv/ nad, přes
acceptable /ək'sept.ə.b|/ přijatelný, vhodný
accident /'æksɪdənt/ nehoda, neštěstí
agonal /'əg.əʊ.nəl/ agonální, týkající se agónie
alert /ə'lɜːt/ bdělý, čilý, zvýšená ostražitost, stav pohotovosti, varovat
amount /ə'maʊnt/ množství, objem, částka
application /ˌæp.lɪ'keɪ.ʃən/ aplikace, použití, využití

artery /'ɑːtərɪ/ tepna
beneficial /ˌben.ɪ'fɪʃ.əl/ prospěšný, blahodárný
benefit /'ben.ɪ.fɪt/ prospěch, užitek, mít užitek
blade /bleɪd/ čepel
blood /blʌd/ **pressure** /'preʃ.ər/ krevní tlak
bundle /'bʌn.dl/ svazek
C-spine, cervical /sə'vaɪ.kəl/ **spine** / spaɪn/ krční páteř
capable /'keɪ.pə.b|/ schopný, způsobilý, zdatný
cardiac /'kɑː.di.æk/ srdeční
caring /'keə.rɪŋ/ starostlivý, pečující
cartilage /'kɑː.təl.ɪdʒ/ chrupavka
catheter /'kæθɪtə/ katétr, cévka
cause /kɔːz/ příčina, záležitost, věc, důvod, přimět, způsobit
clear /klɪər/ čistý, jasný, průzračný, očistit, vyprázdnit
compliance /kəm'plaɪ.ənt s/ dodržování, soulad, kompliance, poddajnost, schopnost proměny velikosti a tvaru (např. plíce při vdechu)
compress /kəm'pres/ obklad, stlačit, zmáčknout
considered /kən'sɪd.əd/ považovaný, uvážený
contain /kən'teɪn/ obsahovat, zahrnovat
copious /'kəʊ.pi.əs/ hojný, bohatý
course /kɔːs/ průběh, kúra (léčebná), postup
create /kri:'eɪt/ vytvořit, stvořit, vyvolat

cricoid /ˈkraɪ.kɔɪd/ **cartilage** /ˈkɑː.təl.ɪdʒ/ chrupavka prstencová, nejspodnější chrupavka hltanová

current /ˈkʌr.ənt/ proud, současný, aktuální

damaged /ˈdæm.ɪdʒd/ poškozený

deal with /dɪəl/ řešit, zabývat se

decompress /ˌdiː.kəmˈpres/ snížit tlak

decompression /ˌdiː.kəmˈpreʃ.ən/ dekomprese, snížení tlaku

diffused /dɪˈfjuːst/ rozptýlený, roztroušený, rozšířený, nejasný, neohraničený

diffusion /dɪˈfjuː.ʒən/ difuze, pronikání

digital /ˈdɪdʒ.ɪ.təl/ digitální

directly /daɪˈrekt.li/ přímo, okamžitě

director /daɪˈrek.tər/ vedoucí, šéf

drop /drɒp/ poklesnout, snížit, klesnout, spadnout, pokles, kapka, upustit na zem

dyspnoea /dɪs.pniː.ə/ dyspnoe, dušnost, porucha dýchání

efficient /ɪˈfɪʃ.ənt/ efektivní, účinný

eject /ɪˈdʒekt/ vyhodit, prudce vyvrhnout

elasticity /ˌɪl.æsˈtɪs.ɪ.ti/ elasticita, pružnost

elderly /ˈel.dəl.i/ postarší, starší

enroute /ˌɒnˈruːt/ cestou, během cesty

epigastrium /ˌepɪˈɡæs.tri.əm/ nadbřišek

equal /ˈiːkwəl/ stejný, rovnat se (čemu)

escape /ɪˈskeɪp/ únikový, utéct, uniknout, uprchnout

exceed /ɪkˈsiːd/ převládat, přesahovat (míru), převýšit, přesáhnout

excellent /ˈek.səl.ənt/ vynikající

excretion /ɪkˈskriː.ʃən/ exkrece, vyměšování, vylučování

exert /ɪɡˈzɜːt/ vyvíjet, uplatnit, vyvinout (tlak)

expiration /ˌek.spəˈreɪ.ʃən/ vypršení, uplynutí

extraction /ɪkˈstræk.ʃən/ extrakce, vynětí

extubate /eks.tjʊ.beɪt/ extubovat

facilitate /fəˈsɪl.ɪ.teɪt/ usnadnit, ulehčit

failure /ˈfeɪ.ljə/ porucha, selhání, závada, výpadek, neúspěch, nezdar, neschopnost

faint /feɪnt/ slabý, tlumený, malátný, na omdlení

finding /ˈfaɪndɪŋ/ závěr, zjištění, nález

found /faʊnd/ nalezený

full /fʊl/ plný, úplně

geriatric /ˌdʒer.iˈæt.rɪk/ geriatrický

glottic /ˈɡlɒt.ɪk/ hlasivkový

gradually /ˈɡræd.jʊ.li/ postupně

grunt /ɡrʌnt/ chrčet, chrochtat

hyperresonance /ˌhaɪ.pə.ˈrez.ən.əns/ nadměrná zvučnost

hypertrophy /haɪˈpɜː.trə.fi/ hypetrofie, zvětšení, zbytnění, zvětšení orgánu

impact /ˈim.pækt/ dopad, náraz, úder, účinek, vliv, výsledek, dopadat, natlačit

impending /ɪmˈpen.dɪŋ/ blížící se, bezprostředně hrozící, nastávající, budoucí imperative /ɪmˈper.ə.tɪv/ nezbytně nutný, zcela nezbytný

improper /ɪmˈprɒp.ər/ nesprávný, nestandardní, nezákonný

improvement /ɪmˈpruːv.mənt/ zlepšení

inadequate /ɪˈnæd.ɪ.kwət/ nedostatečný, neschopný

increasingly /ɪnˈkriː.sɪŋ.li/ stále více, čím dál tím víc (jaký)

indicate /ˈɪn.dɪ.keɪt/ indikovat, označit, ukazovat

infant /ˈɪnfənt/ nemluvně, kojenec, malé dítě, dítě do 1 roku

injury /ˈɪndʒərɪ/ úraz

inspiration /ˌɪn.spɪˈreɪ.ʃən/ inspirace, vdechnutí, vdech

intercostal /ˌɪn.təˈkɒs.təl/ interkostální, mezižeberní

intermittent /ˌɪn.təˈmɪt.ənt/ občasný, přerušovaný

intrathoracic /ˌɪn.trə.θɔːˈræs.ɪk/ intratorakální, nitrohrudní

jugular /ˈdʒʌg.jə.lər/ vein / veɪn/ jugulára, krční žíla

lie /laɪ/ spočívat, ležet

limited /ˈlɪm.ɪ.tɪd/ limitovaný, omezený, malý

low-pitched /ˌləʊˈpɪtʃt/ hluboký, tlumený

lower /ˈləʊ.ə/ airways /ˈeə.weɪz/ dolní dýchací cesty

midaxillary /mɪd.ækˈsɪl.ər.i/ střed podpaží

mistaken /mɪˈsteɪ.kən/ mylný, nesprávný, chybný

needle /ˈniː.dl̩/ jehla, střelka

negative /ˈneg.ə.tɪv/ bez nálezu onemocnění

neutral /ˈnjuː.trəl/ neutrální, nestranný

nonrebreather /ˌnɒn.rəbrə.ðər/ mask / mɑːsk/ dýchací maska s jednocestnou klapkou, vydechnutý oxid uhličitý je vyloučen a není znovu vdechován

notice /ˈnəʊtɪs/ zpozorovat, povšimnout si

observe /əbˈzɜːv/ pozorovat, sledovat, dodržovat

occasional /əˈkeɪʒənəl/ příležitostný, občasný

opening /ˈəʊ.pən.ɪŋ/ otevření, otvor

oriented /ˈɔːrɪəntɪd/ orientovaný

orthostatic /ˌɔː.θəˈstætɪk/ ortostatický, ve vzpřímené poloze

partially /ˈpɑː.ʃəl.i/ částečně, zčásti

past /pɑːst/ za, minulý, dřívější

percussion /pəˈkʌʃ.ən/ poklep, perkuse

pericardial /ˌper.ɪˈkɑːdi.əl/ perikardiální, týkající se osrdečníku

pole /pəʊl/ sloup, stožár, telefonní ap.

posterior /pɒsˈtɪə.ri.ər/ posteriorní, zadní

precaution /prɪˈkɔː.ʃən/ opatrnost, preventivní opatření, bezpečnostní opatření, předběžné opatření

produce /prəˈdjuːs/ způsobit, vyvolat, zapříčinit

prolonged /prəˈlɒŋd/ prodloužený, dlouhotrvající, vleklý

pulsus /pʌls.əs/ paradoxus/ ˈpær.ə.dɒks.əs/ paradoxní

puls, tep, jehož vlny jsou při nádechu menší než při výdechu, patologickým se stává např. při tamponádě srdce či perikarditidě

purpose /ˈpɜː.pəs/ účel, záměr, mít v úmyslu

pursed /pɜːsd/-**lip** /lɪp/ našpulené rty

radial /ˈreɪ.di.əl/ radiální, vřetenní

receive /rɪˈsiːv/ přijmout

remain /rɪˈmeɪn/ vytrvat, zbývat, zůstat

reposition /ˌriː.pəˈzɪʃən/ přemístit, přesunout, posunout

respond /rɪˈspɒnd/ reakce, odpověď

rib /rɪb/ žebro

scenario /sɪˈnɑː.ri.əʊ/ scénář, možný vývoj

seal /siːl/ utěsnit, zalepit, neprodyšně uzavřít

sentence /ˈsen.təns/ věta

shift /ʃɪft/ posunovat, přemístit, přesun, směna

short /ʃɔːt/ **of st** nedostávat se, chybět

sinus /ˈsaɪ.nəs/ sinus, dutina

sniffing /snɪf.ɪŋ/ čichání

sodium bicarbonate /ˌsəʊ.di.əm. baɪˈkɑː.bən.ət/ hydrouhličitan sodný, soda

space /speɪs/ prostor, mezera, vzdálenost

spinal /ˈspaɪ.nəl/ **cord** /kɔːd/ mícha

straight /streɪt/ přímo, přímý, rovný

strike /straɪk/ (struck, struck) zasáhnout, postihnout, udeřit

successfully /səkˈses.fə.li/ úspěšně

suffer /ˈsʌf.ər/ trpět, utrpět, zhoršit se

suspected /səˈspek.tɪd/ suspektní, domnělý podezřelý

swiftly /ˈswɪft.li/ rychle, pohotově

swollen /ˈswəʊ.lən/ oteklý, zduřelý

syncope /ˈsɪŋ.kə.pɪ/ synkopa, přechodné náhlé bezvědomí v důsledku omezení krevního přísunu do mozku

systolic /sɪsˈtɒl.ɪk/ systolický, týkající se systoly

tamponade /tæm.pəˈneɪd/ tamponáda, stlačení srdce tekutinou nahromaděnou v perikardu

tension /ˈtent.ʃən/ **pneumothorax** /ˌnjuː.məˈθɔː.ræks/ tenzní pneumotorax, vzduch v pohrudniční dutině

terminal /ˈtɜː.mɪ.nəl/ konečný, smrtelný, konečné stádium nemoci, umírající pacient

tidal /ˈtaɪdəl/ **volume** /ˈvɒljuːm/ objem vzduchu při nádechu, dechový objem, objem vzduchu nadechnutého či vydechnutého při jednom dechu

tolerate /ˈtɒl.ər.eɪt/ tolerovat snášet

top /tɒp/ navršit, navýšit, vrchol, vrchní část

tracheobronchial /trə.ki.əˈbrɒŋ. ki.əl/ tracheobronchiální, týkající se průdušnice a průdušek

transport /ˈtræn.spɔt/ transport, doprava

trap /træp/ past, nástraha, zachycovat

under /ˈʌn.dər/ pod, podle, v souladu

underneath /ˌʌn.dəˈniːθ/ hned pod čím, bezprostředně pod

upon /əˈpɒn/ na, za, ihned po

utilize /ˈjuː.tɪ.laɪz/ použít, uplatnit

vein /veɪn/ žíla

venous /ˈviː.nəs/ **return** /rɪˈtɜːn/ žilní návrat

visualization /ˌvɪʒ.u.əl.aɪˈzeɪ.ʃən/ vizualizace, zviditelnění, představa

vocal /ˈvəʊkəl/ **cords** /kɔːdz/ hlasivky

warning /ˈwɔː.nɪŋ/ **sign** /saɪn/ varovné znamení

whimper /ˈwɪmpə/ naříkat, skuhrat

withhold /wɪðˈhəʊld/ zadržet, odebrat

within /wɪˈðɪn/ uvnitř, v rámci

Part 2
Cardiology

Unit I

I

What is the correct _____ at which you should _____ chest compressions on an _____ victim of cardiac arrest? 100 times per minute.*

> speed, adult, perform

2

Hypocalcaemia and hypomagnesaemia would ____ _____ result in:
- decreased cardiac conduction
- increased myocardial irritability*
- decreased cardiac contractility
- decreased myocardial automaticity

Hypocalcaemia results in decreased _____ and increased myocardial irritability. Hypomagnesaemia results in increased myocardial _____.

> contractility, irritability, MOST likely

3

The protective sac surrounding the heart is the:
- myocardium
- septum
- endocardium
- pericardium*

The pericardium is the fibroserous sac enclosing the heart that is composed of two layers, the _____ and the parietal _____. The _____ is the middle layer of the walls of the heart. The _____ is the inner walls of the heart that separate the right and left _____ of the heart from the ventricles. The endocardium is the _____ layer of the heart.

> epicardium, myocardium, innermost, pericardium, septum, atria

4

In a patient experiencing chest pain, the presence of jugular venous distension while sitting at a 45° angle indicates right heart compromise.

The _____ _____ reflect the pressure within _____ circulation. Normally, the jugular veins are not _____ in a patient sitting or standing. JVD present at a 45° angle indicates that pressure in the right side of the heart is elevated and indicates right heart _____.

> distended, systemic, compromise, jugular veins

5

Signs and symptoms associated with _____ _____ include distant heart tones, JVD, and:
- pulse _____
- hypotension*
- wheezing
- delayed _____ _____

Beck's triad includes _____, distant heart tones, and JVD. This triad of symptoms can aid in the diagnosis of cardiac tamponade.

pericardial tamponade, hypotension, paradoxus, capillary refill

6

Which term best describes the following definition? Disease of arterial vessels marked by _____, _____, and loss of elasticity in the arterial walls.
- atherosclerosis
- arterionecrosis
- arteriosclerosis*
- angina

_____ is the most common form of arteriosclerosis, usually involving medium-sized and large arteries.

Arterionecrosis is the destruction (_____) of the arteriole.

Angina is chest _____ associated with a deficiency of oxygen supply to the heart muscle.

thickening, hardening, necrosis, discomfort, Atherosclerosis

7

The volume of blood _____ from the left _____ into the _____ system each minute is called:
- preload
- cardiac output*
- afterload
- stroke volume

ventricle, arterial, ejected

8

The _____ against which the heart must pump is called:
- afterload*
- blood pressure
- preload
- cardiac output

_____ is defined as the pressure within the ventricles at the end of diastole.

Blood pressure is defined as pressure that __ _____ on the walls of the arteries.

resistance, is exerted, Preload

9

The _____ of blood ejected from the heart in one cardiac _____ is called:
- cardiac output
- stroke volume*
- preload
- _____

contraction, afterload, amount

10
Nitroglycerin has all of the
following properties:
- prevents vasospasm*
- is a _____*
- decreased preload*
_____ is a vasodilator;
it works against _____ and
decreased preload.

Nitroglycerin, vasodilator,
vasospasm

11
Your patient with ventricular
tachycardia is lethargic,
diaphoretic, and ____ and has
vomited once. His vital signs
are as follows: BP, 54/P; pulse,
184; respirations, 14. Describe
your management of this
patient. ABCs, high-flow oxygen,
cardioversion.*
ABCs and high-flow oxygen
are indicated for this patient,
and _____ needs to be
performed because the patient is
in _____ _____with a
pulse.

cardioversion, ventricular
tachycardia, pale

12
You respond to a 76-year-old
man with syncope. He is sitting
upright in the bathroom when

you arrive. He stated that he was
having a bowel movement when
he _____ ___. Based on the
information provided, you suspect
the cause of the patient's syncope
is:
- digitalis toxicity
- an atrial dysrhythmia
- vasovagal episode*
- underlying myocardial
  ischaemia
Your patient's history should
lead you to the _____ __
a vasovagal episode. Having a
_____ _____ or bearing down
to have a bowel movement can
_____ the vagus nerve and
slow down the heart rate enough
to cause dizziness/syncope.

bowel movement, conclusion of,
stimulate, blacked out

13
All of the following are considered
anginal equivalents:
- diaphoresis, syncope,
  _____*
- dyspnoea, palpitations,
  _____*
- fatigue, dizziness,
  _____*

dizziness, palpitations, syncope

14
You respond to a possible
_____ ____. On arrival, you
find bystander CPR in progress

on a male patient in his thirties. Your first action should be to stop bystander CPR to assess ABCs.* Bystander CPR is a courageous effort to ____ _ ____ and is important in the chain of survival, but there are times when the bystander performs CPR _____. As an EMS provider, you must ____ _____ CPR and verify a patent airway, the absence of breathing, and pulselessness when you arrive on the scene.

save a life, stop bystander, drowning call, inappropriately

15
All of the following are treatable causes of _____ _____ _____:
* hypothermia, hypovolaemia, cardiac _____, acidosis*
* acidosis, _____ thrombosis, pulmonary _____*
* _____ pneumothorax, hyperkalaemia, coronary thrombosis*

Other _____ _____ of PEA are hypoxia, hypokalaemia, and drug overdose.

treatable causes, tension, coronary, pulseless electrical activity, tamponade, embolism

16
How often should you _____ rescue breaths for a child who is _____? 12 to 20 breaths ___ _____.*

per minute, provide, apnoeic

17
What is the _____ ____ of chest compressions to ventilations while _____ two-person CPR on an adult with an advanced airway in place? 30 _____ to 2 ventilations.*

compressions, performing, proper rate

18
You respond to a shopping mall for a possible cardiac arrest. When you arrive, you find a male patient in his seventies in _____ _____. The mall security officers have an ___ _____. The AED is in the process of _____ _ _____. Your first response should be to allow the AED to deliver the initial shock.*
The best treatment for a shockable rhythm is defibrillation. If an AED is in the process of delivering a shock, _____ it to do so.

delivering a shock, cardiac arrest, AED attached, allow

19

Which signs/symptoms are considered atypical presentation of myocardial ischaemia?
- Lower-extremity pain, _____ pain, abdominal pain*
- _____ pain, _____ pain, sharp or knifelike pain*
- nausea, dizziness, palpitations*

Shoulder, reproducible, epigastric

20

A dissecting aortic aneurysm may produce which of the following signs/symptoms?
- a ripping or tearing pain sensation*
- ____ in the abdomen
- the same _____ _____ in each arm
- respiratory distress

A classic description of pain associated with a _____ _____ _____ is a ripping or tearing sensation.

dissecting aortic aneurysm, blood pressure, pain

21

You are evaluating a male patient with _____ __ a tearing sensation and epigastric pain. He tells you that the pain

began two hours ago after eating lunch. He says he has never _____ any pain like this. He rates the pain as a 10 and states that it is _____ into his back and shoulder. Based on the information provided, you suspect the pain may be the _____ __:
- a myocardial infarction
- a hiatal hernia
- an aortic aneurysm*
- gastric oesophageal reflux disease

result of, complaints of, radiating, experienced

Vocabulary I

ABCs /ˌeɪ.biːˈsiː/ ABC resuscitace

advanced /ədˈvɑːnt st/ pokročilý

AED, Automated /ˈɔː.tə.meɪ.tɪd/ **External** /ɪkˈstɜː.nəl/ **Defibrillator** /ˌdiːˈfɪb.rɪ.leɪ.tər/ automatický externí defibrilátor

afterload /ˌɑːf.tər.ˈləʊd/ afterload, dotížení, napětí vyvinuté ve stěně srdeční komory během systoly, vysoký a. zatěžuje srdeční sval, zvyšuje spotřebu kyslíku, zhoršuje prokrvení myokardu a může přispívat k srdečnímu selhání

allow /əˈlaʊ/ dovolit, poskytnout, umožnit

angina /ænˌdʒaɪ.nə/ angína, silná svíravá bolest

anginal /ænˌdʒaɪ.nəl/ anginální, silná, svíravá bolest

aortic /eɪˈɔː.tɪk/ aneurism /ˌæn.jʊə.rɪ.zəm/ výduť srdečnice

arterial /ɑːˈtɪərɪəl/ tepenný

arterionecrosis /ɑːˌtɪə.rɪə.neˈkrəʊ.sɪs/ arterionekróza, nekróza arterií

arteriosclerosis /ɑːˌtɪə.ri.əʊ.skləˈrəʊ.sɪs/ arterioskleróza, tvrdnutí tepen

atherosclerosis /ˌæθ.ə.rəʊ.skləˈrəʊ.sɪs/ ateroskleróza, arterioskleróza, kornatění tepen

atrium pl atria /ˈeɪ.tri.əm/ atrium, srdeční předsíň

attach /əˈtætʃ/ připojit, přilepit se, nalepit se

atypical /ˌeɪˈtɪp.ɪ.kəl/ netypický, neobvyklý

automacity /ɔːˈtɒm.ə.sɪt.i/ automacie, stereotypní, někdy periodicky se opakující děj

back /bæk/ záda, páteř

bear /beər/ down /daʊn/ tlačit, vyřítit se, ležet svou vahou na

black out /ˈblæk.aʊt/ ztratit vědomí, omdlít

bowel /ˈbaʊ.əl/ movement /ˈmuː.mənt/ vyprázdnění stolice:

capillary /kəˈpɪl.ər.i/ refill /ˈriː.fɪl/ zpětné plnění kapilár

cardiac /ˈkɑː.dɪˌæk/ output /ˈaʊtˌpʊt/ minutový objem krve vypuzené srdcem

cardioversion /ˌkɑː.di.əˈvɜː.ʃən/ kardioverze, elektrický výboj použitý při léčbě srdečních arytmií

chain /tʃeɪn/ řetěz, řetězec

composed /kəmˈpəʊzd/ of složený z

compromise /ˈkɒmprəˌmaɪz/ oslabit, ohrozit, vydat v nebezpečí, zhoršit, kompromis

conclusion /kənˈkluː.ʒən/ závěr, úsudek

conduction /kənˈdʌk.ʃən/ vedení, přenos, kondukce tepla, elekrického proudu

contractility /ˌkən.trækˈtɪ.lə.ti/ kontraktilita, stažitelnost

coronary /ˈkɒr.ən.ər.i/ koronární, věnčitý

courageous /kəˈreɪ.dʒəs/ odvážný, statečný

defibrillation /diːˌfɪb.rɪˈleɪ.ʃən/ defibrilace, léčebný úkon, kterým se zruší fibrilace komor, použití elektrického výboje, který na čas „vymaže" veškerou chaotickou srdeční činnost a umožní nástup pravidelnějšího rytmu, výkon zachraňující život

deficiency /dɪˈfɪʃ.ənt.si/ deficit, nedostatek, nedostatečnost

diaphoresis /ˌdaɪ.ə.fəˈriː.sɪs/ diaforéza, pocení

diastole /daɪˈæs.tə.li/ diastola, ochabnutí srdeční svaloviny po předchozí kontrakci (systole)

digitalis /ˌdɪdʒ.ɪˈteɪ.lɪs/ digitalis, náprstník bot.

discomfort /dɪˈskʌmp.fət/ obtíž, nepříjemné pocity, mírná bolest, nepohoda, znepokojení

dissecting /daɪˈsekt.ɪŋ/ aortic / eɪˈɔː.tɪk/ aneurysm /ˈæn.jʊə.rɪ.zəm/ disekující aneurysma aorty, podélné „odlepení" stěny tepny, rozpolcení aortální stěny,

ve stěně aorty vzniká neúplná
trhlina
distant /'dɪs.tənt/ vzdálený,
odměřený, nepřístupný
drowning /'draʊn.ɪŋ/ tonutí,
utopení
dysrhythmia /dɪs'rɪθ.mɪə/
dysrytmie, porucha rytmu
effort /'ef.ət/ snaha, úsilí
eject /ɪ'dʒekt/ vyhodit, prudce
vyvrhnout
elasticity /ˌɪl.æs'tɪs.ɪ.ti/ elasticita,
pružnost
elevated /'el.ɪ.veɪ.tɪd/ vysoký,
zvýšený
embolism /'embə.lɪzəm/ embolie,
náhlé zablokování krevní cévy
embolus pl emboli /'em.bə.ləs/
embolus, vmetek, krevní
sraženina
enclose /ɪn'kləʊz/ uzavřít, obklopit
endocardium /ˌen.də'kɑː.di.əm/
endokard, srdeční nitroblána
epigastric /ˌepɪ'gæs.trɪk/
epigastrický, nadbřiškový
episode /'ep.ɪ.səʊd/ epizoda,
záchvat
equivalent /ɪ'kwɪv.əl.ənt/
ekvivalent, protějšek, obdoba,
stejný, rovnající se čemu
exert /ɪg'zɜːt/ vyvíjet, uplatnit,
vyvinout (tlak)
experience /ɪk'spɪə.ri.ənt s/
zkušenost, prožít, zažít, prožívat,
prodělat, ucítit
fatigue /fə'tiːg/ únava, oslabení,
vysílení, vyčerpání, unavit se

fibroserous /ˌfaɪ.brə'sɪə.rəs/
fibroserózní, týkající se vláknité a
serózní blány
harden /'hɑː.dən/ ztvrdnout,
ztuhnout
hiatal /haɪ'eɪ.təl/ **hernia** /'hɜː.ni.ə/
hiátová hernie neboli hiátová kýla
je vysunutí (herniace) z horní
části žaludku do hrudníku přes
trhliny nebo zeslabení bránice
hiatus /haɪ'eɪ.təs/ otvor, mezera
hypocalcaemia /ˌhaɪ.pəʊ.kæl'siː.
mi.ə/ hypokalcemie, nedostatek
vápníku v krvi
hypomagnesaemia /ˌhaɪ.pəʊ.ˌmæg.
nə'siː.mi.ə/ hypomagnezemie,
nedostatek hořčíku v krvi
hypotension /ˌhaɪ.pəʊ'ten.tʃən/
hypotenze, nízký tlak
hypothermia /ˌhaɪ.pəʊ 'θɜː.mi.ə/
hypotermie, nízká tělesná teplota,
podchlazení
inappropriately /ˌɪn.ə'prəʊ.pri.ət.li/
nepatřičně, nevhodně
initial /ɪ'nɪʃəl/ počáteční, výchozí
inner /'ɪn.ər/ vnitřní
irritability /ˌɪr.ɪ.tə'bɪl.ɪ.ti/
iritabilita, dráždivost, podráždění,
podrážděnost, nedůtklivost
ischaemia /ɪs'kiː.mɪ.ə/ ischémie,
místní nedokrvenost tkáně
jugular /'dʒʌg.jə.lər/ jugulární,
hrdelní, krční, týkající se hrdla
knife /naɪf/ nůž, pobodat, říznout
layer /'leɪ.ə/ vrstva, úroveň,
poloha
like /laɪk/ podobný čemu
marked /mɑːkt/ zřetelný, výrazný

medium /miː.di.əm/ **-sized** /saɪzd/ středně velký

middle /ˈmɪd.l̩/ prostřední

muscle /ˈmʌsəl/ sval

myocardial /maɪ.əˌkɑː.di.əl/ myokardiální, týkající se srdeční svaloviny

myocardium /ˌmaɪ.əˈkɑː.di.əm/ myokard, srdeční svalovina

necrosis /neˈkrəʊsɪs/ nekróza, odumření, místní odumírání tkáně

officer /ˈɒf.ɪ.sər/ referent, důstojník

OPA, Oropharyngeal /ˈɔː.rə ˌfəˈrɪn. dʒi.əl/ **Airway** /ˈeə.weɪ/ zařízení používané k udržení otevřených horních dýchacích cest

output /ˈaʊtˌpʊt/ výdej, objem, výkon

overdose /ˈəʊ.və.dəʊs/ nadměrná dávka, předávkování

parietal /pəˈraɪə.təl/ parietální, temenní

patent /ˈpeɪ.tənt/ průchodný

pericardial /ˌper.ɪˈkɑː.di. əl/ perikardiální, týkající se osrdečníku

pericardium /ˌper.ɪˈkɑː.di.əm/ osrdečník, perikard

pneumothorax /ˌnjuːməʊˈθɔːræks/ pneumotorax, hrudní plynatost, vzduch v pohrudniční dutině hrudní

preload /ˌpriːˈləʊd/ preload, předpětí, předtížení, náplň srdeční komory na konci diastoly, enddiastolický objem, zvyšování p. je jedním z kompenzačních mechanismů při srdečním selhání

presence /ˈprez.ənt s/ účast, přítomnost (osoby, věci ap.), zevnějšek

proper /ˈprɒpə/ pořádný, náležitý, vlastní, samotný

protective /prəˈtek.tɪv/ ochranný, ochrana

pulseless /pʌls.ləs/ bez pulzu

pulselessness /pʌls.ləs.nəs/ nepřítomnost pulzu

radiate /ˈreɪ.di.eɪt/ vyzařovat, rozbíhat se (paprskovitě)

rate /reɪt/ ohodnotit, řadit

reflect /rɪˈflekt/ odrážet

reflux /ˈriːˌflʌks/ zpětný tok, zpětné proudění

reproducible /ˌriː.prə.djuːsɪ.bl̩/ opakující se

rip /rɪp/ trhat, rvát

sac /sæk/ váček, vak

security /sɪˈkjʊə.rɪ.ti/ bezpečnost, ostraha, zajištění, zabezpečení

sensation /senˈseɪ.ʃən/ pocit, cit, čití, dojem, vjem, vnímání

separate /ˈsep.ər.ət/ oddělený, samostatný

septum /ˈsep.təm/ přepážka

sharp /ʃɑːp/ ostrý předmět, prudký, náhlý

shockable /ˈʃɒk.ə.bl̩/ umožňující úder (defibrilátor)

shopping /ˈʃɒp.ɪŋ/ **mall** /mɔːl/ nákupní středisko

shoulder /ˈʃəʊl.dər/ rameno

state /steɪt/ stav, uvádět, prohlašovat

stroke /strəʊk/ **volume** /ˈvɒl.juːm/ tepový objem, objem krve, který srdce vypudí při jednom srdečním stahu tepu, systole

supply /səˈplaɪ/ zásobovat, doplnit, potřeby, zásoby

surround /səˈraʊnd/ obklopovat

survival /səˈvaɪ.vəl/ přežití

systemic /sɪˈstem.ɪk/ systemický, týkající se těla jako celku

tearing /ˈteər.ɪŋ/ prudký

tension /ˈten.ʃən/ tenze, napětí, tlak, tonus

thicken /ˈθɪk.ən/ tloustnout, zhušťovat se

thrombosis /θrɒmˈbəʊ.sɪs/ trombóza, srážení krve v cévách za živa

toxicity /tɒkˈsɪs.ɪ.ti/ toxicita, jedovatost

treatable /triːt.ə.bļ/ léčitelný

underlying /ˌʌndəˈlaɪ.ɪŋ/ skrytý, pod povrchem, základní, spodní

upright /ˈʌp.raɪt/ vzpřímeně, vertikálně, svisle

vagus /ˈvaɪ.gəs/ pl gi bloudivý nerv, X. hlavový nerv

vasodilator /ˌvaɪ.zə.daɪˈleɪ.tər/ vazodilátor, vyvolávající rozšíření cévy

vasospasm /ˌvaɪ.zəʊˈspæzm/ vazospasmus, stažení svalové stěny cév se zúžením průsvitu

vasovagal /ˌvaɪ.zəʊˈvæg.əl/ vazovagální, popisující působení n. vagus na krevní oběh

ventricle /ˈven.trɪ.kļ/ ventrikl, komora, srdeční, mozková, tělní dutina, žaludek

vomit /ˈvɒm.ɪt/ zvracet, zvracení

Unit 2

I

Before providing rescue breathing to an _____ victim, you must check for breathing. You do this by looking, listening, and feeling the_____ through the victim's nose or mouth.*
When performing CPR to an adult in _____ _____, it is important to allow the chest to fully recoil between _____.*

> airflow, compressions, unresponsive, cardiac arrest

2

You are performing ___ on an elderly woman in cardiac arrest. After the patient has been _____ and proper ET tube placement has been confirmed, you should _____ asynchronous CPR while ventilating the patient at a rate of 8 to 10 breaths/minute.*
After an advanced airway is placed, cycles of CPR are no longer delivered. Give _____ chest compressions without pauses for breaths. Give 8 to 10 breaths per minute.

> intubated, perform, continuous CPR

3

Stimulation of the vagus nerve may result in:

- vasodilatation
- an increase in heart rate
- a decrease in heart rate*
- an increase in cardiac output

Stimulation of the _____ nerve can occur in many ways. When _____, a decrease in _____ ____ may be observed.

> vagus, stimulated, heart rate

4

A rapid heart rate or_____ heartbeat may cause the patient to experience a sensation _____ _____ as:

- palpitations*
- dysrhythmia
- fainting
- anxiety

Another common term to describe this _____ is 'fluttering'.

> commonly known, irregular, sensation

5

Your patient is complaining of back and flank pain described as a tearing sensation. Inspection of the abdomen reveals a pulsatile mass. Treatment includes gentle handling and rapid transport.*
____ ___ _____ pain described as a tearing sensation and a _____ abdominal mass are classic signs of an abdominal _____ _____. Gentle handling

and rapid transport to the hospital is essential once the diagnosis is made.

> Back and flank, pulsating, aortic aneurysm

6

The presence of pulmonary congestion indicated by abnormal lung sounds such as crackles (rales) in a patient complaining of chest pain may indicate:
- hypotension
- increased vagal tone
- increased stroke volume
- left ventricular failure*

Left ventricular failure occurs when the heart fails as an effective forward pump, which causes ____ _____ of blood into pulmonary _____.
When the back pressure becomes high enough, it forces the blood into the capillaries of the alveoli, resulting in _____ _____.
Adventitious lung sounds such as crackles are commonly present in _____ ventricular failure.

> back pressure, pulmonary congestion, left, circulation

7

An unwanted ____ _____ of dopamine administration includes:
- increased myocardial oxygen demand*
- _____ depression

- ventricular _____
- dilation of renal _____ at high doses

> respiratory, dysrhythmias, vessels, side effect

8

A 70-year-old woman remains in _____ following 10 minutes of well-coordinated ___, intubation, IV, and several rounds of _____. There are no obvious causes that would explain her cardiac arrest. At this point, it would be MOST appropriate to consider ceasing resuscitative efforts.*

> CPR, medications, asystole

9

You arrive on the scene of a 56-year-old male patient who developed chest pain while mowing the lawn on a hot August day. He states the pain has subsided after a few minutes of ____. Your assessment shows that he is alert and _____; BP, 148/92; pulse, 48; and respiration of 20. His skin is warm and moist. He has no past medical history and takes no medications. Treatment should include transport for evaluation.*
Transport for evaluation must be considered for this patient. A _____ ____ of 48 while

mowing the lawn on a hot August day should be a concern. With the presence of chest pain, you should suspect an _____ cardiac origin and transport.

> rest, oriented, underlying, bradycardic rate

10
Your patient is a 47-year-old male who is experiencing paroxysmal junctional tachycardia. He called EMS because of a sensation of

_____ ___ _____.

There is no previous history of heart disease. The ventricular rate is approximately 130 per minute, BP is 100/70 and falling, and respirations are 32 and shallow. What should you do? Attempt vagal manoeuvres to slow the heart rate down.*
Because the patient does not seem to be tolerating the rapid heart rate well, vagal _____ should be attempted first, followed by _____ _____ if necessary. If the heart rate increases or the patient becomes _____, synchronized _____ may be indicated.

> cardioversion, manoeuvres, unstable, palpitations and light-headedness, pharmacological therapy

11
What is the effect of parasympathetic stimulation on the heart? A decreased rate and increased stroke volume.*
Parasympathetic stimulation through the _____ _____ acts to decrease the heart rate; this paradoxically _____ stroke volume because the longer time interval between contractions allows the _____ to fill more efficiently.

> increases, ventricles, vagus nerve

12
What does pulse pressure refer to? _____ between the systolic and diastolic readings.*
Pulse pressure _____ __ the difference between the _____ ___ _____ blood pressure readings. A _____ pulse pressure indicates increasing diastolic pressure and decreasing systolic pressure. _____will stop once blood pressures come together.

> Perfusion, narrowing, diastolic and systolic, Difference, refers to

13
The presence of pulmonary congestion indicated by abnormal lung sounds such as crackles (rales) in a patient complaining

of chest pain may indicate left ventricular failure.*
Left ventricular failure occurs when the heart fails as an effective forward pump, which causes ____ _____ of blood into pulmonary _____.
When the back pressure becomes high enough, it forces the blood into the capillaries of the alveoli, resulting in _____ _____.
Adventitious lung sounds such as crackles are commonly present in _____ ventricular failure.

> back pressure, pulmonary congestion, left, circulation

14
Cardiogenic shock can result in all of the following: _____, respiratory failure, and an elevated heart rate.*
_____ _____ is the most severe form of pump _____ that often results in dysrhythmias, hypotension, respiratory failure, and possibly organ failure. The heart rate is initially elevated as the body attempts to _____ for the shock.

> compensate, Cardiogenic shock, failure, dysrhythmias

15
This patient is exhibiting the signs and symptoms of which of the following diseases?

- chronic bronchitis
- emphysema
- congestive heart failure*
- status asthmaticus

This patient is exhibiting the classic signs and symptoms of _____ _____ _____. His history of AMI indicates that he may have _____ _____ to the heart and raises the possibility that he is now having an _____ _____ of failure.
What medication should be used for this patient? Morphine sulphate.*
Oxygen, morphine, nitroglycerin, and furosemide are all used in the treatment of ___ _____.

> CHF patients, permanent damage, acute episode, congestive heart failure

16
What does a prolonged sinus tachycardia accompanying an acute _____ _____ suggest?

- Cardiogenic shock may develop.*
- Damage of the heart is minimal.
- Hypervolaemia is the _____ _____.
- The diagnosis of MI is incorrect.

In a patient with acute MI, sinus tachycardia _____

that cardiogenic shock may develop.

suggests, underlying cause, myocardial infarction

17
How should you _____ the patient to check for jugular vein distension?
- _____ flat on his or her back
- _____ upright near 90°
- _____ up in anatomical position
- seated at a 45° angle*

Check for jugular vein distension with the patient _____ at a 45° angle. Most patients will have observable jugular veins when supine.

elevated, position, sitting, lying, standing

18
What does a prolonged sinus tachycardia accompanying an acute _____ _____ suggest?
- Cardiogenic shock may develop.*
- Damage of the heart is minimal.
- Hypervolaemia is the _____ _____.
- The diagnosis of MI is incorrect.

In a patient with acute MI, sinus tachycardia _____ that cardiogenic shock may develop.

suggests, underlying cause, myocardial infarction

19
What does a carotid artery bruit indicate?
- good peripheral _____
- obstruction of blood flow*
- jugular vein _____
- congestive heart failure

_ _____, noisy blood flow in a vessel indicates partial obstruction due to _____ build-up or the presence of an _____.

embolus, plaque, A bruit, perfusion, distension

20
_____ _____ are used to treat paroxysmal supraventricular tachycardia.*
Paroxysmal supraventricular _____ (PSVTs) may be _____ by vagal manoeuvres, such as the Valsalva manoeuvre or ice-water _____.

managed, Vagal manoeuvres, immersion, tachycardia

21
In which situation would you _____ having the patient

perform a Valsalva manoeuvre to slow the heart rate?

- male, age 34, paroxysmal junctional tachycardia*
- male, age 68, idioventricular escape rhythm
- female, age 74, _____ ventricular contractions
- female, age 39, ventricular tachycardia

When PJT is caused by stress or excessive _____ _____ in a patient with no history of heart disease, the Valsalva manoeuvre can be successful at _____ the heart rate.

---

caffeine intake, slowing, premature, consider

Vocabulary 2
adventitious /ˌæd.vənˈtɪʃ.əs/ nahodilý, vyskytující se na nesprávném místě
airflow /ˈeə.fləʊ/ proud vzduchu
alveolus pl alveoli /ˌæl.viˈəʊ.ləs/ plicní sklípek
anxiety /æŋˈzaɪ.ə.ti/ úzkost, strach, obava
asynchronous /eɪˈsɪŋ.krə.nəs/ asynchronní, nesoudobý, nesoučasný
asystole /ə.sɪs.tə.lɪ/ asystola, asystolie, uvolnění srdeční svaloviny, zástava srdeční činnosti
backpressure /ˌbækˈpreʃ.ər/ zpětný tlak

beat /biːt/ tlouci, úder
bruit /bruːt/ šum, šelest
buildup /ˈbɪld.ʌp/ vytvořit, narůstat, hromadit se, nárůst, hromadění, zvětšení objemu
caffeine /ˈkæf.iːn/ kofein
capillary /kəˈpɪl.ər.i/ kapilára
cardioversion /ˌkɑː.di.əˈvɜː.ʃən/ kardioverze, elektrický výboj použitý při léčbě srdečních arytmií
carotid artery / kəˌrɒt.ɪdˈɑː.tər.i/ karotida, krkavice, krční tepna
cease /siːs/ přestat, ustat, zastavit se
commonly /ˈkɒm.ən.lɪ/ obvykle, běžně
compensate /ˈkɒm.pən.seɪt/ kompenzovat, vyvážit, vyrovnat, vyrovnat se
confirmed /kənˈfɜːmd/ potvrzený
congestion /kənˈdʒes.tʃən/ ucpání, zácpa
congestive /kənˈdʒes.tɪv/ městnavý, působící ucpávání
continuous / kənˈtɪn.ju.əs/ nepřetržitý, neustálý, pravidelný
CPR, Cardiopulmonary /ˌkɑː. di.əʊˈpʊl.mə.nə.ri/ **Resuscitation** / rɪˌsʌs.ɪˈteɪ.ʃən/ kardiopulmonární resuscitace
demand /dɪˈmɑːnd/ požadavek, žádat, požadovat
diastolic /daɪˈæs.tə.lɪk/ diastolický
dopamine /ˈdəʊ.pə.miːn/ dopamin, chemická látka, která umožňuje přenos impulsů v mozku
effective /ɪˈfek.tɪv/ efektivní, účinný
effort /ˈef.ət/ snaha, úsilí

embolus pl emboli /'em.bə.ləs/ embolus, vmetek, krevní sraženina

emphysema /ˌemp.fə'si:.mə/ emfyzém, rozedma (plic), rozšíření tkání plynem nebo vzduchem

escape /ɪ'skeɪp/ únikový, utéct, uniknout, uprchnout

essential /ɪ'sen.tʃəl/ základní, důležitý, hlavní

evaluation /ɪˌvæl.ju'eɪ.ʃən/ ohodnocení, ocenění, zhodnocení, vyhodnocení

fail /feɪl/ selhat, neuspět

failure /'feɪ.ljə/ porucha, selhání, závada, výpadek, neúspěch, nezdar, neschopnost

faint /feɪnt/ slabý, tlumený, malátný, na omdlení, ztratit vědomí, omdlít

fall /fɔ:l/ (fell, fallen) padnout, padat k zemi, pád

flank /flæŋk/ bok, slabina, strana

flat /flæt/ plochý, rovný

flutter /'flʌt.ər/ chvění, míhání, kmitání srdečních komor nebo síní

force /fɔ:s/ síla, účinnost, nutit, zatlačit

forward /'fɔ:.wəd/ přední, dopředu

gentle /'dʒen.tl/ jemný

handling /'hænd.lɪŋ/ manipulace

heart /hɑ:t/ **rate** /reɪt/ srdeční frekvence

hypervolaemia /ˌhaɪ.pə.vo'li:.mi.ə/ hypervolemie, nadbytek cirkulující krve

idioventricular /ˌɪd.i.əʊ.ven'trɪk.jə.lər/ idioventrikulární, týkající se pouze srdečních komor

immersion /ɪ'mɜ:.ʃən/ ponoření, potopení

intake /'ɪn.teɪk/ příjem, přísun

junction /'dʒʌŋk.ʃən/ uzel, křížení, spojení

junctional /'dʒʌŋk.ʃən.əl/ **tachycardia** /ˌtæk.ɪ'kɑ:.di.ə/ tachykardie vznikající v atrioventrikulárním uzlu při srdeční frekvenci vyšší než 75 úderů za minutu

light-headedness /ˌlaɪt'hed.ɪd.nəs/ malátnost

manoeuvre /mə'nu:.vər/ manévr

moist /mɔɪst/ mokrý, vlhký (vzduch)

observable /əb'zɜ:.vəbəl/ pozorovatelný, znatelný

obvious /'ɒb.vi.əs/ zjevný, jasný, zřejmý, očividný, samozřejmý, nápadný

paradoxically /ˌpær.ə'dɒk.sɪ.kəl.i/ paradoxně

parasympathetic /'pær.əˌsɪm.pə'θet.ɪk/ parasympatický, týkající se autonomího nervstva s opačným účinkem než sympatikus

paroxysmal /ˌpær.ɒk.'sɪz.məl/ paroxyzmální, záchvatový

past /pɑ:st/ minulý, dřívější

perform /pə'fɔ:m/ vykonat, provést, udělat, fungovat

perfusion /pə'fju:.ʒən/ perfuze, promývání, zásobování orgánů tekutinou

plaque /plɑːk/, /plæk/ plát, destička

premature /ˈprem.ə.tʃər/ předčasný, nedonošený, předčasně narozený

pulmonary /ˈpʊl.mə.nə.ri/ **congestion** /kənˈdʒes.tʃən/ překrvení plic

pulsatile /ˈpʌlsəˌtaɪl/ **mass** /mæs/ pulzatilní hmota

reading /ˈriː.dɪŋ/ odečet, údaj

recoil /rɪˈkɔɪl/ zarazit se, ucuknout

refer /rɪˈfɜːr/ mluvit o kom/čem, odkázat se, odvolávat se na co, svěřit, odkázat, poslat ke specialistovi

renal /ˈriː.nəl/ renální, ledvinový

round /raʊnd/ kolem, kulatý, obchůzka

sensation /senˈseɪ.ʃən/ pocit, cit, čití, dojem, vjem, vnímání, smyslové vnímání

shallow /ˈʃæl.əʊ/ mělký

side /saɪd/ **effect** /ɪˈfekt/ vedlejší účinek

status /ˈsteɪ.təs/ **asthmaticus** /æsθˈmæt.ɪk.əs/ status asthmaticus, těžký a prolongovaný záchvat bronchiálního astmatu se závažnou poruchou dýchání, změnami v parciálním tlaku krevních plynů a ve vnitřním prostředí

stroke /strəʊk/ **volume** /ˈvɒl.juːm/ tepový objem, objem krve, který srdce vypudí při jednom srdečním stahu tepu, systole

subside /səbˈsaɪd/ polevit, zmírnit

supine /ˈsuː.paɪn/ ležící naznak, ležící na zádech, tváří vzhůru, klidný

supraventricular /ˈsuː.prə.venˈtrɪk.jə.lər/ supraventrikulární, ležící nad srdeční komorou

systolic /sɪsˈtɒl.ɪk/ systolický, týkající se systoly

treatment /ˈtriːt.mənt/ léčení, ošetření

unstable /ʌnˈsteɪ.b|/ nestabilní, nestálý

unwanted /ʌnˈwɒn.tɪd/ nechtěný, nežádoucí

vagal /ˈveɪ gəl/ vagální, vztahující se k nervus vagus

Valsalva /vælˈsæl.və/ **manoeuvre** /məˈnuː.vər/ med. Valsalvův manévr, přetlakování uší ucpáním nosu a zatlačením vzduchu do uší

vasodilatation /ˌveɪ.zə.daɪ.ləˈteɪ.ʃən/ vazodilatace, rozšíření cév

ventricular /venˈtrɪk.jə.lər/ ventrikulární, komorový

vessel /ˈves.əl/ céva

Part 3
Medical emergencies

Respiratory; neurology; endocrinology; allergies/ anaphylaxis; gastroenterology; urology; environmental; behavioural; toxicology

Unit I

I

A sharp type of pain that travels along a definitive neural route is termed:

- peritonitis
- somatic pain*
- referred pain
- visceral pain

Dull, _____ _____ pain that originates in the walls of the _____ _____ is termed visceral pain.*

Pain that originates in a _____ other than where it is felt is known as referred pain.*

poorly localized, region, hollow organs

2

In a patient with _____ ____, assessment of the abdomen should be performed in the following order: inspect, auscultate, palpate, percuss.* _____ is the obvious first step since you are going to look before you do anything. _____ may not provide

much useful information, but if you are going to auscultate, it must be performed before palpation. _____ is the third step. You can gain a lot of information through palpation. _____ (if performed) is the last assessment step.

Auscultation, Percussion, Palpation, Inspection, abdominal pain

3

When ventilating a patient via an _____ ____, the amount of air flowing into the lungs will be reduced if there is increased airway resistance.*

Airway resistance resulting from _____, bronchoconstriction, or increased ____ production can cause increased _____ _____, resulting in a decrease in the amount of air flowing into the _____.

mucus, oedema, airway resistance, endotracheal tube, lungs

4

One ____ of Glasgow Coma Scale _____ is:

- pupillary response and size
- respiratory rate
- heart rate
- motor response*

57

The Glasgow Coma Scale measures eye opening and verbal response and ____ _____.

| motor response, measures, area |

5
____ injuries are tissue _____ that occur directly at the point of ____:
- concussion
- contrecoup
- coup*
- epidural

| disruptions, impact, Coup |

6
Why is it important to limit the time ___ _____ a patient's airway?
- The ____ ____ level will decrease.*
- Bradycardia can develop.*
Suctioning removes oxygen from the airway and can cause vagal stimulation resulting in _____. Adults should not be suctioned for longer than 10-15 seconds. _____ patients should not be suctioned for longer than 5 seconds.

| for suctioning, Paediatric, bradycardia, blood oxygen |

7
A syndrome that develops as a complication of an illness such

as multisystem _____, severe sepsis, or ____ _____ is termed:
- adult respiratory distress syndrome (____)*
- pneumonia syndrome (PS)
- chronic obstructive pulmonary disease (COPD)
- congestive heart failure (CHF)
ARDS is a form of _____ _____ that occurs as a response to a wide variety of lung injury insults.

| toxic inhalation, ARDS, pulmonary oedema, trauma |

8
An expression of _____ _____ of abnormal lung cells is best termed:
- pulmonary disease
- chronic bronchitis
- lung cancer*
- viral pneumonia
____ _____ is an excessive and uncontrolled growth of _____ ____.

| Lung cancer, cancerous cells, uncontrolled growth |

9
A 49-year-old male with COPD is tired, confused, and in severe respiratory distress. His _____

_____ _____ is most likely caused by:
- carbon dioxide excretion
- hypoxia*
- tachypnoea

_____ can affect the _____ at the cellular level, resulting in a decreased mental status.

> brain, altered mental status, Hypoxia

10
A diagnostic device for measuring forced _____ is a:
- pulse oximeter
- capnometer
- peak flow meter*
- end-tidal CO_2 detector

The peak _____ ____ _____ measures the amount of air a patient can forcefully exhale with ___ _____.

> respiratory flow meter, one breath, exhalation

11
Which device would be most effective in determining if an endotracheal tube is placed in the stomach? End-tidal CO_2 detector.*
This instrument measures the _____ __ _____ of carbon dioxide in the sampled gas at the tip of the _____ ____. It can be used as an assessment tool to help determine proper endotracheal tube _____.

> endotracheal tube, placement, presence or absence

12
The process of ___ _____ between that alveoli and the pulmonary capillary bed is termed:
- ventilation
- diffusion*
- perfusion
- osmosis

_____ is the process of gas molecules moving across a ____ _____ from a _____ _____ of molecules to a lower concentration.

> higher concentration, Diffusion, gas exchange, cell membrane

13
____ _____ of albuterol administration include:
- hypotension and bradycardia
- pallor and sedation
- tachycardia and tremor*
- respiratory depression

Administration of albuterol can stimulate the _____ nervous system, resulting in an increased ____ ____ and _____.

> tremor, Side effects, sympathetic, heart rate

14

Upper respiratory infections (___) are more severe in:
- patients with asthma or COPD*
- patients with HIV infection*

Patients with ___-_____ respiratory disease or who are _____ are more prone to URI.

immunocompromised, pre-existing, URI

15

Predisposing factors _____ to the development of pneumonia are:
- alcoholism*
- cigarette smoking*
- extremes of age*

Chest pain may be a symptom of a problem but is not a _____ _____ in itself. Extremes of age, cigarette smoking, and alcoholism are all predisposing factors to the _____ __ pneumonia.

predisposing factor, development of, contributing

16

A patient is anxious and has been breathing rapidly and deeply for the past 45 minutes. You can expect his blood _____ _____ level to be:
- elevated
- decreased*
- normal
- acidotic

Rapid, deep breathing can result in _____ _____ of carbon dioxide, leading to _____ _____.

respiratory alkalosis, excess elimination, carbon dioxide

17

When the entire lobe of a lung is filled with infection and cellular debris, it is termed:
- pleural disease
- mild aspiration
- consolidation*
- haemoptysis

The _____, _____, and _____ can fill up the lung, creating consolidation.

infection, debris, fluid

18

You find a morbidly obese 42-year-old patient lying _____ in his bed. He is in marked respiratory distress and is able to speak only in two-word sentences. What should you do FIRST? Sit him up or place him on his side.*

Morbidly obese patients in respiratory distress should be sat up or placed __ _____ ____. When a morbidly obese patient

is supine, his or her own ____
_____ can often impair the
mechanics of _____. This is
known as Pickwickian syndrome.

> respiration, body weight, on their
> side, supine

19
You are called to attend to an
18-year-old male who is having
a severe asthma attack. He is
awake and alert but appears
very tired. His vital signs are as
follows: blood pressure, 158/90;
pulse, 132; respiratory rate, 32
and extremely laboured. Upon
auscultation of his chest you
note breath sounds heard only
in the _____ _____ with very little
wheezing _____.
This is significant because it
shows bronchoconstriction with
air trapping.*
This _____ _____ results
in decreased ___ _____ in the
lungs and can lead to profound
hypoxia.
His fatigue is significant in that
it tells you he is in danger of
respiratory failure.*
_____ in this situation indicates
that the patient is becoming
tired. This is an ominous sign of
_____ respiratory failure and
the development of _____
_____. He is tachycardic at a rate
of 132 beats per minute and has
pale and diaphoretic skin.

What is causing these signs?
Hypoxia and the release of
epinephrine and norepinephrine.*
Both hypoxia and anxiety cause
activation of the _____
nervous system and the
_____ of epinephrine and
norepinephrine, which causes
diaphoresis, elevation of the heart
rate (tachycardia), and peripheral
vasoconstriction (pale skin).
Why is he able to talk only in
_____, _____ _____? His tidal
volume is inadequate for him to
speak in full sentences.*
Because of the air trapping, he
does not have enough air (tidal
volume) available to speak.
Which _____ will assist
__ _____ his airways?
Administration of a nebulized
beta-2 agonist.*
A nebulized beta-2 agonist (such
as albuterol) delivered by a mask
or handheld device using 5-10
LPM of oxygen can assist in
bronchodilation.
What medication can
be administered into the
subcutaneous tissues to help
_____ his respiratory
distress? Epinephrine 1:1,000,
0.3 mg.*
_____ epinephrine is an
option to treat cases of severe
asthma because of its beta-2
agonist properties.

air exchange, alleviate, release, Subcutaneous, serious condition, upper lobes, respiratory arrest, bilaterally, pending, intervention, short, broken phrases, in dilating, sympathetic, Fatigue

20

A disease that results from the _____ of the walls of the _____ and lessens the amount of surface area for ___ _____ is termed:

- emphysema*
- chronic bronchitis
- asthma
- pneumonia

gas exchange, alveoli, destruction

Vocabulary I

acidotic /əˈsɪd.ə.tɪk/ kyselý, o aminokyselinách

activation /ˌæk.tɪˈveɪ.ʃən/ aktivace, zapnutí

alcoholism /ˈæl.kə.hɒl.ɪ.zəm/ alkoholismus

alkalosis /ˌælkəˈləʊ.sɪs/ alkalóza, zvýšený výskyt zásaditých látek v těle

alleviate /əˈliː.vi.eɪt/ zmírnit, zmenšit

altered /ˈɔːltəd/ změněný

appear /əˈpɪər/ zdát se, jevit se, vypadat, objevit se

aspiration /ˌæspɪˈreɪʃən/ aspirace, dýchání

assist /əˈsɪst/ asistovat, pomáhat

attend /əˈtend/ účastnit se, věnovat se, pečovat, starat se

auscultate /ˈɔː.skəl.teɪt/ poslouchat, vyšetřit poslechem

auscultation /ˌɔː.skəlˈteɪ.ʃən/ auskultace, vyšetření poslechem

bradycardia /ˌbræd.ɪˈkaː.di.ə/ bradycardie, zpomalená srdeční činnost

bed /bed/ lůžko (anat.)

beta-2 agonist /ˈbiː.tə.tuː/ **agonists** /ˈæg.ə.nɪsts/ beta-2 agonisté, uvolňují a otevírají dýchací cesty, které se během astmatického záchvatu zužují, astma „uvolňovače" nebo bronchodilatátory

bilaterally /ˌbaɪˈlæt.ər.ə.li/ bilaterálně, dvoustranně

blood /blʌd/ krev

break /breɪk/ (broke broken) zlomit, rozbít

bronchoconstriction /ˌbrɒŋ.kəʊ. kənˈstrɪk.ʃən/ zúžení průdušek

cancer /ˈkænt.sər/ rakovina

cancerous /ˈkæn.sər.əs/ rakovinný

capillary /kəˈpɪl.ər.i/ **bed** /bed/ místo propojení kapilár tepének a žilek

capnometer /kæpˈɒm.ɪ.tər/ kapnometr, analyzátor respiračních plynů jednotlivých dechů pro kontrolu intubace

capnometry /kæpˈnɒm.ə.tri/ měření koncentrace oxidu uhličitého ve vzduchu

cell /sel/ buňka

cellular /ˈsel.jʊ.lər/ buněčný

concussion /kənˈkʌʃ.ən/ otřes mozku
confused /kənˈfjuːzd/ zmatený, popletený
consolidation /kənˌsɒl.ɪˈdeɪ.ʃən/ upevnění, konsolidace, sloučení
contrecoup /ˈkɒn.trə.kuːp/ zpětný odraz, zpětná síla (vyvolávající např. pohmoždění na opačné straně)
contribute /kənˈtrɪb.juːt/ přispět, přispívat, darovat, podílet
COPD, Chronic /ˈkrɒnɪk/ **Obstructive** /əbˈstrʌk.tɪv/ **Pulmonary** /ˈpʊl.mə.nə.ri/ **Disease** /dɪˈziːz/ chronické obstruktivní onemocnění plic
coup /kap/ mrtvice, záchvat
debris /ˈdeb.riː/, /ˈdeɪ.briː/ trosky, úlomky, pozůstatky, poškozená tkáň, buněčný odpad, zbytky, nečistota
deeply /ˈdiːp.li/ hluboce, zhluboka
definitive /dɪˈfɪn.ɪ.tɪv/ definitivní, konečný
destruction /dɪˈstrʌk.ʃən/ destrukce, zkáza, zničení
development /dɪˈvel.əp.mənt/ vývoj, vznik
device /dɪˈvaɪs/ zařízení, vybavení, přístroj
diaphoretic /ˌdaɪ.ə.fəˈret.ɪk/ diaforetický, opocený
diffusion /dɪˈfjuː.ʒən/ difuze, pronikání
disruption /dɪsˈrʌp.ʃən/ disrupce, trhlina, porušení, protržení, porucha, otevření rány

distress /dɪˈstres/ nouze, tíseň, utrpení, strádání, bolest, úzkost, strach
dull /dʌl/ tupý, pomalý, tlumený
elevate /ˈel.ɪ.veɪt/ zvednout
end /end/ **-tidal** /ˈtaɪ.d əl/ týkající se respiračního vzduchu, hodnota CO_2 na konci výdechu, $ETCO_2$
entire /ɪnˈtaɪə/ celý, úplný, veškerý
epidural /ˌepɪˈdjʊərəl/ epidurální, umístění nad durou
epinephrine /ˌepɪˈnef.riːn/ epinefrin (US), hormon vylučovaný nadledvinou, adrenalin
excessive /ekˈses.ɪv/ nadměrný, přílišný, nepřiměřený
exchange /ɪksˈtʃeɪndʒ/ výměna
excretion /ɪkˈskriː.ʃən/ exkrece, vyměšování, vylučování
exhale /eksˈheɪl/ vydechnout, vydechovat
expression /ɪkˈspreʃ.ən/ projev, vyjádření, výraz, výraz tváře
extreme /ɪkˈstriːm/ extrém, krajnost, nejvyšší bod
fatigue /fəˈtiːg/ únava, oslabení, vysílení, vyčerpání, unavit se
fill /fɪl/ naplnit, zaplnit
forced /fɔːst/ nucený, násilný
forcefully /ˈfɔːs.fəl.i/ silně, energicky
gain /geɪn/ získat, nabýt
gas /gæs/ plyn
Glasgow /ˌglɑːz.gəʊ/ **Coma** /ˈkəʊ.mə/ **Scale** /skeɪl/ Glasgowská škála kómatu
growth /grəʊθ/ růst, vývoj

haemoptysis / hiːˈmɒ.ptɪ.sɪs/ hemoptýza, vykašlávání krve

hand-held /ˈhændheld/ přenosný, ruční

hollow /ˈhɒl.əʊ/ prázdný, vpadlý, propadlý

hypoxia /haɪˈpɒk.sɪə/ hypoxie, nedostatečné zásobování tkání kyslíkem

immunocompromised /ˌim.jə.nəʊˈkɒm.prə.maɪzd/ s ohroženou imunitou

impact /ˈɪm.pækt/ dopad, náraz, úder, účinek, vliv, výsledek, dopadat, natlačit

impair /ɪmˈpeər/ oslabit, poškodit, narušit, zhoršit, oslabit, omezit funkci

inhalation /ˌɪn.həˈleɪ.ʃən/ vdechování, nádech

inspect /ɪnˈspekt/ prohlédnout, prozkoumat

inspection /ɪnˈspek.ʃən/ prohlédnutí, prohlídka, kontrola, vyšetřování nemocného pohledem

insult /ˈɪn.sʌlt/ poškození tělesného orgánu, tkáně, urazit, slovně napadnout

intact /ɪnˈtækt/ intaktní, netknutý, nedotčený, neporušený

laboured /ˈleɪ.bəd/ obtížný, namáhavý

lessen /ˈles.ən/ zmenšit, zmírnit, zmenšit se

lobe /ləʊb/ lalok, lalůček

localized /ˈləʊ.kəl.aɪzd/ umístěný

look /lʊk/ pohled, vypadat, budit dojem

measure /ˈmeʒ.ər/ opatření

mechanic /mɪˈkænɪk/ mechanismus

mechanics /məˈkæn.ɪks/ mechanika

membrane /ˈmem.breɪn/ membrána, blána, blána kryjící tělesnou část, orgán ap.

mental /ˈmen.təl/ **status** /ˈsteɪtəs/ duševní stav

mild /maɪld/ mírný, klidný, slabý, lehký

molecule /ˈmɒl.ɪ.kjuːl/ molekula

morbidly /ˈmɔːbɪd.li/ chorobně, patologicky

motor /ˈməʊ.tər/ motorický, pohybový

moving /ˈmuːvɪŋ/ pohyblivý

multisystem /ˈmʌl.tɪˈsɪs.təm/ vícesystémový

nebulized /ˈneb.jə.laɪzd/ nebulizovaný, ve spreji

neural /ˈnjʊə.rəl/ neurální, nervový

norepinephrine /nɔrˌep.əˈnef.rɪn/ norepinefrin, noradrenalin, hormon a neurotransmiter

occur /əˈkɜːr/ objevit se, nastat, přihodit se, vyskytovat se, nacházet se, existovat

oedema /ɪˈdiː.mə/ edém, otok

ominous /ˈɒmɪnəs/ zlověstný, hrozivý

option /ˈɒpʃən/ možnost, volba

order /ˈɔː.dər/ pokyn, příkaz, nařízení, pořadí

originate /əˈrɪdʒ.ɪ.neɪt/ vzniknout, vytvořit

osmosis /ɒzˈməʊ.sɪs/ osmóza, samovolné pronikání molekul rozpouštědla z méně koncentrovaného roztoku do roztoku koncentrovanějšího

oxygen /ˈɒk.sɪ.dʒən/ kyslík

pallor /ˈpæl.ər/ bledost, sinalost

palpate /ˈpæl.peɪt/ provádět palpaci, vyšetřovat pohmatem

palpation /pælˈpeɪ.ʃən/ palpace, pohmat, prohmatávání

peak /piːk/ **flow** /fləʊ/ **meter** /m.ɪ.tər/ výdechoměr, pomůcka pro měření vrcholu výdechové průtokové rychlosti, což je největší možné vydechnutí plícemi po co největším možném vdechu

pending /ˈpen.dɪŋ/ brzký, bezprostředně hrozící

percuss /pəˈkʌs/ proklepat, vyšetřit poklepem

percussion /pəˈkʌʃ.ən/ poklep, perkuse

perfusion /pəˈfjuː.ʒən/ perfuze, promývání, zásobování orgánů tekutinou

peritonitis /ˌper.ɪ.təˈnaɪ.tɪs/ peritonitida, zánět pobřišnice

Pickwickian /pɪkˈwɪk.i.ən/ **syndrome** /ˈsɪndrəʊm/ Pickwikův syndrom, břišní obezita, která omezuje možnost dýchacích pohybů bránice

placement /ˈpleɪs.mənt/ umístění, rozmístění

pleuric /ˈpluə.rɪk/ **disease** /dɪˌziːz/ onemocnění pohrudnice

point /pɔɪnt/ **to** /tə/ ukázat, namířit, upozornit

poorly /ˈpɔː.li/ chabě, nevalně, nemocný

pre-existing /ˌpriː.ɪgˈzɪs.tɪŋ/ dřívější, již existující

predispose /ˌpriː.dɪˈspəʊz/ predisponovat, učinit náchylný

proper /ˈprɒpə/ vhodný, pořádný, náležitý, vlastní, samotný

property /ˈprɒp.ə.ti/ majetek, vlastnictví, vlastnost, charakter materiálu

pulse /pʌls/ **oximeter** /ˈɒk.sɪ.m.ɪ.tər/ pulzní oximetr

pupillary /pjuː.pɪl.ər.i/ pupilární, zornicový

referred /rɪˈfɜːd/ **pain** /peɪn/ přenesená bolest, bolest pociťovaná v jiném místě než kde je její příčina

region /ˈriː.dʒən/ oblast, krajina

release /rɪˈliːs/ propustit, povolit, vypouštět, uvolňovat

remove /rɪˈmuːv/ odstranit, vyjmout, svléknout si

resistance /rɪˈzɪs.tənt s/ rezistence, odpor, odolnost

response /rɪˈspɒns/ odpověď, reakce

route /ruːt/ cesta, trasa

sample /sɑːmp|/ vzorek, ukázka

sedation /sɪˈdeɪ.ʃən/ uklidňující lék

sepsis /ˈsep.sɪs/ sepse, otrava krve, zaplavení organismu bakteriemi

size /saɪz/ velikost

somatic /səˈmæt.ɪk/ somatický, tělesný, tělový

subcutaneous /ˌsʌb.kjʊˈteɪ.ni.əs/ subkutánní, podkožní

surface /'sɜ:.fɪs/ povrch, hladina, zevnějšek, vynořit
sympathetic /ˌsɪm.pə'θet.ɪk/ týkající se sympatického nervového systému
syndrome /'sɪn.drəʊm/ syndrom
tachypnoea /ˌtæk.ɪp.'niː.ə/ tachypnoe, zrychlené dýchání
tired /'taɪəd/ unavený, vyčerpaný
tissue /'tɪʃ.uː/, /'tɪs.juː/ tkáň
tool /tuːl/ nástroj, pomůcka, prostředek
trap /træp/ past, nástraha, zachycovat
tremor /'trem.ər/ třes, chvění

uncontrolled /ˌʌn.kən'trəʊld/ nekontrolovatelný, neovladatelný, neřízený
variety /və'raɪə.ti/ rozmanitost, různost, různorodost
ventilation /ˌven.tɪ'leɪ.ʃən/ dýchání
via /'vaɪə/ přes, prostřednictvím
visceral /'vɪs.ər.əl/ viscerální, útrobní, vnitřní
weight /weɪt/ váha, hmotnost

Unit 2

I

Patients with chronic obstructive pulmonary disease (____) often breathe through pursed lips to increase pressure in the lungs. This method of breathing helps in preventing alveolar collapse.*

_____-___ breathing technique helps _____ _____ within the airways (even during exhalation) to support _____ _____ that have been damaged as a result of disease. In COPD, changes in the bronchioles that can result in significant air trapping include:

- inflammation*
- bronchospasm*
- increased mucus production*

All of these pathologies impair the flow of air through the _____ ____.

---

bronchial tree, maintain pressure, Pursed-lip, bronchial walls, COPD

2

A 64-year-old male presents with increased dyspnoea. He has a barrel chest, is thin, and is pink in colour. Clubbing of the fingers is present. Wheezes and rhonchi are present bilaterally in ___ _____, and pursed-lip breathing is noted. Vital signs are as follows: blood pressure, 162/92; pulse, 118 beats per minute; respiratory rate, 22.

This patient's _____ suggests that he is most likely suffering from COPD.*

The wheezes auscultated bilaterally indicate narrowing of the airways.*

Oedema and bronchoconstriction are examples of problems that can _____ ___ _____.

The rhonchi _____ bilaterally indicate excessive mucus in the larger airways.*

_____ are rattling sounds with a low pitch and snoring quality that is usually associated with _____ mucus or other material in the larger airways.

The clubbing of the fingers is associated with respiratory disease.*

_____ is a deformity produced by the growth of soft tissue about the _____ ___ _____. It is associated with _____ cardiac or respiratory disease.

The ____ _____ of this patient's skin is a result of an excess of circulating red blood cells.*

As a part of the body's own _____ _____, a chronic state of low blood oxygen levels will cause an increased production of ___ _____ _____ (polycythaemia) that give the patient's skin a pink colour.

fingers or toes, Rhonchi, red
blood cells, pink colour, all lobes,
compensatory, appearance,
mechanism, Clubbing, chronic,
excessive, auscultated, narrow
the airway

3
A 19-year-old male is found
breathing very rapidly. His
roommate tells you he has been
having a stressful time lately
and recently lost his job. The
patient is _____, alert, and very
anxious. You note that he has
spasms of his _____ ___ ____.
Vital signs are as follows: blood
pressure, 130/78; pulse rate, 116;
respiratory rate, 44 and regular.
He takes no medications and has
no past medical problems.
Hyperventilation resulting from
pure anxiety leads to:
- respiratory acidosis
- respiratory alkalosis*
- a decreasing blood pH
- hepatic failure
Hyperventilation can result in
an excess elimination of _____
_____, leading to respiratory
alkalosis.
Spasms of the hands and feet are
termed carpopedal spasms.*
_____ decreases blood
calcium levels, which leads to
hypocalcaemia. This results in
_____ ___ _____ of the feet
and hands.

In this situation, it is important to
consider that he has a serious
medical problem.*
Since hyperventilation ___ ____
a true medical emergency such
as a _____ _____, it is
important to consider that this
patient has a serious medical
problem.

fingers and feet, can mask,
pulmonary embolism, cramping
and spasms, Alkalosis, carbon
dioxide, awake

4
Your EMS team is dispatched
to care for a 39-year-old female
with difficulty breathing. She is
awake and appears _____
and_____. She tells
you she had sudden onset
of shortness of breath and a
sense of doom while typing
on her computer keyboard.
Her vital signs are as follows:
blood pressure, 148/92; radial
pulse is strong at 124 beats per
minute; respiratory rate, 36 per
minute and shallow. Her skin is
pale, cool, and dry. She denies
having chest pain or any health
problems.
Your patient's _____ _____
reading is 89% on room air.
This indicates that she has
hypoxaemia.*
_ _____ _____ is used as an
assessment tool. A patient with a

pulse oximetry value of less than 90% with no apparent cause or past medical history is considered to be moderately hypoxic and needs _____-____ _____ administration.
What is significant about her apprehension and sense of doom? It may indicate a threat to life.*
A patient who alerts you to his or her sense of doom should be taken ____ _____. There are numerous reports of patients who have 'sensed' a problem and later suffered a catastrophic event including a _____ __ ____.
During your interview, you find that the patient takes _____ _____ pills and has had left calf _____ for two days with no history of trauma to the area.
This information leads you to suspect a pulmonary embolus.*
A history of taking birth control pills combined with signs and symptoms that include a _____ ___ _____ lower extremity suggest deep vein thrombosis.
This predisposes the patient to developing _____ _____.
You interpret her cardiac rhythm as atrial _____ with a rapid ventricular response.*
Management of her condition would include all of the following:
• being on alert for _____ arrest*

• monitoring the cardiac rhythm*
• _____ intravenous access*

very seriously, threat to life, tenderness, fibrillation, establishing, pulse oximetry, high-flow oxygen, pulmonary embolus, A pulse oximeter, birth control, painful and inflamed, cardiac, restless, apprehensive

5
A 23-year-old healthy male who has been _____ by another person has a pulse rate of 146 and a respiratory rate of 32.
These vital signs _____ that his sympathetic nervous system is activated.*
Sympathetic nervous system _____ causes pupillary dilation and will _____ the pulse and respiratory rate.

stimulation, increase, threatened, indicate

6
Stroke, or _____ _____, can be compared to a heart attack in that:
• In both cases, _____ _____ causes tissue damage.*
• _____ can be beneficial in treating certain heart and brain attacks.*

Both heart attack and brain attack cause organ tissue damage due to the interruption of blood flow. Studies show that thrombolytic agents used to treat heart attack patients can be effective in treating occlusive strokes.

brain attack, Thrombolytics, oxygen deprivation

7

A 30-year-old suddenly developed a 2- to 3-minute grand mal seizure. On the scene you find an _____ ___ _____ patient. After inserting an oropharyngeal airway, applying high-flow oxygen, and assisting ventilations with a bag-valve mask, the patient's pulse oximetry reading is 90%. His skin is pale and moist. It is important to consider:
- a paralyzed diaphragm
- transport to a hospital
- endotracheal intubation*
- placement of a nasopharyngeal airway

A _____ _____ reading of 90% in a person who is on high-flow oxygen indicates _____ _____. Intubation should be considered.

moderate hypoxia, pulse oximetry, unconscious and unresponsive

8

A 30-year-old suddenly developed a 2- to 3-minute grand mal seizure. On the scene you find an unconscious and unresponsive patient with the following vital signs: BP, 178/100; pulse, 50 and regular; respiratory rate, 32 and irregular. He has no history of substance abuse but has complained of headaches for the past two weeks. His blood glucose registers 110.

You suspect that his problem is most likely the result of:
- hypoglycaemia
- a structural lesion*
- hyperglycaemia
- atrial fibrillation

_____ _____, such as brain tumours and intracerebral bleeds, can press on and _____ brain tissue. This can cause seizures and a number of other illnesses.

Two minutes after inserting an _____ _____, applying high-flow oxygen, and assisting his ventilations with a ___-_____ ____, the patient's pulse oximetry reading is 90%. His skin is pale and moist.
It is important to consider immediate endotracheal intubation*
A pulse oximetry _____ __ 90% in a person who is on high-flow

oxygen indicates moderate hypoxia. Intubation should __ _____.

It is important to avoid excessive hyperventilation because it can decrease the blood PaO_2 to dangerously low levels.*

Excessive _____ of a patient with increasing intracranial pressure can decrease the blood arterial carbon dioxide to dangerous levels.

The patient is now exhibiting decorticate posturing to _____ _____.

These signs indicate a lesion at or above the upper brainstem.*

Decorticate posturing (_____) indicates a lesion at or above the _____. Decerebrate posturing (_____), however, results from a lesion within the brainstem.

Structural lesions, brainstem, painful stimuli, oropharyngeal airway, flexion, extension, hyperventilation, reading of, be considered, bag-valve mask, destroy

9

A 27-year-old patient is complaining of persistent headache, fatigue, and pain upon flexion of his neck. He has had a chronic fever of 100 °F (37.8 °C) for the past two days.

His complaints lead you to suspect meningitis.*

Headache with fever, fatigue, and pain ____ _____ of the neck are all _____ signs and symptoms of meningitis.

In treating this patient, you would wear gloves and place a mask on yourself and the patient.*

Universal _____ include the use of _____ ___ _ ____ by the care provider as well as putting a mask on the patient, which significantly reduces the chance of exposure to the pathogen.

precautions, gloves and a mask, upon flexion, suspicious

10

You have a patient with metastatic brain cancer. He opens his eyes __ ____ and answers questions with _____ _____. When you start an IV in his left arm, he withdraws from the IV needle piercing the skin.

You would _____ his Glasgow Coma Scale: 9.*

You should always have a Glasgow Coma Scale chart available __ _____ in your ___ _____. This patient has a GCS score of 9: eye opening = 2, verbal response = 3, motor response = 4.

calculate, incomprehensible sounds, EMS practice, to reference, to pain

II

Which of the following are signs/symptoms of an acute cerebrovascular accident?

- _____ of the speech*
- facial ____*
- drooling*
- weak ____ _____ on the affected side*

---
slurring, motor response, droop

I2

You are called to a local restaurant for a patient exhibiting bizarre behaviours and shouting obscenities. He is pale, diaphoretic, and _____ any past _____ _____.
Which intervention should be most appropriate? Finger stick to check blood glucose.*
A _____ _____ ____ is a quick ____ to rule out hypoglycaemia, which could be the cause of this patient's _____. Any patient with an _____ ____ of consciousness should be tested for hypoglycaemia.

---
altered level, glucose finger stick, denies, behaviour, medical problems, tool
---

I3

You are called to assist a 25-year-old known Type I diabetic patient who is complaining of abdominal pain, _____, and

_____. His glucometer reading is 510.
The highest _____ _____ for this patient is to correct fluid volume deficit.*
This patient has diabetic _____ and is likely to be profoundly _____ because excess glucose acts as an osmotic diuretic. Fluid replacement with normal saline should be started _____.

---
dehydrated, ketoacidosis, immediately, vomiting, lethargy, treatment priority
---

I4

A patient's _____ reads 66. You may encounter all of the following symptoms of hypoglycaemia:

- _____ mental status*
- bizarre behaviour*
- hunger*

The signs and symptoms of hypoglycaemia are many and varied. Altered mental state including _____, bizarre behaviour, or _____ is often the most important and early _____ of a problem. Other signs/symptoms may include diaphoresis, tachycardia, _____, and headache. ____ may be present in severe cases.

glucometer, agitation, Coma, irritability, altered, indicator, weakness

15

You receive a call to the home of a 66-year-old male with a _____ __ weakness. The patient is cooperative but continues to ask you the same questions over and over again. You are concerned because he has developed _____ _____ over the past 5 minutes and is now diaphoretic.

Your next action is to establish IV and obtain a _____ _____ for a blood glucose test.*

With a presentation of confusion and diaphoresis, you should be thinking of _____.

Blood sample, hypoglycaemia, increased confusion, complaint of

16

When the body is not able to use glucose as a _____ _____ __ _____, adipose cells begin _____ ____, resulting in ketoacidosis.*

This ___-_____ metabolism results in a rise of blood ketones, which can lead to _____.

ketoacidosis, breaking down, primary source of energy, fat-based

17

Signs and symptoms of Graves' disease include agitation, emotional changes, insomnia, ___ _____, weight loss, and _____.

You must be familiar with signs and symptoms of the most common _____ _____.

Graves' disease is the result of thyrotoxicosis (excessive thyroid hormones).

endocrine disorders, heat intolerance, exophthalmos

18

A male patient has ingested 30 levothyroxine tablets that belonged to his mother. You recognize this medication as a thyroid replacement hormone. You attach the ECG monitor and observe a sinus tachycardia of 140 with a corresponding pulse rate. Treatment would include expedited transport for definitive care.*

_____ _____ is a true medical emergency that requires _____ _____ to definitive care. Drug therapy that will block the effects of the _____ _____ of thyroid hormone is required.

expedited transport, toxic level, Thyroid storm

19

A patient with Cushing's _____ would MOST likely present with:

• ketoacidosis
• hypoglycaemia*
• decreased urination
• acute hyperactivity

_____ is associated with Cushing's syndrome due to _____ cortisol levels.

excessive, Hypoglycaemia, syndrome

20

You are caring for a 78-year-old female patient who has a long history of _____ (Cushing's syndrome). She is complaining of left-side weakness. You are assigned to establish an IV line and obtain a blood sample for _____ _____ testing. You should take great care with venipuncture in this patient because hyperadrenalism leads to easy bruising and a delay in healing.* Long-term effects of hyperadrenalism lead to paper-thin (almost transparent) skin that can be easily _____ __ ____. The disease process also results in _____ _____.

hyperadrenalism, delayed healing, bruised or torn, blood glucose

Vocabulary 2

abuse /ə'bjuːz/ zneužívání, týrání
access /'æk.ses/ přístup, vstup
accident /'æksɪdənt/ nehoda, neštěstí
act /ækt/ jednat, činit, působit, jednat podle, řídit se
adipose /'æd.ɪ.pəʊs/, /-pəʊz/ tukový
affect /ə'fekt/ ovlivnit, ovlivňovat, působit, postihnout, zasáhnout
agitation /ˌædʒ.ɪ'teɪ.ʃən/ nervozita, rozrušení, vzrušení, znepokojení
alveolar /ˌæl.vi'əʊ.lər/ alveolární, sklípkový
apparent /ə'pær.ənt/ zřejmý, patrný, jasný
appearance /ə'pɪə.rənt s/ vzhled, zjev, zevnějšek, objevení se
apprehension /æp.rɪ'hen.ʃən/ obava, strach, předtucha
atrial /'eɪ.tri.əl/ **fibrillation** /ˌfaɪ.brɪ'leɪ.ʃən/ fibrilace srdečních předsíní, porucha srdečního rytmu
attach /ə'tætʃ/ připojit, přilepit se, nalepit se
barrel /'bær.əl/ sud, barel
behaviour /bɪ'heɪ.vjə/ chování, jednání, reakce
beneficial /ˌben.ɪ'fɪʃ.əl/ prospěšný, blahodárný
birth /'bɜːθ/ **control** /kən'trəʊl/ **pill** / pɪl/ antikoncepční pilulka
bizarre /bɪ'zɑːr/ bizarní, divný, podivný
blade /bleɪd/ lopatka
bleed /bliːd/ krvácet, krvácení

blood /blʌd/ **sample** /'sɑːm.pļ/ vzorek krve

brainstem /'breɪn.stem/ mozkový kmen

break /breɪk/ **down** /daʊn/ porucha, porušení, havárie, defekt, zhroutit se, nevydržet

bronchial /'brɒŋ.ki.əl/ **tree** /triː/ průduškový strom

bronchiole /'brɒŋ.ki.əʊl/ průdušinka

bronchospasm /ˌbrɒŋ.kəʊ.'spæz.əm/ bronchospasmus, křeč průdušek

bruise /bruːz/ modřina, podlitina

calcium /'kæl.si.əm/ vápník, kalcium

calculate /'kælkjʊˌleɪt/ vypočítat, spočítat, spoléhat na co

calf /kɑːf/ lýtko

care /keə/ péče, starost, dohled, pozornost

care /keə/ **provider** /prə'vaɪ.dər/ ošetřovatel, pečovatel

carpopedal /ˌkɑː.pə'pɪːd.əl/ karpopedální, týkající se zápěstí a nohy

case /keɪs/ případ, daná situace

catastrophic /ˌkæt.ə'strɒf.ɪk/ katastrofální, tragický

chart / tʃɑːt/ graf, diagram, schéma, nákres

check /tʃek/ kontrolovat, zkontrolovat, kontrola

clubbing /'klʌb.ɪŋ/ paličkovité prsty

collapse /kə'læps/ zhroutit se, kolaps

coma /'kəʊ.mə/ kóma, hluboké bezvědomí

compare /kəm'peər/ porovnat, srovnat

compensatory /ˌkɒm.pən'seɪt.ə ri/ kompenzační

concern /kən'sɜːn/ zájem, starost, obavy, znepokojení

confusion /kən'fjuːʒən/ zmatek, záměna

cool /kuːl/ chladný, studený

cooperative /kəʊ'ɒp.ər.ə.tɪv/ spolupracující, vstřícný

corresponding /ˌkɒr.ɪ'spɒn.dɪŋ/ odpovídající

cortisol /'kɔː.tɪ.sɒl/ kortizol, glukokortikoidní hormon vylučovaný nadledvinami

cramp /kræmp/ křeč

decerebrate /dɪˌser.ə'breɪt/ **posturing** /'pɒs.tʃər.ɪŋ/ decerebrační postavení, vnitřní rotace horních končetin s flexním postavením rukou

decorticate /ˌdi.ko:ti'keɪt/ **posturing** /'pɒs.tʃər.ɪŋ/ dekortikační postavení (rigidita), při zvýšeném nitrolebním tlaku, následkem ischemie mozku nebo poškození hemisfér, změny postavení končetin, flexe loktů, zápěstí a prstů a extenze dolních končetin

deep /diːp/ hluboký, dlouhý

definitive /dɪ'fɪn.ɪ.tɪv/ definitivní, konečný

dehydrated /ˌdiː.haɪ'dreɪ.tɪd/ dehydratovaný, odvodněný

delay /dɪ'leɪ/ zdržet, odkládat, odložit, zpozdit, zpoždění

deny /dɪ'naɪ/ zapřít, popřít

diabetic /ˌdaɪəˈbet.ɪk/ **ketoacidosis** /ˈkiːtəʊˌæs.ɪˈdəʊ.sɪs/ diabetická ketoacidóza, acidóza způsobená nadměrným množstvím ketolátek v krvi

diaphoresis /ˌdaɪ.ə.fəˈriː.sɪs/ diaforéza, pocení

diaphragm /ˈdaɪ.ə.fræm/ bránice, přepážka

dilation /daɪˈleɪ.ʃən/ dilatace, rozšíření, roztažení

dispatch /dɪˈspætʃ/ vyslat, poslat, odeslat, odeslání

diuretic /ˌdaɪ.jʊəˈret.ɪk/ diuretický, močopudný lék

doom /duːm/ zkáza, zánik

drool /druːl/ slintat, sliny tekoucí z úst

droop /druːp/ viset, klesat vysílením, sklonit hlavu

emergency /ɪˈmɜː.dʒənt.si/ naléhavá nutnost, pohotovost

emotional /ɪˈməʊ.ʃən.əl/ emocionální, citový

encounter /ɪnˈkaʊntə/ setkat se, setkání, zkušenost

endocrine /ˈen.də.krɪn/ endokrinní, s vnitřní sekrecí

establish /ɪˈstæb.lɪʃ/ navázat, založit, vytvořit

event /ɪˈvent/ událost, případ, akce

exhibit /ɪgˈzɪb.ɪt/ ukázka, projevit, projevovat příznaky

exophthalmos /ˌeks.ɒfˈθæl.məs/ exoftalmus, vystouplé oko

expedite /ˈek.spə.daɪt/ urychlit

extension / ɪkˈsten.tʃən/ natažení, prodloužení, rozšíření

facial /ˈfeɪ.ʃəl/ obličejový, lícní

familiar /fəˈmɪl.i.ər/ **with** /wɪð/ seznámený, dobře známý

fat-based /fæt.beɪst/ tukový

fibrillation /ˌfaɪ.brɪˈleɪ.ʃən/, /ˌfɪb.rɪˈleɪ.ʃən/ fibrilace srdečních komor

fingerstick /ˈfɪŋ.gə.stɪk/ píchnutí do prstu

flexion /flek.ʃən/ flexe, ohnutí, ohyb, ohýbání

glucometer /ˌgluːkəˈm.ɪ.tər/ glukometr

grand mal /ˌgrɑːndˈmæl/ velký epileptický záchvat

Graves' /greɪvz/ **disease** /dɪˈziːz/ Gravesova-Basedowova nemoc, autoimunitní onemocnění štítné žlázy provázené její hyperfunkcí

heal /hiːl/ hojit, léčit, vyléčit se, zahojit

hepatic /hepˈæt.ɪk/ hepatický, jaterní

hyperactivity /ˌhaɪ.pərˈæk.tɪv.ɪ.ti/ hyperaktivita

hyperadrenalism /ˌhaɪ.pər.ædˈri.nəl.ɪzm/ hyperadrenalismus, zvýšená sekrece adrenalinu

hypocalcaemia /ˌhaɪ.pəʊ.kælˈsiː.mi.ə/ hypokalcemie, nedostatek vápníku v krvi

hypoxaemia /ˌhai.pɒkˈsiː.mi.ə/ hypoxemie, snížené množství kyslíku v krvi

immediate /ɪˈmiː.di.ət/ bezprostřední, okamžitý

incomprehensible /ɪnˌkɒm.prɪˈhen.sɪ.b̩l/ nesrozumitelný

inflamed /ɪnˈfleɪmd/ zanícený

inflammation /ˌɪn.fləˈmeɪ.ʃən/ zánět
insertion /ɪnˈsɜː.ʃən/ zasazení,
aplikace (vložka)
insomnia /ɪnˈsɒm.ni.ə/ insomnie,
nespavost
interruption /ˌɪn.təˈrʌp.
ʃən/ přerušení, přerušování,
vyrušování
intolerance /ɪnˈtɒl.ər.ənt s/
intolerance, nesnášenlivost
intracerebral /ˌɪn.trəˈser.ə.brəl/
nitromozkový, ležící uvnitř mozku
intravenous /ˌɪn.trəˈviː.nəs/
intravenózní, nitrožilní
irritability /ˌɪr.ɪ.təˈbɪl.ɪ.ti/
iritabilita, dráždivost, podráždění,
podrážděnost, nedůtklivost
IV, intravenous /ˌɪn.trəˈviː.nəs/
intravenózní, nitrožilní
ketoacidosis /ˈkiː.təʊˌæ.ɪˈdəʊ.sɪs/
ketoacidóza, acidóza, způsobená
nadměrným množstvím ketolátek
v krvi
ketone /ˈkiː.təʊn/ keton
lesion /ˈliː.ʒən/ léze, rána, zranění,
poranění, poškození, porucha,
postižené místo
levothyroxine /lev.ɒ.θaɪˈrɒk.sɪn/
levothyroxine, lék na poruchy
štítné žláty
management /ˈmænɪdʒmənt/
řízení, ošetření, léčba
mask /mɑːsk/ maska, maskovat
meningitis /ˌmen.ɪnˈdʒaɪ.tɪs/
meningitida, zánět mozkových
blan, aseptic m. virová
meningitida
mental /ˈmen.təl/ status /ˈsteɪtəs/
duševní stav

metastatic /ˌmet.əˈstæt.
ɪk/ metastatický, týkající se
metastázy
moderately /ˈmɒd.ər.ət.li/ mírně,
přiměřeně
moist /mɔɪst/ mokrý, vlhký
narrow /ˈnær.əʊ/ úzký, těsný,
omezený, zúžit
nasopharyngeal /ˌneɪ.zə.fəˈrɪn.dʒi.
əl/ nazofaryngeální, nosohltatový
note /nəʊt/ zaznamenat, zapsat,
poznámka, vzkaz, zpráva
obscenity /əbˈsen.ɪ.ti/ obscénnost,
sprosté slovo
obtain /əbˈteɪn/ získat, dosáhnout
occlusive /ɒˈkluː.sɪv/ uzavřený
oedema /ɪˈdiː.mə/ edém, otok
onset /ˈɒn.set/ propuknutí, začátek
osmotic /ɒzˈmɒt.ɪk/ pressure /ˈpreʃ.
ər/ osmotický tlak, tlak tekutiny
rozpouštědla na biologické
polopropustné membráně
painful /ˈpeɪn.fəl/ bolestivý,
působící bolest
paralyze /ˈpær.əl.aɪz/ paralyzovat,
ochromit
part /pɑːt/ část, součást, role,
spoluúčast, rozdělit
pathogen /ˈpæθ.ə.dʒən/ patogen,
původce, choroboplodný zárodek
pathology /pəˈθɒl.ə.dʒi/ patologie
persistent /pəˈsɪs.tənt/
perzistentní, trvalý, přetrvávající,
úporný, nepolevující
pH /ˌpiːˈeɪtʃ/ pH kyselost či
zásaditost prostředí
pierce /pɪəs/ propíchnout,
probodnout
pill /pɪl/ pilulka, prášek, tabletka

polycythaemia /ˌpɒl.ɪ.saɪˈθiːm.ɪ.ə/ polycytemie, zmnožení všech krevních elementů v krvi

postural /ˈpɒst.ʃər.əl/ posturální, postojový, týkající se držení těla

posture /ˈpɒs.tʃər/ držení těla, postoj, postavení těla, dát do pozice

practice /ˈpræk.tɪs/ praxe, praktika, postup

predispose /ˌpriː.dɪˈspəʊz/ predisponovat, učinit náchylným

profoundly /prəˈfaʊnd.li/ hluboce, nesmírně

pupillary /pjuː.pɪl.ər.i/ pupilární, zornicový

pure /pjʊər/ čistý, bez příměsí

pursed /pɜːsd/-lip /lɪp/ našpulené rty

radial /ˈreɪ.di.əl/ radiální, vřetenní

rattle /ˈræt.l̩/ rachotit, drnčet

recognize /ˈrekəɡˌnaɪz/ rozpoznat, uznat, ocenit, poznat

red /red/ blood /blʌd/ cell /sel/ červená krvinka

reference /ˈref.ər.ənt s/ doporučení

replacement /rɪˈpleɪs.mənt/ navrácení, náhrada, nahrazení, nové umístění, vrácení

restless /ˈrest .ləs/ neklidný, nepokojný

rhonchus /rong'kəs/ pl. -chi chrapot

rise /raɪz/ zvednout, stoupat

roommate /ˈrʊm.meɪt/ spolubydlící

rule /ruːl/ out /aʊt/ vyloučit

saline /ˈseɪ.laɪn/ slaný, solný roztok, fyziologický roztok

seizure /ˈsiː.ʒə/ křečový stav, záchvat (nemoci), záchvatový

sense /sens/ smysl, pocit, vjem, rozum, chápat, mít smysl

shouting /ˈʃaʊ.tɪŋ/ pokřikování, křičení

show /ˈʃəʊ/ ukázat, zachycovat, jevit, projev

slur /slɜːr/ mumlat opile, ospale apod.

snore /snɔːr/ chrápat, zachrápání

soft /sɒft/ měkký, jemný

source /sɔːrs/ zdroj, příčina

speech /spiːtʃ/ řeč, mluvení

state /steɪt/ stav, uvádět, prohlašovat

structural /ˈstrʌktʃərəl/ konstrukční, stavební

substance /ˈsʌb.stənt s/ substance, látka, hmota

sudden /ˈsʌd.ən/ náhlý, nečekaný

suspicious /səˈspɪʃ.əs/ nedůvěřivý, podezíravý

sustain /səˈsteɪn/ vydržet, snést, utrpět

tenderness /ˈten.də.nəs/ bolestivost, citlivost na dotek

thin /θɪn/ tenký, prořídnout

threat /θret/ hrozba, ohrožení, výhrůžka

thrombolytic /θrɒm.bəˈlɪt.ɪk/ trombolytický, rozpouštějící krevní sraženinu, trombus

thyroid /ˈθaɪə .rɔɪd/ storm /stɔːm/ život ohrožující komplikace zvýšené činnosti štítné žlázy

thyroid gland /ˈθaɪə .rɔɪdˌɡlænd/ štítná žláza, štítný, týkající se štítné žlázy

thyrotoxicosis /ˌθaɪˈrəˌtɒksiˈkəʊ.sɪs/ tyreotoxikóza, otrava způsobená hyperfunkcí štítné žlázy

toe /təʊ/ prst na noze

torn /tɔːn/ roztržený, roztrhaný

transparent /trænˈspær.ənt/ transparentní, průhledný

tumour /ˈtjuː.mər/ tumor, nádor

unconscious /ʌnˈkɒnʃəs/ v bezvědomí

unresponsive /ˌʌn.rɪˈspɒnt .sɪv/ bez reakce, nereagující, netečný

urination /ˌjʊə.rɪˈneɪ.ʃən/ močení

value /ˈvæl.juː/ hodnota, význam, cena

varied /ˈveə.rɪd/ rozmanitý, různorodý, pestrý

vascular /ˈvæs.kjʊ.lər/ vaskulární, cévní

vein /veɪn/ žíla

venipuncture /ˌve.niˈpʌŋk.tʃər/ nabodnutí žíly, puštění žilou

weakness /ˈwiːk.nəs/ ochablost, chatrnost, slabost

weight /weɪt/ **loss** /lɒs/ úbytek váhy

wheeze /wiːz/ sípat, těžce dýchat, sípání

withdraw /wɪðˈdrɔː/ stáhnout, ustoupit, odejít

within /wɪˈðɪn/ uvnitř, v rámci

Unit 3

1

Hyperadrenalism is associated with a high incidence of atherosclerosis including hypertension and stroke.*
_____ is associated with high incidence of atherosclerosis, hypertension, and _____, which are all risk factors for _____.

> stroke, Hyperadrenalism, diabetes

2

A patient experiencing Addisonian crisis may display these signs/symptoms: cardiovascular collapse, hypotension, and hypoglycaemia.*
Presentation of _____ _____ (Addisonian crisis) may include cardiovascular _____, hypotension, and _____. These serious signs/symptoms are attributed to _____ _____ in the water and electrolyte _____ within the body.

> major disturbances, collapse, adrenal insufficiency, hypoglycaemia, balance

3

You have a patient who presents with a whole body rash. There is no complaint of shortness of breath.
What history findings lead you to conclude that ___ ____ is the result of a delayed hypersensitivity reaction? History of taking a new medication for the past seven days.*
A _____ hypersensitivity reaction may occur several hours or even days _____ _____.
Common causes are _____ __ _____. A patient may very well present with the signs/symptoms of allergic reaction several days after starting a new medication.

> after exposure, medications and chemicals, the rash, delayed

4

Urticaria is defined as raised areas or wheals on the skin due to histamine release.*
Raised areas or wheals on the skin associated with _____ reaction and _____ _____ are known as urticaria (_____).

> hives, histamine release, allergic

5

You are called to an elementary school. On arrival, you are directed to a teacher. The class is holding a birthday party for Austin, who turned 10 today. His

mom baked brownies for the party that contained nuts.
The teacher is _____ __ nuts.
She ate brownies 5 minutes ago.
She complains of _____ in her chest that is _____ __ _____ to breathe. She is not able to talk in ____ _____.
Given this information, you suspect the patient is experiencing a severe allergic reaction.*
Her respiratory distress is _____ _____. Her blood pressure is 74/48; pulse, 140; respirations, 40. You decide to administer epinephrine.
The correct ____ ___ _____ are 3-5 ml of 1:10,000 solution IV.*
Because this patient is demonstrating pending cardiovascular and respiratory _____, the administration of _____ epinephrine is indicated.

dose and route, collapse, making it difficult, intravenous, full sentences, allergic to, becoming worse, tightness

6
A patient with severe vomiting presents with the _____ of his eyes dramatically blood red. This is most likely the result of:
- hyphaema
- subconjunctival haemorrhage*
- conjunctivitis
- blunt trauma

A _____ _____ involves rupture of small blood vessels in the subconjunctival space resulting in the white of the eye becoming _____ ___.
This may occur after a _____ _____ or _____ _____.
While it looks dramatic, this type of haemorrhage usually clears without _____ and rarely causes any residual problems.

strong sneeze, intervention, scleras, excessive vomiting, subconjunctival haemorrhage, blood red

7
You arrive on the scene of a 30-year-old male lying on the ground. According to a bystander, the patient was on top of a ladder changing a light bulb. After he stuck his hand in the light fixture, he was attacked by yellow jackets that had a nest in the fixture. The patient then jumped from the top of the ladder to escape the bees. You estimate his fall to the ground to be 8 feet. He has numerous yellow jacket _____ on his left arm and neck.
The patient is unconscious and _____. As you assess his airway and breathing, you observe a respiratory rate of 8 per minute with deep _____

respirations, _____ muscle use, and obvious inspiratory stridor with each breath. Management of this patient's airway would include C-spine immobilization, assist ventilations, and immediate endotracheal intubation.*
With the possibility of spine injury, proper precautions must be taken. Assessment of the chest reveals no obvious trauma. You note equal but distant lung sounds with _____ on auscultation.
You suspect the respiratory distress to be from bronchial constriction _____ __ anaphylactic reaction.*
Based on the presence of bee stings and the absence of obvious _____ _____ causing the respiratory distress, you should suspect severe _____ _____ secondary to anaphylactic shock.

accessory, stings, gasping, wheezing, bronchial constriction, unresponsive, secondary to, chest trauma

8
You are assessing a patient with acute right lower-quadrant pain. You suspect acute appendicitis. A _____ ____ of pain from _____ located one or two inches above the anterior iliac crest in a direct line with the umbilicus is known as McBurney's point.*
The presence of _____ _____ in this patient represents peritoneal irritation.*
Rebound tenderness is pain on release of the examiner's hand, allowing the patient's abdominal wall to return to its normal position and is usually associated with _____ _____.
This assessment finding can be present in other abdominal conditions and is not _____ __ appendicitis.

specific to, rebound tenderness, common site, appendicitis, peritoneal irritation

9
Your patient states that he has experienced right upper-quadrant pain and right shoulder pain for the last seven days.
The patient is ____, _____, and in obvious discomfort. He has a bounding pulse rate of 132. He states that this episode of pain began after eating fried onion rings with hot mustard sauce.
You suspect his _____ ____ ____ is caused by stress response to the body and sympathetic nervous system activation.*
You notice that he has pain with _____ under the right costal margin.
This is known as Murphy's sign.*

Murphy's sign is pain caused when an _____ _____ is palpated by pressing under the right costal margin.
With the information gathered you suspect:

- pancreatitis
- appendicitis
- cholecystitis (inflammation of the gallbladder)*
- diverticulitis

---

elevated heart rate, inflamed gallbladder, palpation, pale, diaphoretic

---

10

A 39-year-old male patient is lying on a couch, covered with several blankets. He has a garbage can next to him that has a small amount of vomitus in it. He has a past _____ _____ of alcoholism.
The patient _____ __ severe epigastric pain that _____ into his back and shoulders. His _____ is softly distended, and he will not allow you to palpate it due to the pain. He states that he took his temperature 30 minutes ago and it was 104.2 °F (40.1 °C). BP is 86/42; pulse, 138; respirations, 20.
You suspect the patient is _____ ____ pancreatitis.*
His history of alcoholism and presentation should lead you to suspect severe _____.

Eighty per cent of all cases of pancreatitis are associated with alcoholism.
You suspect his vital signs are a result of septic shock from the disease process.*
His BP of 86/42 and pulse of 138 lead you to believe a _____ _____ is present. His temperature of 104.2 °F (40.1 °C) may indicate _____. Severe pancreatitis is associated with septic shock, and when present, it has a high _____ ____.

---

suffering from, abdomen, mortality rate, medical history, sepsis, pancreatitis, complains of, radiates, shock state

---

11

You respond to a 21-year-old male with a complaint of vomiting after he drank an excessive amount of alcohol. He is _____, _____, and experiencing excessive dry heaves at this time. You note the presence of specks of blood on the toilet. He has no history of GI problems and takes no medications.
You suspect the_____ is the result of a Mallory-Weis tear.*
An _____ ___ or laceration that _____ ____ excessive vomiting is known as a Mallory-Weis tear. While you may suspect this type of injury, it is difficult to be 100% certain. Do

not ____ ___ more serious causes of upper GI bleeding.

---

potassium, overaggressive dialysis, Bradycardia, hypotension

---

bleeding, alert, results from, oriented, rule out, oesophageal tear

---

12

Maroon or tarry-coloured _____ indicates:
- peritonitis
- bowel obstruction
- the presence of partially digested blood*
- alcoholism

_____ is dark, tarry, ____-_____ stool that indicates the presence of _____ _____ blood.

---

partially digested, stool, Melena, foul-smelling

13

_____ and _____ following an Overaggressive dialysis treatment are MOST indicative of:
- hypovolaemia
- hypokalaemia*
- hyperkalaemia
- air embolism

_____ _____ treatment can lead to a reduction of _____ (hypokalaemia). This is likely to be seen immediately after dialysis treatment.

14

What treatment for the care of a patient who is suffering from complications of dialysis is correct? To prevent _____ of the problem, start an IV only if ordered by medical control.* Fluid administration in dialysis patients should be under the _____ _____ of medical control. Dysrhythmias are _____ and, if present, are generally caused by electrolyte _____. To prevent accidental damage to the shunt, a BP should never be assessed on the arm with the

_____.

---

imbalances, direct authority, common, shunt, exacerbation

15

You arrive on the scene of a 54-year-old female patient who is unable to urinate. She states that she had outpatient surgery in which she received anaesthesia. She presents in severe discomfort and has a _____ _____ bladder that is noticeable on inspection of the abdomen. This patient's situation is a true medical emergency.*
The _____ __ _____ is a true medical emergency because a full, distended bladder

is _____ _____ for the patient. Definitive care usually requires insertion of a _____ _____, which is not common in the prehospital setting. EMS treatment is primarily supportive.

inability to urinate, urethral catheter, firmly distended, extremely painful

16

A 42-year-old male presents with severe pain in the left flank area with no history or signs of trauma. The patient has excruciating _____ pain with intermittent vomiting.

What problem would you suspect as the cause of the patient's discomfort?

- abdominal aortic aneurysm
- appendicitis
- gallbladder attack
- renal calculi*

_____ _____ of flank pain, excruciating colicky pain, and _____ are considered classic signs and symptoms of _____ _____ (kidney stones).

Treatment for this patient would be IV fluids and morphine.* _____ ____ should be focused on comfort and support. Give nothing by mouth and establish IV line for medication administration. An antiemetic may

be indicated, and ____ _____ is important.

Note: While there may be concern about the use of pain medication in 'undiagnosed' abdominal pain or that administration of pain medication may ____ _____ and make in-hospital assessment more difficult, the use of morphine is not _____ in renal calculi.

vomiting, Sudden onset, mask symptoms, contraindicated, pain management, renal calculi, colicky, Prehospital care

17

You are transporting a patient who is _____ ___ _____ of methamphetamine. The patient, who is clearly anxious, has a BP of 176/92, a pulse of 146, and respiration of 24. The patient suddenly becomes _____ and begins thrashing around, trying to ___ ___ the stretcher.

You should administer intramuscular haloperidol.* A benzodiazepine such as a haloperidol should be used to control anxiety caused by _____ _____. Chemical restraints are a widely accepted prehospital treatment.

stimulant abuse, get off, violent, under the influence

18

A skin rash, a metallic taste in the mouth, and explosive diarrhoea are MOST indicative of:

- lead poisoning
- cyanide poisoning
- arsenic poisoning*
- mercury poisoning

_____ is the second leading cause of acute _____ _____. Symptoms are a metallic taste in the mouth, explosive _____, and severe _____ pain.

> abdominal, diarrhoea, Arsenic, metal poisoning

19

You are called to attend to a 61-year-old female complaining of headache, vomiting, abdominal pain, and ___ __ _____. She has recently been using a gas home-heating device to warm up her bedroom. Her sister lives next door, and they always eat every meal together. The patient cannot get out of bed, saying she is ___ _____. She appears to be sleeping now.

Upon assessing the patient you note that she can speak clearly, moves all extremities slowly, and has a blood pressure of 164/86, pulse regular at 104, and respiratory rate at 18 with normal effort. She has not eaten since last evening when she ate dinner with her sister. Her sister, however, feels fine.

The patient's condition suggests carbon monoxide poisoning.* The ____-_____ _____ in the bedroom, the patient's signs and symptoms, and the fact that her sister is not sick should lead you to suspect carbon monoxide poisoning.

Her pulse oximetry is 99%. This can be misleading because pulse oximetry is inaccurate in certain cases of _____.*

Because carbon monoxide binds readily with the _____ molecule, the _____ _____ reading can read normal even though the patient may be hypoxic.

What treatment is most important? Provide high-flow oxygen.*

_____ high-flow oxygen is essential in patients with _____ _____ poisoning.

> loss of coordination, carbon monoxide, Providing, poisoning, haemoglobin, home-heating device, too tired, pulse oximetry

20

Physical assessment findings, signs, or symptoms that support your suspicion that a patient is _____ ___ _____ of alcohol or drugs include chest pain and dysrhythmias, confusion

and polyuria, dilated pupils and anxiety, and constricted pupils and respiratory depression.*
Chest ____ and dysrhythmias are typical signs/symptoms of cocaine abuse.
_____ and polyuria represent alcohol use.
Dilated _____ and anxiety represent evidence of hallucinogens.
_____ pupils and respiratory depression are the result of opiates.

Confusion, Constricted, under the influence, pain, pupils

Vocabulary 3
abrupt /əˈbrʌpt/ náhlý, neočekávaný, prudký
accessory /əkˈses.ər.i/ akcesorní, přídatný
accumulate /əˈkjuː.mjʊ.leɪt/ akumulovat, nashromáždit se
Addison's disease /ˈæd.ɪ.sənz. dɪˌziːz/ Addisonova nemoc, nedostatečnost kůry nadledvin
allow /əˈlaʊ/ dovolit, poskytnout, umožnit
anaphylactic /ˌæn.ə.fɪˈlæk.tɪk/ anafylaktický, vztahující se k anafylaxi
aneurysm /ˌæn.jʊə.rɪ.zəm/ aneuryzma, výduť, místní abnormální rozšíření krevních cév, zvláště arterií, vrozený defekt cévní stěny

anterior /ænˈtɪə.ri.ər/ přední, předchozí
anti-emetic /ˌæn.tɪ.ɪˈmet.ɪk/ antiemetický, antiemetikum, lék proti nevolnosti a zvracení
appendicitis /əˌpen.dɪˈsaɪ.tɪs/ zánět slepého střeva
arsenic /ˈɑː.sən.ɪk/ arzén
asymmetrical /ˌeɪ.sɪˈmet.rɪk.əl/ asymetrický, nesouměrný
attack /əˈtæk/ útok, napadení, záchvat
attribute /ˈæt.rɪ.bjuːt/ přičítat, přisuzovat, symbol
awareness /əˈweə.nəs/ povědomí, vědomí, vnímavost, uvědomování si
balance /ˈbæl.əns/ vyrovnávat, rovnováha
bee /biː/ včela
bind /baɪnd/ (bound, bound) spojit, vázat, vazba
bladder /ˈblæd.ər/ měchýř
blood /blʌd/ **vessel** /ˈves.əl/ krevní céva
blunt / blʌnt/ tupý, oblý, přímý
bound /baʊnd/ skákat, běžet
brownie /ˈbraʊ.ni/ sušenka
bulb /bʌlb/ žárovka
C-spine, cervical /səˈvaɪ.kəl/ **spine** / spaɪn/ krční páteř
campus /ˈkæm.pəs/ areál univerzity
carbon monoxide /ˌkɑː.bən.məˈnɒk. saɪd/ oxid uhelnatý
cessation /sesˈeɪ.ʃən/ skončení, zastavení, ustání
chemical /ˈkem.ɪ.kəl/ chemický, chemická látka

cholecystitis /ˌkəʊ.lɪ.sɪˈstaɪ.tɪs/ cholecystitida, zánět žlučníku

colicky /ˈkɒl.ɪ.ki/ trpící kolikou, kolikový

comfort /ˈkʌm.fət/ pohodlí, uklidnění, utěšit, poskytnout útěchu

complaint /kəmˈpleɪnt/ stížnost, nemoc, neduh, potíž

conclude /kənˈkluːd/ usoudit, dojít k závěru

conditioning /kənˈdɪʃ.ən.ɪŋ/ udržování kondice, cvičení, navykání si

conjunction /kənˈdʒʌŋk.ʃən/ spojení, kombinace

conjunctivitis /kənˌdʒʌŋk.tɪˈvaɪ.tɪs/ zánět očních spojivek

constricted /kənˈstrɪkt.ɪd/ zúžený, stáhnutý

copperhead /ˈkɒp.ər.hed/ jedovatý had, jed ničí červené krvinky

costal /ˈkɒs.təl/ žeberní

cottonmouth /ˈkɒt.ən.maʊθ/ ploskolebec vodní, druh jedovatého hada

Crohn's disease /ˈkrəʊnz.dɪˌziːz/ Crohnova nemoc, regionální enteritida

cyanide /ˈsaɪə.naɪd/ kyanid

daydream /ˈdeɪ.driːm/ být duchem nepřítomný, snění za bílého dne

delayed /dɪˈleɪd/ zpožděný, odložený

demonstrate /ˈdem.ən.streɪt/ předvádět, vyložit, ukázat, dokázat, dát najevo

direct /daɪˈrekt/ nasměrovat, zamířit, řídit, dohlížet

disc /dɪsk/ ploténka (meziobratlová), kotouč

discomfort /dɪˈskʌmp.fət/ obtíž, mírná bolest, nepohoda, znepokojení

discontinuation /ˌdɪs.kənˌtɪn.juˈeɪ.ʃən/ ukončení, zastavení

distant /ˈdɪs.tənt/ vzdálený, odměřený, nepřístupný

distend /dɪˈstend/ roztáhnout se, zduřet

disturbance /dɪˈstɜː.bənt s/ nepokoj, výtržnost, porucha

diverticulitis /ˌdaɪ.və.tɪk.jʊˈlaɪ.tɪs/ divertikulitida, zánět divertikulu

dose /dəʊs/ porce, dávka, příděl

drizzle /ˈdrɪz.əl/ mrholit, mžení

drowsy /ˈdraʊ.zi/ ospalý, mátožný

dysphasia /disˈfeɪ.zɪə/ dysfázie, porucha řeči

electrolyte /ɪˈlek.trə.laɪt/ elektrolyt, roztok, který vede elektřinu

equal /ˈiːkwəl/ stejný, rovnat se (čemu)

escape /ɪˈskeɪp/ únikový, utéct, uniknout, uprchnout

essential /ɪˈsen.t ʃəl/ základní, důležitý, hlavní

estimate /ˈes.tɪ.meɪt/ odhad, odhadnout

exacerbation /ɪɡˌzæsəˈbeɪʃən/ zhoršení, ztížení

examiner /ɪɡˈzæm.ɪ.nər/ vyšetřovatel, zkoušející

excruciating /ɪkˈskruː.ʃi.eɪ.tɪŋ/ nesnesitelný, mučivý

expectorate /ɪkˈspek.tər.eɪt/ vykašlávat (hlen)

experience /ɪkˈspɪə.ri.ənt s/ zkušenost, prožít, zažít, prožívat, prodělat, ucítit

eyebrow /ˈaɪ.braʊ/ obočí

fibrillate /ˈfaɪ.brɪ.leɪt/ fibrilovat, jednotlivá vlákna srdečního svalu nebo jejich skupiny se stahují samostatně, fibrilace komor bez léčby vede rychle k smrti

finding /ˈfaɪndɪŋ/ závěr, zjištění, nález

fire fighter /ˈfaɪə‚faɪ.tər/ hasič

fixture /ˈfɪks.tʃər/ příslušenství, vybavení

focused /ˈfəʊkəst/ cílený, zaměřený, soustředěný

foul /faʊl/ odporný

frown /fraʊn/ zamračit se, zamračený pohled

gallbladder /ˈgɔːlˈblæd.ər/ žlučník

garbage /ˈgɑː.bɪdʒ/ **can** /kæn/ popelnice

gasp /gɑːsp/ lapat po dechu, zalapat po dechu

gather /ˈgæð.ər/ shromáždit, získat, zjistit, dozvědět se

goblet /ˈgɒb.lət/ sklenka, pohárek

goof /guːf/ **around** /əˈraʊnd/ blbnout, dělat kraviny

ground /graʊnd/ zem, podlaha, území

haemorrhage /ˈhem.ər.ɪdʒ/ krvácení, vnitřní krvácení

hallucinogen /həˈluː.sɪ.nə.dʒen/ halucinogen, prostředek na vyvolání halucinace

heave /hiːv/ zvedat se (žaludek), dávit

histamine /ˈhɪs.tə.miːn/ histamin

hives /haɪvz/ kopřivka

humidity /hjuːˈmɪd.ɪ.ti/ vlhkost

hyperkalaemia /‚haɪ.pə.kæˈliː.mi.ə/ hyperkalemie, nadbytek draslíku v krvi

hypersensitivity /‚haɪ.pə.‚sen.sɪˈtɪv.ɪ.ti/ hypersensitivita, přecitlivělost

hyphaema /haɪ.θe.mə/ hyféma, krev v přední komoře oční před duhovkou

hypokalaemia /‚haɪ.pəʊ.kæˈliː.mi.ə/ hypokalemie, nedostatek draslíku v krvi

hypovolaemia /‚haɪpəʊ.vəˈlː.mi.ə/ hypovolemie, nízký objem krve v těle

iliac /ˈɪl.i.æk/ **crest** /krest/ kyčelní hřeben

imbalance /‚ɪmˈbæl.ənt s/ nerovnováha, nevyrovnanost

immobilization /ɪ‚məʊ.bəl.aɪˈzeɪ.ʃən/ imobilizace, znehybnění, fixace

inaccurate /ɪˈnæk.jʊ.rət/ nepřesný

inattentiveness /‚ɪn.əˈten.tɪv.nəs/ nepozornost

incidence /ˈɪnt .sɪ.dənt s/ výskyt, počet případů, četnost nemoci ap.

influence /ˈɪnflʊəns/ vliv, účinek

inguinal /ˈɪŋ.gwɪ.nəl/ ingvinální, tříselný

insertion /ɪnˈsɜː.ʃən/ zasazení, aplikace (vložka)

inspiratory /ɪnˈspaɪə.rə.tər.i/ inspirační, vdechový

insufficiency /‚ɪn.səˈfɪʃ.ən.si/ nedostatečnost

intermittent /ˌɪn.təˈmɪt.ənt/ občasný, přerušovaný

intervention /ˌɪn.təˈven.ʃən/ intervence, zákrok, zakročení, zásah

intramuscular /ˌɪn.trəˈmʌs.kjʊ.lər/ intramuskulární, nitrosvalový

irritation /ˌɪr.ɪˈteɪ.ʃən/ podráždění

jerk /dʒɜːk/ trhnout, škubnout, cuknutí, trhnutí, škubnutí

ladder /ˈlæd.ər/ žebřík

lead /led/ olovo

light-headed /ˌlaɪtˈhed.ɪd/ malátný, mající závrať, zmámený

major /ˈmeɪ.dʒə/ hlavní, významný, větší, velký, důležitý, významnější, závažný, převážný

Mallory-Weis /ˈmæl.ər.i-vaɪs/ **syndrome** /ˈsɪn.drəʊm/ Malloryho-Weissův syndrom, stav charakterizovaný krvácením z lineárních ruptur v oblasti ezofagogastrické junkce, vzniká při silném zvracení, někdy u alkoholiků, jedna z příčin hematemeze

margin /ˈmɑː.dʒɪn/ okraj, pokraj, lem, lemovat

maroon /məˈruːn/ kaštanově hnědý

medication /ˌmed.ɪˈkeɪ.ʃən/ medikace, léky

melaena /məˈliː.n.ə/ melena, černě zabarvená stolice natrávenou krví

mercury /ˈmɜː.kjʊ.ri/ rtuť

metallic /məˈtæl.ɪk/ kovový

methamphetamine /ˌmeθ. æmˈfet.ə.mi:n/ metamfetamin, též

pervitin, syntetické stimulancium z řad amfetaminů

mimic /ˈmɪm.ɪk/ napodobovat

misleading /ˌmɪsˈliː.dɪŋ/ zavádějící, klamný, mylný

mortality /mɔːˈtæl.ə.ti/ mortalita, úmrtnost

Murphy's /ˈmɜː.fiz/ **sign** /saɪn/ Murphyho příznak, pacient je vyzván k nádechu při hluboké palpaci pod pravým žeberním okrajem, při choleocystitidě ucítí bolest

mustard /ˈmʌs.təd/ hořčice

nerve / nɜːv/ nerv

nest /nest/ hnízdo, uhnízdit se

nondiscernible /ˌnɒn.dɪˈsɜː.nɪ.bļ/ nerozeznatelný, neviditelný

note /nəʊt/ zaznamenat, zapsat, poznámka, vzkaz, zpráva

noticeable /ˈnəʊ.tɪ.sə.b| / patrný, zjevný, nápadný

numerous /ˈnjuː.mə.rəs/ početný

obvious /ˈɒb.vi.əs/ zjevný, jasný, zřejmý, očividný, samozřejmý, nápadný

onion /ˈʌn.jən/ cibule (zelenina)

onset /ˈɒnˌset/ propuknutí, začátek

outermost /ˈaʊ.tə.məʊst/ nejvzdálenější (od středu)

outpatient /ˈaʊt.peɪ.ʃənt/ ambulantní pacient

outpouching /ˈaʊt.paʊtʃ.ɪŋ/ posunutí části tkáně zevnitř navenek, vytvoření váčku

palsy /ˈpɔːl.zi/ obrna, ochrnutí, paralýza

pancreatitis /ˌpæŋ.kri.əˈtaɪ.tɪs/ pankreatitida, zánět slinivky břišní

partially /'pɑː.ʃəl.i/ částečně, zčásti

pending /'pen.dɪŋ/ brzký, bezprostředně hrozící

peritoneal /ˌper.ɪ.tə'ni.əl/ peritoneální, pobřišniční

peritonitis /ˌper.ɪ.tə'naɪ.tɪs/ peritonitida, zánět pobřišnice

periumbilical /ˌper.ɪ.ʌm'bɪl.ɪ.kəl/ periumbilikální, ležící kolem pupku

petit mal /ˌpə'ti'mæl/ malý epileptický záchvat

phlegm /flem/ hlen

pill-rolling /'pɪlˌrəʊ.lɪŋ/ **tremor** /'trem.ər/ klidový třes palce a prstů ruky u Parkinsonovy choroby

pit viper /'vaɪpə/ chřestýšovec, had

polyuria /ˌpɒl.ɪ'jʊə.rɪ.ə/ polyurie, nadměrné močení

potassium /pə'tæs.i.əm/ draslík

precaution /prɪ'kɔː.ʃən/ bezpečnostní opatření

presume /prɪ'zjuːm/ předpokládat, domnívat se

pupil /'pjuːpəl/ zornička

radiate /'reɪ.di.eɪt/ vyzařovat, rozbíhat se (paprskovitě)

raise /reɪz/ vytáhnout, zvýšit, zvýšení, zvednout, zřídit

rash /ræʃ/ vyrážka

rebound /ˌriː'baʊnd/ **tenderness** /'ten.dər.nəs/ zvýšená bolestivost při náhlém uvolnění tlaku

release /rɪ'liːs/ propustit, povolit, vypouštět, uvolňovat

renal /'riː.nəl/ **calculi** /'kæl.kjʊ.laɪ/ ledvinové kameny

residual /rɪ'zɪd.ju.əl/ residuální, zbylý, zbytkový

restraint /rɪ'streɪnt/ restrikce, zamezování, omezení, překážka, zabezpečení v autě

reveal /rɪ'viːl/ odhalit, prozradit, objevit

ring /rɪŋ/ kruh, kroužek, prstenec, kruhový otvor

rough /rʌf/ drsný, hrubý

route /ruːt/ cesta, trasa

rule /ruːl/ **out** /aʊt/ vyloučit

rupture /'rʌp.tʃər/ ruptura, protržení, zlomení, kýla, výhřez

sclera /'sklɪə.rə/ skléra, oční bělmo

search /sɜːtʃ/ **for** /fɔː/ hledat

secondary /'sek.ən.dri/ sekundární, druhotný, vedlejší

sheet /ʃiːt/ prostěradlo, útržek, plátek, list, vrstva

shunt /ʃʌnt/ posunout, přesunout, zkrat, posunutí, odklonit se od směru, umělá cesta pro odklonění tekutiny

side /saɪd/ strana, bok, vedlejší

site /saɪt/ místo, poloha, plocha, oblast, umístění, být umístěn

slipper /'slɪp.ər/ bačkora, trepka

snake /sneɪk/ had

sneeze /sniːz/ kýchnout, kýchnutí

soaked /səʊkt/ nasáklý, promáčený

soccer /'sɒk.ər/ fotbal

specific /spə'sɪf.ɪk/ specifický, konkrétní, přesný

speck /spek/ skvrnka

spell /spel/ doba, (krátké) období

stagnate /stæg'neɪt/ stagnovat, váznout

state /steɪt/ stav, uvádět, prohlašovat

stick /stɪk/ (stuck, stuck) uvíznout

sting /stɪŋ/ štípnutí, bodnutí, žihadlo

stonelike /'stəʊn.laɪk/ kameni podobný

stool /stu:l/ stolice, výkaly

strenuous /'stren.ju.əs/ namáhavý, vysilující

stretcher /'stretʃə/ nosítka pro zraněné

stridor /straɪd.ər/ stridor, pískavý zvuk při ztíženém dýchaní

subconjunctival /ˌsʌbˌkɒn.dʒaŋk.'tɪ.vəl/ subkonjunktivální, podspojivkový

succession /sək'seʃ.ən/ řada, série

suffer /'sʌf.ər/ trpět, utrpět, zhoršit se

supportive /sə'pɔ:.tɪv/ nápomocný, podporující

surgery /'sɜ:.dʒər.i/ chirurgie, chirurgický zákrok

suspect /sə'spekt/ mít podezření, domnívat se

suspicion /sə'spɪʃən/ podezření, podezírání

tarry /'tær.i/ térový, dehtový

tear /teər/ protržení, trhlina, trhat, odtrhnout

telephone /'tel.ɪ.fəʊn/ telefon, telefonní

temporal /'tem.pər.əl/ temporální, spánkový

tepid /'tep.ɪd/ vlažný, vlahý

thrash /θræʃ/ bít, tlouci

tightness /'taɪt.nəs/ tíseň, těsnost, napětí

umbilicus /ʌm'bɪl.ɪ.kəs/ pupek

unaware /ˌʌn.ə'weər/ netušící, neuvědomující si

urethra /jʊə'ri:.θrə/ močová trubice

urinate /'jʊə.rɪ.neɪt/ močit

urticaria /ˌɔ:.tɪ'keə.ri.ə/ kopřivka

valuable /'væl.jʊ.bļ/ cenný, hodnotný

varix /ˌveə.rɪks/ pl varices / 'vær.ɪ.si:z/ varix, křečová žíla, krevní městka

vertebral /'vɜ:.tɪ.brəl/ vertebrální, obratlový, páteřní

violent /'vaɪələnt/ agresivní, prudký, silný, násilný

voluntary /'vɒləntərɪ/ dobrovolný, vůlí ovladatelný

wheal /wi:l/ napuchlina, šrám, podlitina

white /waɪt/ oční bělmo

yellow jacket /'jel.oʊˌdʒæk.ɪt/ vosa, včela

Unit 4

1

These statements about delirium tremens are true:

- DTs can occur from either an _____ discontinuation or _____ of alcohol after prolonged use.*
- DTs are characterized by a decreased level of consciousness and _____.*
- There is _____ _____ associated with DTs.*

significant mortality, abrupt, ingestion, hallucinations

2

All of the following are signs and symptoms of _____ _____:

- salivation*
- lacrimation*
- urination*

SLUDGE is a helpful mnemonic to remember signs of poisoning: S = salivation, L = lacrimation, U = urination, D =_____, G = GI (_____) upset, E =_____. Other symptoms of organophosphate poisoning include _____, bradycardia, anxiety, and _____ _____.

bronchoconstriction, defecation, visual disturbances, organophosphate poisoning, emesis, gastrointestinal

3

The patient is conscious but slow to respond and appears highly intoxicated. He asks for help and falls to the floor. His appearance is pale and diaphoretic with a blood pressure of 90/64, pulse of 144, and respiration of 36. You note that the porch is covered in ground-coffee emesis.
This patient is most likely suffering from ruptured oesophageal varices.*
The patient's past _____ _____ and _____ should lead you to the conclusion of ruptured _____ _____.
His appearance and vital signs indicate shock.*
This patient __ _____ shock as evidenced by his _____ pulse rate (144), evidence of _____ (pale and moist skin), and his ability to maintain his _____ _____.
Treatment of this patient should include close monitoring of airway _____, administration of _____ oxygen, establishment of intravenous access, and treatment for shock.*
As always, the airway is your priority. You must protect the

airway and prevent _____ of emesis. Supplemental oxygen, _____ intravenous access, and treatment for shock are required.
During transport to the hospital, your patient has several additional episodes of vomiting. It starts as coffee-ground _____ that quickly changes to bright red blood. He is less responsive with intermediate periods of _____. Blood pressure is 82/64, pulse 148, respirations 40.
You know that his vital signs and change in mental status indicate decompensated shock.
His condition is _____, and rapid transport is necessary.*

is experiencing, blood pressure, medical history, supplemental, emesis, aspiration, patency, establishing, serious, syncope, elevated, vasoconstriction, presentation, oesophageal varices

4
The MOST common and _____ ____ of pit viper _____ is rapidly developing oedema around the bite area.*
Pit vipers include rattlesnakes, copperheads, and cottonmouths. Rapidly developing oedema around the ____ ____ can occur in as little as 15 minutes.

envenomation, bite area, reliable sign

5
Minute respiratory _____ is best described as the _____ __ ___ moved in and out of the ____ in 1 minute.*

lungs, volume, amount of air

6
You respond to the local college campus soccer field for a 20-year-old female patient with a complaint of severe muscle cramps. The temperature is 88 °F (31.1 °C) with high humidity. The patient had just finished a strenuous workout when the cramps began. Her skin is hot to touch, and she is sweating profusely.
You suspect this patient is suffering:
- heatstroke
- heat exhaustion
- heat cramps*
- exercise-induced fatigue

___ _____ are acute painful spasms of the voluntary muscles following _____ activities in a ___ _____.
Treatment should include oral hydration if the patient is able to take fluids.*
Treatment for heat cramps include _____ the patient from the hot environment and

administering oral _____ _____ or sport drinks for hydration. If oral fluids cannot be administered because of nausea, __ __ ____ of normal saline may be needed.

> removing, Heat cramps, an IV line, strenuous, saline solution, hot environment

7

Your ambulance is assigned to stand by at a building fire. The outside temperature is 103 °F (39.4 °C) and the _____ are wearing full protective clothing. Approximately 30 minutes into the incident, a firefighter has collapsed, and you are _____ to care for him. The patient is a 36-year-old male in good physical condition. He appears anxious and complains of nausea and a headache. He is _____ profusely with cool, clammy skin. BP is 116/48, radial pulse is 150 and weak, respirations are 36 and shallow, and temperature is 101.2 °F (38.3 °C).

This patient's signs/symptoms indicate:

- heatstroke
- heat exhaustion*
- heat stress
- heat fatigue

Profuse sweating with cool and clammy skin; tachycardia; rapid, shallow respiration; and a body temperature over 99.8 °F (37.7 °C) indicates ____ _____.

Treatment for this patient should include removing clothing, establishing IV of normal saline, and placing in air conditioning.* The patient is now apprehensive. _____ reveals a BP of 78/30; pulse, 154; respirations, 36 and shallow. You are unable to take another temperature because he is not cooperating. His skin is extremely hot to touch and has stopped sweating. Online medical control has requested that you start rapid active cooling. This can be achieved by covering the patient in a sheet that has been soaked in tepid water.* This patient has progressed from ___ _____ to _____ as indicated by severe apprehension, hypotension, hot skin, and the cessation of sweating.

Overcooling of a heatstroke patient may cause a reflex hypothermia. Shivering may result, which can lead to a rise in core temperature; 102 °F (38,9 °C) should be used as a target temperature to prevent overcooling.*

> heat exhaustion, Reassessment, sweating, heat exhaustion, firefighters, assigned, heatstroke

8

You are called for a 62-year-old male with a _____ __ severe abdominal pain. He is lying as still as possible in his bed.
Upon inspection of the abdomen, you find _____ in the periumbilical area. This is known as Cullen's sign.*

- This _____ finding may indicate intraabdominal haemorrhage.*

---
assessment, ecchymosis, complaint of

9

You are called by the local police department to help search for an elderly man with Alzheimer's disease who wandered away from his home. It is 11.30 p.m. and he has been missing for three hours. It is 3 °C outside with a light drizzle. The man is wearing pyjamas and slippers. At 4.30 a.m. the patient is located lying behind a pile of wood five blocks from his home. He is unconscious, unresponsive, apnoeic, and pulseless. His skin is cold to the touch, and his muscles are _____. His core body temperature is 32 °C.
Initial treatment should include CPR.*
CPR is indicated even if _____ __ ____ are present.

Hypothermic patients cannot be presumed dead until a core body temperature of 34 °C has been achieved and _____ _____ are still unsuccessful. You are considering the administration of cardiac medication for this patient. IV medication may be administered but spaced at longer-than-standard intervals.* ____ _____ is reduced so administered medication such as epinephrine or lidocaine ___ _____ to toxic levels. In addition, administered drugs may retain in the _____ _____. When the patient is rewarmed and peripheral circulation resumes, a large toxic bolus of medication may be delivered to the central circulation. Care during transportation for this patient should include all of the following: avoiding rough handling due to cardiac irritability, protecting against further ____ ____, and transporting in a horizontal position.*

---
heat loss, resuscitation efforts, Drug metabolism, may accumulate, peripheral circulation, signs of death, rigid
---

10

You are called to attend to a patient who fell 7 feet (2.13 m) from a porch and landed on

his head. He is_____,
has erratic respirations, and is
bleeding from a ___ _____. Your
first action to manage the airway
would be:
- nasotracheal intubation
- head-tilt, chin-lift
- jaw thrust*
- to initiate in-line traction
  with intubation

The modified ___ _____ is the
easiest and safest method to
manage the airway immediately.

jaw thrust, head wound, unresponsive

11

You are having lunch with your
nephew J. and his friend S. You
notice that S. appears to have
periods of inattentiveness and
daydreaming. During these
spells, his eyelids _____, and
he appears to be _____ __ his
surroundings. You ask J. if he has
ever noticed this before. J. says
he has been 'goofing around' like
this for a week now.
These signs indicate S. may have
petit mal seizure disorder.*
_____ ___, or absence, seizure
is characterized by a brief loss
of awareness for 10-30 seconds.
This type of seizure occurs in
_____ and usually disappears
after 20 years of age.

childhood, unaware of, flutter, Petit mal

12

A 58-year-old female has a
history of smoking two packs of
cigarettes per day. She suffers
from frequent upper respiratory
infections with a _____
_____ and expectorates white,
thick _____. She most likely is
suffering from:
- asthma
- congestive heart failure
- chronic bronchitis*
- bronchiolitis

Years of exposure to _____
_____ (e.g. cigarettes)
can result in an increase in
the number of goblet cells in
the bronchial system with an
increased _____ __ _____.

production of mucus, toxic irritation, productive cough, phlegm

13

A 66-year-old female is unable to
get out of bed. She responds to
verbal stimuli with clear speech,
her smile is asymmetrical, she
cannot move her left leg, and
she weakly moves her left arm.
Her skin is warm but pale. Vital
signs are as follows: BP, 162/88;
pulse, 110 beats per minute
and irregular; respiratory rate,
22 per minute with lung sounds

clear bilaterally. A blood glucose reading is 130 mg/dl. The cardiac monitor shows a very irregular, narrow complex tachycardia with no identifiable P waves.
Damage of what body system __ _____ movement of the left side of her body?

- cardiovascular system
- central nervous system*
- pulmonary system
- endocrine system

An asymmetrical smile in conjunction with the inability to move her left leg and weakness of her left arm indicate injury to the patient's _____ _____ _____ (CNS)

The patient's _____ smile is most likely a direct result of damage to cranial nerve VII.

A patient's ability to smile, _____, lift eyebrows, and _____ ___ _____ is controlled by cranial nerve VII.*

Why was it important to obtain a blood glucose reading on this patient? Hypoglycaemia can mimic stroke.*

Patients who are hypoglycaemic can exhibit signs and symptoms similar to a stroke.

Her cardiac rhythm is atrial fibrillation.*

_____ _____ is an irregular, narrow complex rhythm with nondiscernible P waves.

This cardiac rhythm makes her more prone to the development of:

- diabetes
- emboli*
- brain tumours
- cardiogenic shock

As the atria fibrillate, they also dilate. This allows for blood to _____ in the atria and can lead to ____ _____.

A family member states that she was fine one hour ago when he talked to her on the telephone. This is important information because it establishes a reference point for the onset of symptoms.*

Studies suggest that there is a three-hour window between the time of onset of symptoms and the time of thrombolytic intervention for treatment to be _____. Establishing a _____ _____ for the onset of symptoms is critical.

is affecting, Atrial fibrillation, reference point, asymmetrical, effective, central nervous system, stagnate, clot formation, frown, wrinkle the forehead

14

You are called to attend to a 51-year-old male who fell in his living room. His wife states that he has been very depressed and has not eaten or drunk anything for the past twenty-four hours. You notice the patient has a stone-like face, _____ _____, and is exhibiting 'pill-rolling' _____. These are all signs of:

- multiple sclerosis
- Bell's palsy
- Parkinson's disease*
- vertebral disc disease

In managing this patient, it is important to start an intravenous line, determine a blood glucose level, and apply a cardiac monitor.*

Starting an intravenous line will allow access for medications if necessary. _____ the blood glucose level will show if the altered mental status is due to hypoglycaemia, and applying a _____ _____ will determine if there is a rhythm disturbance.

cardiac monitor, Determining, muscular rigidity, movements

15

Your EMS unit is called to attend to a 79-year-old female who experienced an abrupt onset of facial drooping, dysphasia, and marked _____. Upon examination, she is now alert and oriented, _____ clear, and moves all extremities well. Vital signs are normal.

Your assessment findings _____ ___ to suspect transient ischemic attack.*

Since her signs and symptoms_____ _____ and she has no neurological deficit, she most likely suffered a _____ ischemic attack. TIA is considered a significant _____ ____ for the development of a _____.

stroke, hemiparesis, warning sign, disappeared rapidly, lead you, speech, transient

16

Ecchymosis in the _____ ____ associated with intraabdominal _____ is known as:

- peritonitis
- Cullen's sign
- Mallory-Weiss ____
- Grey Turner's sign*

sign, flank area, haemorrhage

17

Small outpouchings of mucosal and submucosal tissue that push through the outermost layer of the _____ is known as:

- Crohn's _____
- inguinal hernia
- _____ colitis
- diverticulitis*

disease, ulcerative, intestine

18

A peak flow value of 100 (l/min.) shows:

- normal _____
- mild severity
- moderate _____
- severe respiratory compromise*

A ____ ____ of 100 (l/min.) is very low; 400-650 l/min. is the normal range.

| peak flow, value, severity |

19

In differentiating between syncope and a grand mal seizure, you know that syncope:

- often begins in a standing position*
- presents with jerking motions during

  _____

- causes the patient to remain drowsy following the event
- is often _____ by aura

_____ usually occurs when the person is in the _____
_____. It can begin with dizziness or feeling light-headed or can occur without warning.

| standing position, Syncope, unconsciousness, preceded |

20

A seizure characterized by a rapid ____ _____ or auras that include unusual smells, tastes, or sounds is termed:

- simple partial seizure disorder
- _____ ___ seizure disorder
- pseudoseizure _____
- complex partial seizure disorder*

A complex partial seizure disorder can present in many ways since they usually _____ in the temporal lobe of the brain. They are usually of _____ _____, and while patients experience a loss of contact with their surroundings, they do not lose motor tone.

| short duration, originate, disorder, mood change, petit mal |

21

Your EMS team is called to a patient in her mid thirties who is having a generalized motor seizure. Bystanders inform you that she has been seizing continually for the past 10 minutes. You note that the patient __ _____ violently, is diaphoretic, and is slightly cyanotic.

This prolonged seizure is specifically termed:

- petit mal seizure disorder
- grand mal seizure disorder
- complex seizure disorder
- status epilepticus*

_____ _____ is two or more generalized motor seizures occurring in succession and is a life-threatening emergency situation. The most valuable early intervention is to use bag-valve mask assistance with 100% oxygen.*
Air exchange is poor during a generalized motor seizure. It is extremely important to protect the airway from obstruction and deliver 100% oxygen using a bag-valve mask for _____ _____.

Administration of the medication terminated her seizure activity. Now you should be alert for which of the following side effects?
• respiratory depression*
• hyperglycaemia
• hypertension
• fever
Valium (_____) is a sedative and anticonvulsant that depresses seizure activity in the brain. A side effect of Valium is respiratory depression.

Status epilepticus, respiratory assistance, diazepam, is shaking

Vocabulary 4
abrupt /əˈbrʌpt/ náhlý, neočekávaný, prudký
accumulate /əˈkju:.mjʊ.leɪt/ akumulovat, nashromáždit se
asymmetrical /ˌeɪ.sɪˈmet.rɪk.əl/ asymetrický, nesouměrný
awareness /əˈweə.nəs/ povědomí, vědomí, vnímavost, uvědomování si
campus /ˈkæm.pəs/ areál univerzity
cessation /sesˈeɪ.ʃən/ skončení, zastavení, ustání
colitis /kə.lɪ.tɪs/ kolitida, zánět tlustého střeva
conclude /kənˈklu:d/ usoudit, dojít k závěru
conditioning /kənˈdɪʃ.ən.ɪŋ/ udržování kondice, cvičení, navykání si
conjunction /kənˈdʒʌŋk.ʃən/ spojení, kombinace
copperhead /ˈkɒp.ər.hed/ jedovatý had, jed ničí červené krvinky
daydream /ˈdeɪ.dri:m/ být duchem nepřítomný, snění za bílého dne
discontinuation /ˌdɪs.kənˌtɪn.juˈeɪ.ʃən/ ukončení, zastavení
disturbance /dɪˈstɜ:.bənt s/ nepokoj, výtržnost, porucha
diverticulitis /ˌdaɪ.vəˌtɪk.juˈlaɪ.tɪs/ divertikulitida, zánět divertikulu
drizzle /ˈdrɪz.əl/ mrholit, mžení
drowsy /ˈdraʊ.zi/ ospalý, mátožný
dysphasia /disˈfeɪ.zɪə/ dysfázie, porucha řeči
expectorate /ɪkˈspek.tər.eɪt/ vykašlávat (hlen)

experience /ɪkˈspɪə.ri.ənt s/ zkušenost, prožít, zažít, prožívat, prodělat, ucítit

eyebrow /ˈaɪ.braʊ/ obočí

fibrillate /ˈfaɪ.brɪ.leɪt/ fibrilovat, jednotlivá vlákna srdečního svalu nebo jejich skupiny se stahují samostatně, fibrilace komor bez léčby vede rychle k smrti

fire fighter /ˈfaɪə‚faɪ.tər/ hasič

frown /fraʊn/ zamračit se, zamračený pohled

goblet /ˈgɒb.lət/ sklenka, pohárek

goof /guːf/ **around** /əˈraʊnd/ blbnout, dělat kraviny

humidity /hjuːˈmɪd.ɪ.ti/ vlhkost

inattentiveness /‚ɪn.əˈten.tɪv.nəs/ nepozornost

inguinal /ˈɪŋ.gwɪ.nəl/ ingvinální, tříselný

intervention /‚ɪn.təˈven.ʃən/ intervence, zákrok, zakročení, zásah

irritation /‚ɪr.ɪˈteɪ.ʃən/ podráždění

jerk /dʒɜːk/ trhnout, škubnout, cuknutí, trhnutí, škubnutí

light-headed /‚laɪtˈhed.ɪd/ malátný, mající závrať, zmámený

mimic /ˈmɪm.ɪk/ napodobovat

nondiscernible /‚nɒn.dɪˈsɜː.nɪ.bl̩/ nerozeznatelný, neviditelný

onset /ˈɒn‚set/ propuknutí, začátek

outermost /ˈaʊ.tə.məʊst/ nejvzdálenější (od středu)

outpouching /ˈaʊt.paʊtʃ.ɪŋ/ posunutí části tkáně zevnitř navenek, vytvoření váčku

palsy /ˈpɔːl.zi/ obrna, ochrnutí, paralýza

partially /ˈpɑː.ʃəl.i/ částečně, zčásti

petit mal /‚pəˈtiˈmæl/ malý epileptický záchvat

phlegm /flem/ hlen

pill-rolling /ˈpɪl‚rəʊ.lɪŋ/ **tremor** / ˈtrem.ər/ klidový třes palce a prstů ruky u Parkinsonovy choroby

pit viper /ˈvaɪpə/ chřestýšovec, had

polyuria /‚pɒl.ɪˈjʊə.ri.ə/ polyurie, nadměrné močení

presume /prɪˈzjuːm/ předpokládat, domnívat se

rough /rʌf/ drsný, hrubý

search /sɜːtʃ/ **for** /fɔː/ hledat

sheet /ʃiːt/ prostěradlo, útržek, plátek, list, vrstva

slipper /ˈslɪp.ər/ bačkora, trepka

soaked /səʊkt/ nasáklý, promáčený

soccer /ˈsɒk.ər/ fotbal

spell /spel/ doba, (krátké) období

stagnate /stægˈneɪt/ stagnovat, váznout

state /steɪt/ stav, uvádět, prohlašovat

stonelike /ˈstəʊn.laɪk/ kameni podobný

strenuous /ˈstren.ju.əs/ namáhavý, vysilující

succession /səkˈseʃ.ən/ řada, série

temporal /ˈtem.pər.əl/ temporální, spánkový

tepid /ˈtep.ɪd/ vlažný, vlahý

unaware /‚ʌn.əˈweər/ netušící, neuvědomující si

urinate /ˈjʊə.rɪ.neɪt/ močit

valuable /ˈvæl.jʊ.bl̩ / cenný, hodnotný

varix /ˌveə.rɪks/ pl varices /
ˈvær.ɪ.siːz/ varix, křečová žíla,
krevní městka
vertebral /ˈvɜː.tɪ.brəl/ vertebrální,
obratlový, páteřní
voluntary /ˈvɒləntərɪ/ dobrovolný,
vůlí ovladatelný
workout /ˈwɜːkˌaʊt/ cvičení, trénink
wrinkle /ˈrɪŋkəl/ vráska, záhyb

Part 4
Trauma

Assessment; recognition; and treatment of various traumatic injuries

Unit I

I
You arrive on the scene of a patient who has been stabbed with a knife in the right side of the back. The patient presents with left-sided hemiparalysis and sensory loss. Despite another stab wound to the right abdomen, the patient denies pain. What type of _____ _____ injuries do you suspect?

- compression
- transection
- neurogenic shock
- Brown-Séquard's syndrome*

_____-_____ syndrome is caused by a _____ injury that affects one side of the spinal cord. The damage to the one side results in _____ ___ _____ loss to that side of the body because of the switching of the associated nerves as they enter the spinal cord.

sensory and motor, spinal cord, penetrating, Brown-Séquard's

2
Describe the effects of pericardial tamponade. Cardiac output is reduced, and central venous pressure rises.*
In pericardial _____, the pericardial sack fills with fluid and compresses ___ _____. This impairs _____ _____. The result is a decrease in _____ _____ (the left ventricle cannot effectively fill and pump) and an increase in central venous pressure (venous blood returning to the heart is impaired and the _____ _____ cannot fill or pump effectively).

right ventricle, cardiac output, ventricular filling, tamponade, the heart

3
Your patient rolled a farm tractor over a hill. He has a large puncture wound to his right neck above the clavicle. It appears that the wound is from a tree branch. Moderate bleeding is present. Care for the puncture wound would include:

- application of direct pressure with a bulky trauma dressing
- application of an occlusive dressing*
- application of a sterile dressing
- needle decompression

Application of an _____ _____ is necessary because this is a highly vascular area. An occlusive dressing will prevent air from _____ an injured vessel and the development of an ___ _____.

Which transport position would be appropriate for this patient?
• Trendelenburg position*
• left lateral recumbent
• right lateral recumbent
• prone
The Trendelenburg position would be appropriate to decrease the potential for air _____ into an injured vessel.

A major concern with this type of injury is:
• rib fracture
• clavicle fracture
• flail chest
• oedema*
Oedema is a serious concern because injury to this _____ _____ area of the neck can lead to a rapidly expanding _____. This haematoma can put pressure on other blood vessels, resulting in _____ _____ ____ to the brain, or put pressure on nearby _____ _____, resulting in an airway management nightmare!

| air embolism, decreased blood flow, entering, highly vascular, airway structures, haematoma, aspiration, occlusive dressing |

4
You perform a rapid trauma survey on an MBC (motorbike collision) victim and find him _____ and very pale, with ____ and _____ skin. He has contusions, _____, and diminished breath sounds on the right side of the chest. BP is 74/50; pulse of 140 centrally; no peripheral pulse found at this time; and respirations, 32 and shallow.
What is the most likely cause of these findings? Haemopneumothorax.*
With the information given _____, absent peripheral pulses, and diminished breath sounds on the right with chest trauma on the right a _____ is likely.
An _____ _____ and rapid trauma survey should be completed in what length of time? Less than 3 minutes.*
This patient received an initial assessment and rapid trauma survey to identify all ____ _____.
It is recommended that these assessment steps be _____ in 2 or 3 minutes or less.

> initial assessment, performed, life threats, haemopneumothorax, cool, clammy, crepitus, lethargic, hypotension

5
Which of the following would you expect to cause the greatest _____?
- a hunting knife
- a bullet from a handgun
- a bullet from a rifle*
- an arrow

Ballistics is the study of projectiles in motion. Studies suggest that wounds from _____ _____ are two to four times ____ _____ than handgun bullets due to mass energy and _____.

> velocity, more lethal, rifle bullets, cavitation

6
The next three questions are based on the following scenario: You have arrived on the scene where you find a 50-year-old male who has a large jagged laceration from a chain saw on his medial left upper thigh. Bright red blood is spurting from the wound. Your patient is alert, _____, and anxious, with pale, _____ skin.
What is the priority of care for this patient? Apply a pressure dressing while elevating the left leg.*

This patient is alert and oriented, so he has an _____ airway and is breathing.
Your priority for this patient is circulation, which includes _____ major haemorrhage. Application of a _____ _____ and elevation are necessary.

> pressure dressing, oriented, diaphoretic, intact, stopping

Your rapid _____ _____ reveals an isolated upper leg laceration that is 7 inches (17.8 cm) in length and _____ bright red blood freely. His BP is 110/60; peripheral pulse, 128; respiratory, rate 24; and his GCS is 15. Several components of the circulatory system are essential for adequate _____. These are components of the _____ _____:
- stroke volume and the Frank-Starling mechanism*
- preload and afterload*
- the pump, the fluid, and the container*

Bleeding has been controlled, and your patient is en route to the trauma centre. You instruct your partner to _____ __ _____ and deliver fluid resuscitation.

The most appropriate treatment is a bolus of normal saline or Ringer's lactate solution.*

> circulatory system, profusion, trauma assessment, pumping, establish IV access

7

The next four questions are based on the following scenario: You are on duty at your EMS service when you are called to respond to a car that struck a light pole. As you arrive on the scene, you notice that power lines are down on top of the car. The driver is hanging halfway out of the driver's side window, unconscious, with slow, snoring-type respirations.
What is your first priority? Calling the power company for assistance prior to starting patient care.*
Your safety is the _____ _____.
Do not approach the car until you are notified by the proper officials that the power has been _____
___.

After the patient is removed from the car, a rapid trauma _____ shows a GCS of 9; BP, 178/100; pulse, 56; and respirations, 34 and irregular.
What is your differential diagnosis from this assessment?

- hypoglycaemia
- hyperglycaemia
- Cushing's syndrome*
- CVA

Cushing's or herniation syndrome __ _____ __ hypertension, bradycardia, and erratic respirations.
To manage the airway of this patient appropriately, you would intubate and hyperoxygenate with BVM at a rate of 24 breaths per minute.*
Intubation and _____ _____ are essential. You would hyperventilate this patient because he exhibits signs/symptoms of _____
_____ _____
(Cushing's syndrome).

You have established two large-bore IVs of normal saline. The appropriate rate is enough fluid to maintain stable vital signs.*
The objective of prehospital fluid resuscitation is __ _____ vital signs until the patient arrives at the hospital.

> is manifested by, turned off, to stabilize, supplemental oxygen, first priority, survey, increased intracranial pressure

8

Please state the best clue ___ _____ possible injuries that may be sustained in a motor vehicle collision (___):

- length of skid marks
- debris at the scene
- _____ symptoms
- mechanism of injury*

for determining, patient, MVC

9

A 42-year-old male is the victim of a house fire. He has reddened and blistered areas over most of the anterior chest, abdomen, and anterior surfaces of both arms. Using the rule of nines, estimate the percentage of BSA he has burned: 27% (chest = 9%, abdomen = 9%, anterior surfaces of both arms = 9%).*

Initial treatment for this burn patient would include covering the burn area with dry, bulky _____ and keeping the patient warm.* Manage the burns by _____ them with a dry, bulky dressing. A dressing reduces air movement past sensitive partial-thickness burns, thus reducing pain. Damaged skin loses temperature _____ _____, so it is important to keep the patient covered, even if the environment is not cold.
Medical control has asked that you initiate _____ _____ en route to the hospital: two large-bore catheters are introduced, and a bolus of 0.5 ml of normal saline (NS) for every

kilogram of the patient's weight multiplied by the percentage of BSA is initiated.* Current fluid resuscitation recommends that two large-bore catheters __ _____. When the EMS transport time is less than one hour, a bolus of 0.5 ml of _____ _____ (NS) for every kilogram of the patient's weight multiplied by the percentage of BSA should be initiated.

While transporting your burn patient to the ____ _____, you notice that his voice now sounds _____ and he is making crowing sounds on inspiration. What is the most likely cause? _____ for help while standing inside the burning house.* Risk factors for inhalation injuries associated with burns include standing in the burn environment (__ _____ rise), screaming or yelling in the hot _____ (the ____ _____ allows toxic gases to enter the lower airway), and being trapped in a closed burn environment.

normal saline, environment, hot gases, regulation capacity, dressings, fluid therapy, covering, open glottis, hoarse, be introduced, Screaming, burn centre

10

A burn victim with suspected thermal or chemical airway burns needs close monitoring for signs of _____ _____. Appropriate management would include _____ high-flow oxygen by a _____ mask at 15 litres per minute once the airway has been secured.*

nonrebreather, respiratory
compromise, providing

11

These statements regarding electrical injuries are true:
- Until the power is off, nobody should __ _____ to approach the electrical-burn patient.*
- Patients in cardiac arrest, because of _____, have a high _____ ____ if prehospital intervention is prompt.*
- When treating a victim of a recent lightning strike, the rescuer need not be grounded to prevent electrical shock.*

By the time the victim of a _____ _____ is reached, the electricity will have dissipated. While you may be concerned as long as the storm remains nearby, there is __ _____ of electrical shock from _____ the victim of a lightning strike.

survival rate, electrocution, be
allowed, no danger, lightning
strike, touching

12

The next two questions are based on the following scenario:
You are called to the scene of a 22-year-old man who was playing in a softball tournament. He was hit in the eye with a hard-hit line-drive softball. According to his teammates he was knocked to the ground and had a brief ____ __ _____ that lasted approximately 7 seconds.

While assessing the injured eye, you notice a collection of blood in front of the patient's pupil and iris. What is your differential diagnosis?
- raccoon eye
- retinal detachment
- hyphaema*
- corneal laceration

_____ is a collection of blood in the _____ _____ of the eye due to trauma. This type of injury is a potential threat to the patient's _____ and requires _____ by an ophthalmologist.
How would you transport this patient to the hospital?

Immobilized on a _____ with the head of backboard elevated.* A C-spine injury should be suspected with any injury to the head. Treatment of this patient would include ___ ____ _____. The preferred position of transport of a hyphaema is with the head elevated; therefore, you should _____ the head of the backboard.

backboard, anterior chamber, full body immobilization, elevate, Hyphaema, evaluation, vision, loss of consciousness

13
You arrive on the scene to find a pickup truck that struck a utility pole head-on. The patient is ambulatory on scene. He is alert and oriented to person and place but slow to respond. You note the smell of alcohol on the patient as you speak with him.

You are sent to evaluate the damage to the truck. Which finding would lead you to believe the patient may have a life-threatening injury?
- a deformed dashboard
- a deformed steering wheel*
- the airbag did not deploy
- significant front-end damage

The amount of energy required to deform a steering wheel is significant. Possible ____-_____ injuries from the body striking a steering wheel include flail chest, _____ contusion, _____ ____, tracheal or vascular injuries, _____ contusion, pneumothorax, and solid and hollow organ injury. Bilateral femur fractures may result if an up-and-over path occurred.
It is important to remember that when dealing with an _____ _____, your assessment must be thorough because alcohol can mask signs and symptoms of injury.*
Alcohol is a central nervous system _____. Because of this, alcohol can ____ signs and symptoms of injury. It is important to assess all trauma patients _____, but be especially meticulous when you suspect drug/alcohol use.

aortic tear, pulmonary, depressant, intoxicated patient, thoroughly, mask, life-threatening, myocardial

14
You are called to the scene of a patient who was involved in an altercation at the local pool hall. You find one victim in the back alley anxious and screaming

ENGLISH FOR PARAMEDICS

for your assistance. You notice immediately that he has clammy skin and a dusky appearance. He has a respiratory rate of 40, and his breathing is shallow. He tells you that he has been hit multiple times in the _____, _____, and ____ with a pool stick by two big guys. While assessing his chest, you notice multiple contusions to the right side, with diminished respirations on the right.

What would you suspect?
- cardiac tamponade
- haemothorax
- ruptured diaphragm
- pneumothorax*

With a history of chest trauma, diminished breath sounds, agitation, and increased respiratory rate, along with _____ colour, you should suspect _____.

While en route to the local trauma centre with this patient, you notice that his level of consciousness has decreased and his colour has not improved despite 100% O₂ by nonrebreather mask. He is becoming _____, and his pulse rate is 140. Respiratory rate remains at 40, and his breathing is still shallow. Ongoing assessment reveals _____ neck veins and hyperresonant percussion on the right chest.

Your next course of action would be needle decompression between the second and the third intercostal space in the anterior chest.*
The above symptoms are classic for tension pneumothorax, which is a serious and immediate ____ _____ that requires immediate _____ _____.

life threat, chest, abdomen, back, hypotensive, dusky, pneumothorax, chest decompression, distended

15
A 22-year-old male is found in an alley with multiple stab wounds to the extremities, abdomen, and chest. BP is 82/40; pulse, 142 and weak; respirations, 10. Your exam reveals distended neck veins, equal breath sounds, and a radial pulse that disappears during inspiration. You suspect cardiac tamponade.*
The diagnosis of cardiac tamponade often relies upon symptoms. Hypotension, distended neck veins, and _____ heart sounds are classic symptoms of cardiac tamponade and are known as Beck's triad. If the patient loses his or her _____ _____ during inspiration, it is suggestive of _____ _____ and the presence of cardiac tamponade.

111

As you log-roll the patient to place him on the long spine board, you inspect his back and discover another stab wound just below the right scapula. You observe blood bubbling out of the wound with each breath.
You suspect an open pneumothorax.*
An open pneumothorax (sucking chest wound) includes a _____ or bubbling sound as air moves in and out of the chest wall.
_____ is usually present, and frothing of the blood may occur as the ___ ___ _____ combine.
Priority care for this patient would include closure of the chest wall with an occlusive dressing taped on three sides.*
Treatment of an open pneumothorax includes _____ the chest wall __ _____ of an occlusive dressing that is _____ on three sides.

---

by application, muffled, taped, Bleeding, closing, air and blood, pulsus paradoxus, peripheral pulse, sucking

---

16
You arrive on the scene of a 34-year-old male who was struck by a car. Bystanders tell you the patient was standing on the sidewalk when his neighbour, who was backing out on the driveway,

struck him. Your patient is sitting in the yard with an obvious open tibia/fibula fracture on the right leg.

As you _____ his right upper chest, you notice the patient guarding his shoulder. Closer exam reveals a fractured_____. Complications associated with a fractured clavicle include injury to the:
- carotid artery
- subclavian vein*
- descending aorta
- inferior vena cava

Physical exam concludes that the right clavicle fracture and open right tibia/fibula fracture are his only obvious injuries, but you are concerned because his level of consciousness __ _____ and his heart rate has increased 30 beats per minute. Although his abdomen was unremarkable upon examination, you know that an _____ of severe abdominal trauma is the presence of:
- absent bowel sounds
- back pain
- referred pain to the clavicle
- unexplained shock*
When assessment of a trauma patient does not reveal significant injury, the presence of _____ _____ should

lead you to suspect serious
_____/_____ trauma.

> clavicle, indicator, unexplained
> shock, abdominal/thorax,
> auscultate, is deteriorating

17
A high-velocity bullet passes
through the body. Besides
the direct damage caused by
the _____, what other related
condition could cause harm to the
patient?
- the type of _____ used to
  make the bullet
- the internal opening
  created by cavitation*
- the _____ residue
- the length of the bullet
Cavitation caused by the pressure
wave of the bullet's forces
creates both _____ and
_____ openings within the
tissues. Tremendous forces are
transferred from the _____ of
the bullet to the tissues, causing
damage.

> permanent, metal, bullet,
> gunpowder, temporary, velocity

Vocabulary I
agitation /ˌædʒ.ɪˈteɪ.ʃən/ nervozita,
rozrušení, vzrušení, znepokojení
air bag, airbag /ˈeə.bæg/ airbag,
bezpečnostní nafukovací vak
alley /ˈæl.i/ ulička, průchod

altercation /ˌɔːltəˈkeɪʃən/ ostrý
spor, prudká hádka
ambulatory /ˌæm.bjəˈleɪ.tər.i/
chodící
approach /əˈprəʊtʃ/ blížit se,
přiblížit se, přistoupit, přístup,
cesta, kontakt, snaha o kontakt
postoj
arrow /ˈær.əʊ/ šipka, ukazatel
backboard /ˈbæk.bɔːd/ páteřní
deska
ballistics /bəˈlɪs.tɪks/ balistika
be /biː/ **trapped** /træpd/ být
uvězněný, chycený
bilateral /baɪˈlæt.ər.əl/ bilaterální,
dvoustranný
blister /ˈblɪs.tər/ puchýř
bowel /ˈbaʊ.əl/ střevo, útroby
Brown-Sequard's /braʊn-sei.
kahr/ **syndrome** /ˈsɪn.drəʊm/
Brown-Sequardův syndrom,
soubor příznaků, které se vyvinou
po hemisekci míchy, protětí její
levé nebo pravé poloviny či při
útlaku její poloviny, pacient trpí
stejnostrannou poruchou hybnosti
a vibračního a diskriminačního čití
a poruchou citlivosti pro bolest,
teplo a chlad na straně opačné
bubble /ˈbʌb.l/ bublat, být plný
čeho
bulky /ˈbʌl.ki/ objemný velký,
rozměrný, tlustý
bullet /ˈbʊl.ɪt/ kulka, střela
cardiac /ˈkɑː.dɪˌæk/ **output** /ˈaʊt.pʊt/
minutový objem krve vypuzené
srdcem
cavitation /ˌkæv.ɪˈteɪ.ʃən/ kavitace,
vytváření dutin

113

chain /tʃeɪn/ řetěz, řetězec

chamber /'tʃeɪm.bə/ komora

chest /tʃest/ hrudník, prsa

clammy /'klæm.i/ studeně vlhký, lepkavý

clavicle /'klævɪkəl/ klavikula, klíční kost

closure /'kləʊ.ʒə/ zavření, uzavírka

collection /kə'lekʃən/ nahromadění, soubor, sbírání, sbírka

collision /kə'lɪʒ.ən/ srážka, kolize

component /kəm'pəʊnənt/ složka, součást

compression /kəm'preʃən/ komprese, stlačení, stisknutí, slisování

conclude /kən'kluːd/ usoudit, dojít k závěru

container /kən'teɪ.nər/ nádoba

contusion /kən'tjuː.ʒən/ pohmožděnina, zhmožděnina

corneal /kɔː'ni.əl/ korneální, týkající se rohovky

crepitus /'krep.ɪ.təs/ krepitus, praskot

crow /krəʊ/ kokrhat (kohout)

current /'kʌr.ənt/ proud, současný, aktuální

dashboard /'dæʃˌbɔːd/ přístrojová deska auta

deal with /dɪəl/ řešit, zabývat se

debris /'deb.riː/, /'deɪ.briː/ trosky, úlomky, pozůstatky

decompression /ˌdiː.kəm'preʃ.ən/ dekomprese, snížení tlaku, snížení tlaku vzduchu

deny /dɪ'naɪ/ odmítat, zapřít, popřít, popírat

deploy /dɪ'plɔɪ/ nasadit, rozmístit

depressant /dɪ'pres.ənt/ látka s tlumivým účinkem

descend /dɪ'send/ sestoupit

detachment /dɪ'tætʃmənt/ oddělení, odstup, odloučení

deteriorate /dɪ'tɪə.ri.ə.reɪt/ zhoršit, zhoršovat

diagnosis /ˌdaɪ.əg'nəʊ.sɪs/ diagnóza

diaphragm /'daɪ.ə.fræm/ bránice, přepážka

differential /ˌdɪf.ə'ren.t ʃəl/ různící se, rozdílový

disappear /ˌdɪs.ə'pɪər/ zmizet

dissipate /'dɪs.ɪ.peɪt/ rozptýlit se

down /daʊn/ srazit

dress /dres/ ošetřit, ovázat ránu

driveway /'draɪvˌweɪ/ příjezdová cesta, vjezd

dusky /'dʌs.ki/ tmavý, tlumený o barvě

duty /'djuːtɪ/ služba, povinnost

electrocution /ɪˌlek.trə'kjuː.ʃən/ smrt elektickým proudem

elevation /ˌel.ɪ'veɪ.ʃən/ zvýšení, povýšení

enroute /ˌɒn'ruːt/ cestou, během cesty

erratic /ɪ'ræt.ɪk/ nepředvídatelný, nevypočitatelný

expand /ɪk'spænd/ rozšířit se, zvětšit, roztáhnout

femur pl femora /'fiː.mər/ femur, kost stehenní

fibula pl -ae /'fɪb.jʊ.lə/ fibula, kost lýtková

finding /'faɪndɪŋ/ závěr, zjištění, nález

flail /fleɪl/ **chest** /tʃest/ paradoxní dýchání při zlomenině žeber

flail /fleɪl/ volně se pohybující (bez svalové kontroly)

force /fɔːs/ síla, účinnost, nutit, vyvíjet tlak, přinutit, donutit, zatlačit

Frank-Starlings mechanism / ˈmekəˌnɪzəm/ Frankův-Starlingův mechanismus, zákon, zvýšená náplň srdce na konci diastoly preload zvýší intenzitu srdečního stahu, množství krve vypuzené při následné systole – tepový objem

froth /frɒθ/ pěna, pěnit se

glottis /ˈglɒt.ɪs/ pl glotides glotis, hlasivková štěrbina, nejužší část hrtanu

grounded /graʊnd.ɪd/ uzemněný

guard /gɑːd/ bránit, chránit se

gunpowder /ˈgʌnˌpaʊ.dər/ střelný prach

haematoma pl haematomata / ˌhiː.məˈtəʊ.mə/ hematom, krevní výron, podlitina, modřina

haemopneumothorax /ˈhiː.məˌnjuː. məˈθɔː.ræks/ hemopneumotorax, nahromadění krve a plynu v plicích

handgun /ˈhændˌgʌn/ ruční střelná zbraň, pistole ap.

hang /hæŋ/ viset

hanging /ˈhæŋɪŋ/ zavěšení, pověšení, oběšení

harm /hɑːm/ ublížit, zranit, poškodit, ublížení, zranění

head on /ˌhedˈɒn/ čelně, zepředu, zpříma

hemiparalysis /ˌhem.ɪ.pəˈræl.ə.sɪs/ viz hemiparesis

hemiparesis /ˌhem.ɪ.pəˈriː.sɪs/ hemiparéza, částečné ochrnutí jedné poloviny těla

herniation /ˌhɜː.niˈeɪ.ʃən/ herniace, vysunutí části orgánu mimo jeho přirozené místo, vytvoření kýly

hit /hɪt/ (hit, hit) udeřit, narazit, vrazit

hoarse /hɔːs/ chraplavý, ochraptělý

hollow /ˈhɒl.əʊ/ prázdný, vpadlý, propadlý

hunting /ˈhʌn.tɪŋ/ **knife** /naɪf/ lovecký nůž

hyperglycaemia /ˌhaɪ. pə.glaɪˈsiː.mi.ə/ hyperglykémie, zvýšené množství glukózy v krvi

hyperresonant /ˌhaɪ.pə.ˈrez.ən.ənt/ nadměrně zvučný, rezonující

hyperventilate /haɪ.pəˈven.tɪ.leɪt/ nadměrně rychle dýchat

hyphaema /haɪ.θe.mə/ hyféma, krev v přední komoře oční před duhovkou

indicator /ˈɪn.dɪ.keɪ.tər/ indikátor, ukazatel

inferior /ɪnˈfɪə.ri.ər/ **vena cava** /ˌviː. nəˈkeɪ.və/ dolní dutá žíla

initial /ɪˈnɪʃ.əl/ iniciála, šifra

intact /ɪnˈtækt/ intaktní, netknutý, nedotčený, neporušený

intercostal /ˌɪn.təˈkɒs.təl/ interkostální, mezižeberní

iris /ˈaɪrɪs/ oční duhovka

jagged /ˈdʒæg.ɪd/ rozeklaný, zubatý

knock /nɒk/ srazit, udeřit

laceration /ˌlæsəˈreɪʃən/ lacerace, tržná rána

large /lɑːdʒ/ bore /bɔː/ jehla s velkým průměrem, velká jehla

lateral /ˈlæt.rəl/ laterální, boční, postranní

lethal /ˈliː.θəl/ smrtící, smrtonosný

lightning /ˈlaɪt.nɪŋ/ blesk, elektrický výboj

line /laɪn/ -drive /draɪv/ odpal v basebalu, silný úder, míček letí na nebo lehce nad trajektorií

log /lɒg/ -roll /rəʊl/, logroll přetočit jako jeden celek

maintain /meɪnˈteɪn/ udržovat, uchovat, zachovat

mark /mɑːk/ znak, známka, skvrna, stopa, otisk

meticulous /məˈtɪk.jʊ.ləs/ úzkostlivě pečlivý

motion /ˈməʊʃən/ pohyb, pokynout

motor /ˈməʊ.tər/ motorický, pohybový

muffle /ˈmʌf.l̩/ utlumit, ztlumit, ztišit

multiple /ˈmʌl.tɪ.p|/ násobek, mnohonásobný, mnohočený

multiply /ˈmʌltɪplaɪ/ násobit, rozmnožit

nightmare /ˈnaɪt.meər/ noční můra, zlý sen

nonrebreather /ˌnɒn.rəbrə.ðər/ mask /mɑːsk/ dýchací maska s jednocestnou klapkou, vydechnutý oxid uhličitý je vyloučen a není znovu vdechován

notify /ˈnəʊtɪˌfaɪ/ oznámit, uvědomit, informovat

occlusive /ɒˈkluː.sɪv/ dressing / ˈdres.ɪŋ/ okluzní obvaz, uzavřený obvaz

oedema /ɪˈdiː.mə/ otok

official /əˈfɪʃəl/ úředník, představitel, funkcionář

partial /ˈpɑː.ʃəl/ částečný, dílčí

path /pɑːθ/ cesta, dráha pohybu

pericardial /ˌper.ɪˈkaːdi. əl/ perikardiální, týkající se osrdečníku

physical /ˈfɪz.ɪ.kəl/ tělesný, lékařská prohlídka

pickup /ˈpɪkʌp/ vozidlo s valníkovým nákladním prostorem

pole /pəʊl/ sloup, stožár, telefonní ap.

pool /puːl/ hall /hɔːl/ biliárová herna

pool /puːl/ stick /stɪk/ tágo

potential /pəˈten.ʃəl/ potenciál, možnost, schopnost

power /ˈpaʊə/ line /laɪn/ elektrické vedení

power /ˈpaʊə/ pravomoc, kompetence, elektřina

power /paʊər/ company /ˈkʌm. pə.ni/ elektrická společnost

pressure /ˈpreʃ.ə/ dressing /ˈdres.ɪŋ/ tlakový obvaz

profusion /prəˈfjuː.ʒən/ hojnost, spousta

projectile /prəˈdʒek.taɪl/ projektil, střela, náboj

prompt /prɒmp t/ promptní, okamžitý, pohotový, přimět, dohnat koho k čemu

prone /prəʊn/ na břiše ležící

puncture / ˈpʌŋk.tʃə/ punkce, vpich, otvor propíchnutí, propíchnout
raccoon /rəˈkuːn/ **eyes** /aɪz/ „mývalí oči", zhmožděniny kolem očí
recognition /ˌrek.əgˈnɪʃ.ən/ rozpoznání, zjištění, uznání, pochopení
recumbent /rɪˈkʌm.bənt/ ležící
redden /ˈred.ən/ zčervenat, zrudnout
rescuer/ˈres.kjuː.ər/ zachránce
residue /ˈrez.ɪ.djuː/ reziduum, zbytek
retinal /ˈret.ɪ.nəl/ retinální, sítnicový
rib /rɪb/ žebro
rifle /ˈraɪ.fl̩/ puška, kulovnice
roll /rəʊl/ **over** /ˈəʊ.vər/ překulit se
saline /ˈseɪ.laɪn/ slaný, solný roztok, fyziologický roztok
saw /sɔː/ pila, řezat
scapula /ˈskæp.jʊ.lə/ pl -ae lopatka
scream /skriːm/ křičet, ječet, křik, výkřik, jekot
sensory /ˈsent .sər.i/ smyslový
skid /skɪd/ skluz, smyk
snore /snɔːr/ chrápat, zachrápání
solid /ˈsɒl.ɪd/ pevný, tvrdý, jednolitý
spine /spaɪn/ **board** /bɔːd/ páteřní deska
spurt /spɜːt/ prýštit, tryskat, vystříknutí, proud
stab /stæb/ bodnout
stable /ˈsteɪ.bl̩/ stabilní, stabilizovaný, stálý
steering /ˈstɪər.ɪŋ/ **wheel** /wiːl/ volant

stick /stɪk/ hůl k chůzi
storm /stɔːm/ bouře
strike /straɪk/ (struck, struck) zasáhnout, postihnout, udeřit
strike /straɪk/ úder
subclavian /sʌbˈkleɪv.ɪ.ən/ podklíčkový, uložený pod klíční kostí
suck /sʌk/ sát, odsávat
supplemental /ˌsʌp.lɪˈmen.təl/ doplňkový, dodatečný
surface /ˈsɜː.fɪs/ povrch, hladina, zevnějšek, vynořit se
survey /ˈsɜː.veɪ/ průzkum, přehled, vyšetření, prohlídka, posoudit
survival /səˈvaɪ.vəl/ přežití
sustain /səˈsteɪn/ vydržet, snést, utrpět
switch /swɪtʃ/ prohodit, vyměnit, přepnout
tamponade /tæm.pəˈneɪd/ tamponáda, stlačení srdce tekutinou nahromaděnou v perikardu
tape /teɪp/ lepicí páska, přilepit, zalepit
teammate /ˈtiːm.meɪt/ spoluhráč
tear /teər/ protržení, trhlina
temporary /ˈtempərərɪ/ dočasný, přechodný
tension /ˈtent .ʃən/ **pneumothorax** /ˌnjuːməˈθɔː.ræks/ tenzní pneumotorax, vzduch v pohrudniční dutině
thickness /ˈθɪknɪs/ síla, tloušťka v průřezu
thigh /θaɪ/ stehno
thorax /ˈθɔː.ræks/ hrudník

tibia /'tɪb.i.ə/ pl. -ae holeň, kost holenní
touching /'tʌtʃ.ɪŋ/ dotknutí se
transection /ˌtræn'sek.ʃən/ příčný řez
transfer /træns'fɜːr/ přemístit, přesunout, přesun
tremendous /trɪ'men.dəs/ ohromný, obrovský
Trendelenburg /tren.del.'en. berg/ **position** /pə'zɪʃ.ən/ Trendelenburgova poloha, při níž pacient leží na zádech a jeho pánev je uložena výše než hlava, užívá se při šoku k zlepšení prokrvení životně důležitých orgánů
truck /trʌk/ nákladní auto, kamión
turn /tɜːn/ **off** /ɒf/ odbočit, vypnout
unremarkable /ˌʌn.rɪ'mɑː.kə.bl̩/ nezajímavý, obyčejný
utility /juː'tɪl.ɪ.ti/ služby (veřejné), technická infrastruktura, dodávky vody, doprava

vascular /'væs.kjʊ.lər/ vaskulární, cévní
velocity /vɪ'lɒsɪtɪ/ rychlost
voice /vɔɪs/ hlas, hlasový, vyslovit vyjádřit (názor, mínění)
wave /weɪv/ vlna, kývat, mávnout čím
yell /jel/ ječet, ječení, výkřik

Unit 2

I

You respond to a 25-year-old male involved in an industrial accident. Upon arrival, you see that your patient is trapped in a machine. He has suffered a partial amputation of the right leg just above the knee that is bleeding profusely.
Your first action is to stabilize the machinery.*
Stabilizing the machinery serves two purposes. First, it assures your_____, and second, it will prevent _____ _____ to the patient.

The patient remains _____ in the machine. He is awake, alert, and anxious. His blood pressure is 96/44; pulse, 142; respiration, 26. His skin is pale and moist. He is in what state of shock? Compensated.*
This patient is in _____ _____. His elevated pulse rate (142) and evidence of vasoconstriction (____, _____ ____) is able to maintain his blood pressure despite continued blood loss.

The patient has been freed from the machinery. Direct pressure and elevation do not stop the haemorrhage.

The next step would be to apply pressure at an arterial point proximal to the injury.*
If bleeding still persists after direct pressure and elevation, the next step is to find an _____ _____ _____ proximal to the wound and apply firm pressure.

Despite all efforts to control the bleeding, you are not successful. His pulse is now 52 and very weak. His respirations are 6 and laboured. Blood pressure is 78/30.
This shock state indicates decompensated shock.*
_____ _____ is when the body can __ _____ respond to the _____ blood loss.
This is evident in the scenario by a decreased pulse rate, respirations, and blood pressure.

> Decompensated shock, continued, compensated shock, arterial pulse point, safety, additional injury, pale, moist skin, trapped, no longer

2

You are caring for a 24-year-old male who wrecked his all-terrain vehicle. He states that his handlebar struck him in the stomach. He has _____ ___ _____ in the abdomen, and you suspect bowel rupture.

This condition can lead to peritonitis and the development of serious complications.*
Rupture of the _____ or small bowel that allows digestive enzymes to enter the peritoneal cavity can cause _____, which can lead to infection and

_____ _____.

> serious complications, peritonitis, bruising and tenderness, stomach

3
You are called to the scene of a stabbing. You find one victim lying supine on the ground in a large pool of blood with multiple lacerations to the abdomen.
The scene is secure. Your initial assessment finds a patient responding only to pain with no peripheral pulse and a respiratory rate of 8.
Priority care of this patient would be intubation and fluid resuscitation.*
Priority for this patient who presents with respiratory compromise and hypovolaemia is _____ _____ and _____

_____.

While transporting this patient to the hospital, a large section of bowel protrudes through one of the lacerations.

Your management would be to gently cover the area with _____ _____ and nonadherent material as a dressing.*
Intestines should never be _____ ____ into the abdominal compartment. A moist nonadherent dressing should be gently placed over the bowel to prevent it from drying out because of the risk of _____ _____.

> irreversible damage, moistened gauze, airway support, fluid resuscitation, pushed back

4
You respond to a 'man down' call. When you arrive, you find a 52-year-old male lying on the ground next to a ladder. It is unclear if he was placing the ladder against the house when he came into contact with power lines or if he fell from the top of the ladder.

Examination shows the patient to be unresponsive. He has a rapid, _____ _____ and snoring respirations of 8. BP is 88/42. Treatment should include _____ the airway with a ___ _____ manoeuvre and ventilation with a bag-valve device.*
It is unclear if this patient fell, so you ____ _____ trauma and C-spine injury. A jaw-thrust

manoeuvre and bag-valve mask ventilation is the ____ _____.

jaw-thrust, best choice, must suspect, irregular pulse, opening

5
There are anatomic differences in _____ _____ compared to adults.
When using the rule of nines for _____ _____, what is a correct _____ for a child? The head of a child is 18% compared to 9% of an adult.*

calculating burns, modification, paediatric patients

6
Your patient is a 44-year-old female who was burned when a high-temperature water pipe exploded. She has _____ to the chest, abdomen, _____ right arm, and _____ __ ___ right leg. According to the rule of nines, this patient ___ _____ 36% burns.*
Chest = 9%, abdomen = 9%, entire arm = 9%, front of the leg = 9%.

blisters, entire, has sustained, front of the

7
The next three questions are based on the following scenario:

You are called to the scene of a 60-year-old woman who fell down a flight of stairs. The patient is found to be _____ and oriented, with warm, dry, and pink skin. She is _____ __ a headache and upper-back pain. Her vital signs are as follows: BP, 90/62; pulse, 60; and respiration rate, 20.
Which would be your _____ _____? Neurogenic or distributive shock.*
_____ or distributive shock is recognized by hypotension, bradycardia, and a normal initial appearance.

During your rapid trauma survey, you find that the patient has no sensation below the border of the ribcage.
This would suggest _____ _____ between T4 and T10.* You would suspect injury at the thoracic level.

You have started a large-bore IV of normal saline on this patient. Choose the appropriate solution and rate: normal saline at a rate to maintain a systolic BP of 90.* The objective of prehospital fluid resuscitation is to stabilize vital signs until the patient arrives at the hospital. This patient requires close observation since neurogenic shock does not allow

the body's normal _____ _____ a head injury is
_____ to work. capable of.

Neurogenic, compensatory
mechanisms, initial impression,
spinal pathology, complaining of,
alert

life threat, isolated injuries,
transportation decisions, head
injury

9
Your patient was struck in the
head with a 6-inch-diameter (15
cm) tree branch while trimming a
tree. He complained of dizziness
immediately after the incident but
states he feels fine now. The next
day, he complains of _____
___ _____.
You suspect a subdural
haematoma.*
A _____ _____ is usually
due to rupture of _____ _____
_____. This type of bleeding is
slow, and the _____ of symptoms
___ _____ several hours to develop
after the injury.

8
You are called to the scene of a
mass-casualty incident where you
are responsible for the triage and
_____ _____. Which
of the following patients would be
the first to be transported to the
local trauma centre?
• a 50-year-old man
complaining of knee and
ankle pain
• an 18-year-old female
with a 5-minute lapse of
consciousness after being
struck in the head*
• a 25-year-old female,
eight months pregnant,
with partial-thickness
burns on her arms and
legs covering 5% of her
BSA (body surface area)
• a 32 -year-old male with
a large piece of metal
impaled in his left foot

Of the choices listed, the patient
with a possible ____ _____
should be transported first.
Others are all _____ _____
that do not pose an immediate

onset, subdural haematoma,
small venous vessels, may take,
dizziness and vomiting

10
Which head injury will likely
result in immediate neurological
signs/symptoms with rapid
deterioration?
• concussion
• contusion
• subdural haematoma
• epidural haematoma*

An _____ _____ involves _____ _____. Because the bleeding is arterial, _____ _____ builds rapidly, compressing the _____ and increasing pressure within the skull. As the pressure rapidly builds, the patient will immediately display _____ _____/_____.

> neurological signs/symptoms, cerebrum, arterial vessels, epidural haematoma, intracranial pressure

II

Cushing's reflex includes a sudden _____ in systolic pressure, _____, and:
- erratic (_____ ____) respirations*
- irregular pulse
- increased respirations
- pupil dilation

> bradycardia, increase, usually slow

12

You are called to the scene of a single-car MVC involving a 25-year-old female who is thirty weeks pregnant.
What normal physiological alterations take place during pregnancy that may affect your assessment of this patient?

Decreased blood pressure and increased pulse.*
Normal physiological changes to vital signs during the _____ _____ of pregnancy include _ ____ in blood pressure 1-15 mmHg due to a reduction in peripheral vascular resistance. The ____ ____ will increase 10-20 beats per minute due to an increased maternal blood volume.
Note: The blood pressure will rise back to baseline in the third trimester. Keep these _____ _____ in mind when assessing a pregnant trauma patient.

You ascertain that this patient needs to be transported to the local trauma centre for evaluation. What would be the best technique for the transport? Properly secured to the backboard and tilted to the left side.*
The backboard must be tilted on its ____ ____ 10-15 degrees to prevent _____ _____ syndrome. Tilting the board will allow ___ _____ to displace to the left and _____ compression of the inferior vena cava.
During what month of gestation does the uterus rise out of the pelvic cavity and become more susceptible to blunt trauma? Fifth month.*
After the third month of gestation, the foetus and uterus grow rapidly. After the fifth month of

123

pregnancy, the uterus rises out of the pelvis and is more _____ to injury.

---

normal changes, heart rate, supine hypotension, second trimester, prone, a drop, left side, the uterus, prevent

---

13
A 5-year-old boy fell 10 feet (3 metres) from a jungle gym at school, hitting his head on the ground. Your initial evaluation reveals a child who is lethargic and does not respond appropriately __ _____. His respirations are shallow at a rate of 40 with a _____ ___ ____ radial pulse.
What is your first priority? Rapid C-spine control and airway assistance with BVM and high-flow O₂.*
Injured children can rapidly transition from a state of rapid and laboured breathing to a state of _____ _____, resulting in respiratory arrest. _____ _____ is essential.
One of the most important prognostic indicators of potential CNS injury is history of loss of consciousness.*

Airway management, total exhaustion, rapid and weak, to commands

---

14
You are dispatched to a 77-year-old male patient who has fallen from a ladder while cleaning the gutters. He fell approximately 14 feet (4.3 metres) and struck the ground. He is awake and very anxious. He is having obvious trouble breathing. His pulse is 104; respirations, 34; and blood pressure, 122/76. His wife tells you that he struck his back on the riding lawn mower as he fell. In your assessment, you find crepitus and instability to the left ribcage. ____ _____ are present and equal. Closer assessment reveals paradoxical movement. You suspect:
- tension pneumothorax
- massive haemothorax
- flail chest*
- abdominal aneurysm
Flail chest is three or more _____ ____ that are fractured in two or more places. This segment of the chest is free to move with the pressure changes of respirations.
Paradoxical movement is best described as chest wall movement that is inward with inspiration and outward with expiration.*
Paradoxical chest wall movement associated with flail chest is defined as the motion of a flail

segment _____ __ the normal motion of the chest wall.

Prehospital management for this patient includes:
- a needle decompression midclavicular line
- positive pressure ventilation*
- an occlusive dressing
- chest decompression midaxillary line

Positive pressure ventilation of the patient with a flail chest _____ the mechanism that causes the paradoxical chest wall movement, restores tidal volume, and reduces the pain of chest wall movement.

Your patient is in severe respiratory distress. Reassessment reveals absent lung sounds on the left, _____ _____ to the right, and SpO$_2$ reading of 82%. Immediate treatment must include left-side chest decompression.* The signs and symptoms displayed by this patient are consistent with a left-side _____ _____, and immediate chest decompression is required.

reverses, tracheal deviation, tension pneumothorax, Lung sounds, adjacent ribs, opposite to

15

One of the most common mechanisms of injury in the geriatric population is falls. This statement is true regarding the force required to ____ _ ____ in a geriatric patient: less force is required than in other patients.* _____ is common in the geriatric population. This disease process makes bones much more _____ to hip and other fractures. In _____ _____, a simple action such as sneezing may _____ __ a fracture.

susceptible, severe cases, result in, break a bone, Osteoporosis

16

You are called to the scene of an assault on a 75-year-old woman. She is unresponsive, with blood coming from the back of her head and multiple contusions and skin tears to her knees and arms. She has snoring respirations, a strong radial pulse of 60 beats per minute, and a moderate amount of bright red blood from a large laceration and haematoma in her occipital region.
What is your first priority?
Immediately _____ ___ _-____ and open the airway.* Airway and the C-spine are always a priority before _____ _____.

Why would this patient be more susceptible to severe ___ _____?

- a history of Alzheimer's disease
- dehydration
- Pickwickian syndrome
- decreased size of the brain*

As part of the normal physiologic changes ____ _____, a decrease occurs in brain weight and size. By the age of 80, the brain loses approximately 3.5 ounces (99 grams) in weight.

After completing your rapid trauma assessment on your patient, you find a blood pressure of 99/54, a heart rate of 50, and a respiratory rate of 14 and regular. What is your priority of care? Careful fluid resuscitation.* Fluid resuscitation needs to be carefully administered due to the decreased response of the _____ _____ with age. Reduced circulation and loss of circulatory defence responses, coupled with increased presence of ventricular dysfunction, produce a significant challenge in _____ _____ in the elderly.

managing shock, with aging, stabilize the C-spine, other treatments, head trauma, cardiovascular system

Vocabulary 2

additional /əˈdɪʃ.ən.əl/ dodatečný, další, doplňkový

adjacent /əˈdʒeɪ.sənt/ sousední, přilehlý, vedlejší

affect /əˈfekt/ ovlivnit, ovlivňovat, působit, postihnout, zasáhnout

age /eɪdʒ/ věk, stárnutí, stárnout

alert /əˈlɜːt/ bdělý, čilý

all-terrain vehicle /ˌɔːl.tə.reɪnˈviː.ɪ.kl/ terénní vůz

allow /əˈlaʊ/ dovolit, poskytnout, umožnit

alteration /ˌɒl.təˈreɪ.ʃən/ změna

ankle /ˈæŋ.kl/ kotník

appropriately /əˈprəʊ.pri.ət.li/ vhodně, náležitě, přiměřeně

arrest /əˈrest/ zástava

arterial /ɑːˈtɪə.ri.əl/ arteriální, tepenný

ascertain /ˌæs.əˈteɪn/ zjistit, dopátrat se

assault /əˈsɒlt/ útok, napadení, přepadnout

assure /əˈʃɔːr/ ujistit, zajistit, ubezpečit

baseline /ˈbeɪsˌlaɪn/ základní čára, výchozí bod, východisko

blunt /blʌnt/ tupý, oblý, přímý

border /ˈbɔː.dər/ okraj, hranice

bruising /ˈbruː.zɪŋ/ pohmožděniny, podlitiny

calculate /ˈkælkjʊˌleɪt/ vypočítat, spočítat

capable /ˈkeɪ.pə.bl̩/ schopný, způsobilý, zdatný

cerebrum /sɪˈriː.brəm/ cerebrum, velký mozek

challenge /'tʃæl.ɪndʒ/ čelendž, provokační injekce, vyvolání odezvy

clavicular /klə'vɪkjʊlə/ klavikulární, klíční

command /kə'mɑːnd/ příkaz, ovládnutí, kontrola, velení

compartment /kəm'pɑːt.mənt/ oddělení, prostor, vymezený prostor

compensatory /ˌkɒm.pən'seɪt.ə ri/ kompenzační

complete /kəm'pliːt/ doplnit, dokončit, skončit

compress / kəm'pres/ stlačit, zmáčknout

concussion /kən'kʌʃ.ən/ otřes mozku

condition /kən'dɪʃ.ən/ stav, fyzická kondice, potíže, onemocnění, podmínka

consistent /kən'sɪs.tənt/ with /wɪð/ shodný, odpovídající, v souladu

contusion /kən'tju:.ʒən/ pohmožděnina, zhmožděnina

couple /'kʌp.l/ spojovat dohromady

decrease /dɪ'kriːs/ snížit se, zmenšit, pokles

defence /dɪ'fent s/ obrana, obhajoba, ochrana

despite /dɪ'spaɪt/ navzdory, i přes

deterioration /dɪˌtɪə.ri.ə'reɪ.ʃən/ zhoršení kvality, úpadek

deviation /ˌdi:.vɪ'eɪʃən/ deviace, odchylka, úchylka, vybočení

diameter /daɪ'æm.ɪ.tər/ průměr (kružnice)

digestive /da ɪ'dʒes.tɪv/ trávicí, zažívací

dispatch /dɪ'spætʃ/ vyslat, poslat, odeslat, odeslání

displace /dɪ'spleɪs/ vytlačit, nahradit

distributive /dɪ'strɪbjʊtɪv/ distributivní, rozdělený

dizziness / 'dɪz.ɪ.nəs/ závrať, točení hlavy, mrákotný stav

epidural /ˌepɪ'djʊərəl/ epidurální, umístění nad durou

equal /'iːkwəl/ stejný, rovnat se (čemu)

evident /'ev.ɪ.dənt/ zjevný, očividný, zřejmý

exhaustion /ɪg'zɔ:s.tʃən/ vyčerpání, vyčerpanost

firm /fɜːm/ pevný

flight /flaɪt/ of stairs /steərz/ rameno schodiště mezi patry

foetus /'fi:.təs/ fetus, plod

free /fri:/ svobodný, volný, zbavený, prostý

gauze / gɔːz/ gáza, mul

gently /'dʒent.li/ jemně, mírně

gestation /dʒes'teɪ.ʃən/ gestace, gravidita, těhotenství

gutter /'gʌt.ər/ okap, okapový žlab

handlebar /ˌhæn.dl.bɑ:/ řídítka jízdního kola

impale /ɪm'peɪl/ nabodnout, napíchnout

impression /ɪm'preʃ.ən/ dojem, pocit, znak

indicator /'ɪn.dɪ.keɪ.tər/ indikátor, ukazatel

initial /ɪ'nɪʃəl/ počáteční, výchozí

instability /ˌɪn.stəˈbɪl.ɪ.ti/ nestabilita, labilita

intestine /ɪnˈtes.tɪn/ střevo, trakčník

inward /ˈɪn.wəd/ dovnitř směřující, vnitřní

irreversible /ˌɪr.ɪˈvɜː.sɪ.bļ/ nezvratný

jungle /ˈdʒʌŋ.gl/ **gym** /dʒɪm/ prolézačka na dětském hřišti

laboured /ˈleɪ.bəd/ obtížný, namáhavý

lapse /læps/ uplynulá doba, výpadek, vynechání

lawn mower /ˈlɔːnˌməʊ.ər/ sekačka trávy

maternal /məˈtɜː.nəl/ těhotenský, mateřský

midaxillary /mɪd.ækˈsɪl.ər.i/ střed podpaží

midclavicular /mɪd.kləˈvɪk.jʊ.lər/ týkající se střední části klíční kosti

mind /maɪnd/ mysl, paměť

moisten /ˈmɔɪsən/ navlhčit, zvlhnout

motion /ˈməʊʃən/ pohyb, pokynout

nonadherent /ˌnɒn.ədˈhɪə.rənt/ nepřilnavý

occipital /ɒkˈsɪp.ɪ.təl/ okcipitální, týlní, zátylní

osteoporosis /ˌɒs.ti.əʊ.pəˈrəʊ.sɪs/ osteoporóza, prořídnutí kostí, onem. kosti způsobující úbytek kostní tkáně

outward /ˈaʊt.wəd/ zevní, směřující ven, zevnějšek

paradoxical /ˌpær.əˈdɒk.sɪ.kəl/ paradoxní

persist /pəˈsɪst/ přetrvávat, pokračovat, vytrvat

pipe /paɪp/ trubka, potrubí, trubice

pregnancy /ˈpreg.nən.si/ těhotenství

pregnant /ˈpregnənt/ těhotná

profusely /prəˈfjuːs.li/ hojně, silně

prognostic /prɒgˈnɒs.tɪk/ prognostický, předpovídající

prone /prəʊn/ **to** /tə/ mající sklony, náchylný

protrude /prəˈtruːd/ vyčnívat

proximal /ˈprɒk.sɪ.məl/ proximální, bližší trupu nebo hlavě

push /pʊʃ/ tlačit, posunout, postrčit, strčit, prodrat se

reassessment /ˌriː.əˈses.mənt/ přehodnocení, nové zhodnocení

rib /rɪb/ **cage** /keɪdʒ/ hrudní koš

section /ˈsek.ʃən/ část, úsek, průřez, odříznutí, pitva

secure /sɪˈkjʊə/ zajistit, zabezpečit, upevnit

segment /ˈseg.mənt/ segment, úsek, část, díl, článek orgánu

shock /ʃɒk/ šok, otřes, náraz

skull /skʌl/ lebka

small /smɔːl/ **bowel** /ˈbaʊ.əl/ tenké střevo

subdural /sʌbˈdjʊ.ə.rəl/ subdurální, ležící pod tvrdou plenou mozkovou

supine /ˈsuː.paɪn/ ležící naznak, ležící na zádech, tváří vzhůru, klidný

susceptible /səˈsep.tɪ.bļ/ náchylný, snadno podléhající

sustain /səˈsteɪn/ vydržet, snést, utrpět

tenderness /'ten.də.nəs/
bolestivost, citlivost na dotek
tilt /tɪlt/ naklonit, sklon, sklopit
transition /træn'zɪʃ.ən/ přechod,
změna stavu
triage /'traɪ.ɪdʒ/ rychlé třídění
raněných a nemocných,
stanovení priorit dle naléhavosti
trim /trɪm/ oříznout, ostříhnout,
zkrátit
uterus /'juː.tər.əs/ uterus, děloha

vague /veɪg/ vágní, nejasný,
neurčitý
valve /vælv/ chlopeň, klapka,
ventil
vasoconstriction /ˌveɪ.zə.kən'strɪk.
ʃən/ vazokonstrikce, zúžení cév
wreck /rek/ zcela zničit, obrátit v
trosky

Unit 3

I

You respond to an explosion at a local fireworks production factory. The explosion rocked the ground several blocks away. There are multiple patients.

The mechanism of injury from a blast or explosion can be from three factors: primary, secondary, and tertiary.
The mechanism of injury of a patient who suffers injuries from being struck by material propelled by the blast force is considered a secondary mechanism of injury.*
A _____ _____ of injury from a _____ __ _____ is defined as any injury sustained from being struck by material propelled by the blast force.
The mechanism of injury of a patient being thrown and impacting the ground or other object is considered a tertiary mechanism of injury.*
A tertiary mechanism of injury from a blast or explosion is defined as any injury sustained from _____ _____ and _____ ___ _____ or other objects.

Your first patient is a 43-year-old male with burns over the front of his right arm, upper chest, and the front of his right leg.

Using the rule of nines, what percentage of burns does this patient have? 22.5%.*
Front of right arm = 4.5%, _____ _____ = 9%, front of right leg = 9%.

This patient is hoarse, has singed nasal hair, is coughing up charcoal-coloured sputum, and has developed inspiratory stridor. Treatment should include immediate endotracheal intubation.*
Your concern with this patient is complete _____ _____ secondary to _____ of the airway. Immediate endotracheal intubation is indicated.

impacting the ground, upper chest, swelling, secondary mechanism, blast or explosion, being thrown, airway obstruction

2

The following _____ regarding a Glasgow Coma Scale score 7 is true:

- A perfect GCS score is 15, and a score of 7 represents serious injuries.*
- A score between 9 and 12 indicates _____ injury.
- A score of 8 or below _____ severe head injury.

> moderate, represents, statement

3

You arrive at the scene of a trench collapse. There are three trapped victims who are buried to the mid chest. The rescue will take several hours because they will need to be dug out by hand. Crush syndrome is a significant concern because crush injuries release toxins into the central circulation that can cause:

- alkalosis
- increased renal function
- cardiac dysrhythmias*
- dyspnoea

_____ _____ creates lactic acid due to _____ _____ that takes place within the crushed body part. One of the _____ _____ with releasing a body part that has been crushed for several hours is the release of the lactic acid and other _____ into the circulating _____ _____ that can lead to profound metabolic acidosis. Sodium bicarbonate is indicated in the treatment of crush syndrome.

> Crush syndrome, major concerns, anaerobic metabolism, toxins, blood volume

4

You are called to a scene of a motor vehicle collision

(MVC). During your initial assessment, you find an _____32-year-old male with multiple _____ to his face and head. He has _____ respirations and a weak, _____ peripheral pulse. Your first action would be:

- to control major bleeding
- rapid extrication
- to open the airway with a jaw thrust and immobilize the cervical spine*

Always remember ABCs.

> contusions, snoring, unresponsive, thready

5

Which of the following statements is true regarding _____ ____?

- Always use _____ or neutralizing agents.
- Acid burns are typically more serious than _____ burns.
- Both acids and alkalis cause burns by disrupting cell membranes and damaging tissues on contact.*
- Always _____ a chemical spill from downwind.
- Antidotes and neutralizing agents should _____ be used as they may cause a violent reaction with the contaminants.*

- Alkali burns are typically more severe because of their liquefaction necrosis process.*
- You should approach from upwind.*

approach, chemical burns, antidotes, alkali, never

6
Beck's triad is often associated with pericardial tamponade. It includes distant heart tones, ___ (jugular venous distension), and:
- _____ paradoxus
- hypotension*
- wheezing
- delayed capillary refill

Beck's triad includes _____, distant heart tones, and JVD. This triad of symptoms can aid in the diagnosis of _____ _____.

cardiac tamponade, pulse, hypotension, JVD

7
A stab wound to the stomach or small intestine would cause gastric contents to enter the peritoneal cavity. Presentation would include:
- a rapid onset of cramping pain
- referred pain to the left shoulder
- a gradual onset of pain throughout the _____

- a rapid onset of sharp pain diffused throughout the abdomen*

Injury to the stomach or small bowel that allows digestive enzymes to enter the _____ _____ can cause a rapid development of _____ ____ throughout the abdomen. This is a serious concern because peritonitis can develop and lead to _____ complications.

serious, peritoneal cavity, sharp pain, abdomen

8
Your trauma patient opens her eyes, pulls her hand away when _____, and speaks only in garbled _____.
What is her Glasgow Coma Scale score? 9.*
The score is 9: 2 points for eye _____, 5 points for_____ _____, and 2 points for _____.

motor response, opening, pinched, sounds, speech

9
Your patient is a 34-year-old woman who has been in an automobile _____. Her respiratory rate is 34 with normal chest wall _____, systolic blood pressure is 78, capillary refill is _____, and her Glasgow Coma Scale score is 10.

ENGLISH FOR PARAMEDICS

This patient's Revised Trauma Score is 9.*
Using the _____ Trauma Score, the patient has 3 points for the GCS, 3 points for the _____ blood pressure, and 3 points for the respiratory rate.

Revised, delayed, systolic, expansion, crash

10
You are caring for a female patient who ___ _____ by an automobile. She opens her eyes to voice _____ only, localizes pain when you pinch her arm, and is _____ ___ _____.
Her Glasgow Coma Scale score is 12.*
The GCS score for this patient is 12: 3 points for opening her eyes to _____ _____, 5 points for _____ ____, and 4 points for speaking clearly although the _____ _____ is confused.

verbal stimuli, localizing pain, awake but confused, thought process, was struck, command

11
What is the Glasgow Coma Scale score for a patient who opens her eyes __ _____ to pain, speaks _____, and _____ in response to pain? 8.*
Eye opening = 2, verbal response = 2, motor response = 4.

withdraws, incomprehensibly, in response

12
Your patient, a middle-aged female, was a _____ struck by a car. She opens her eyes only in response to pain and makes __ _____ response; her best motor response is withdrawal in response to pain.
The Glasgow Coma Scale score for this patient is 7.*
Her score of 7 __ _____ __ 2 points for pain, 1 point for verbal response, and 4 points for motor response.

is composed of, pedestrian, no verbal

13
With the START triage method, several _____ _____ are quickly assessed to determine the order to care for and transport patients. According to the START method, which of the following patients would receive _____ _____ to support haemodynamic status without further assessment?
• male, radial pulse present, skin warm and dry
• female, _____ _____ present, capillary refill time 1 sec.
• male, radial pulse present, skin pale and cyanotic*

133

- female, radial pulse present, capillary refill time 0.5 sec.

The START method quickly reviews _____ _____ to determine patient priority: respirations, pulse, and mental status. After respiratory status is assessed, the basis for judging a patient's haemodynamic status is the presence or absence of a radial pulse or _____ _____ and temperature.

vital signs, radial pulse, three categories, skin colour, immediate treatment

14
What does a red tag mean in the METTAG triage system?
- The _____ is dead.
- The victim has critical injuries.*
- The victim has _____ injuries.
- The victim has _____ injuries.

When using the _____ _____ a red tag indicates a patient with _____ injuries who needs rapid transport.

critical, serious, METTAG system, victim, minor

15
Patients who are found in a hazardous-materials _____

should be initially treated in which containment zone? Warm. Major decontamination and treatment for life-threatening _____ should be conducted by properly protected personnel in the _____ _____.

incident, conditions, warm zone

16
You respond to a 41-year-old male who has been injured in an explosion at an illegal chemistry (drug) laboratory. During assessment, you notice a spinal deformity and a possible closed-head injury. Your patient also has ruptured tympanic membranes and signs of sinus injuries.
Which of the following is not a phase of blast injury?
- alpha*
- primary
- secondary
- tertiary impact

_____ _____ _____ is divided into three phases: primary, secondary, and tertiary. The primary phase occurs during the initial air blast and _____ _____. The secondary phase occurs when the patient is ___ __ _____ propelled by the overpressure of the blast wave. The tertiary phase occurs when the victim is _____ ____ from the

blast into the ground or other hard objects.
This patient's sinus injuries most likely occurred during which blast phase?
- alpha
- primary*
- secondary
- tertiary impact

During the primary blast, forces from the pressure wave and initial air blast result in _____ of air-containing organs such as the sinuses, auditory canals, stomach, lungs, and intestines.

Your victim has first- and second-degree burns to his face. These are flash burns from the _____. Witnesses deny that the patient's clothes were __ ____. You should suspect what injury?
- extensive lung tissue burns
- extensive airway burns
- aspiration pneumonia
- limited airway burns*

Often, burns are _____ to the oro- and nasopharynx in the upper airway. _____ stridor or _____ indicates that oedema is developing, which may lead to _____ _____. Flash burns rarely result in _____ airway or lung tissue burns. Aspiration pneumonia is an infectious process that develops following the introduction of a foreign body into the lungs. It is unlikely in this

scenario, and if it has occurred, there will be no signs of infection yet.

During your assessment, you notice a rigid, very tender abdomen. If this injury occurred in the secondary phase, it would be due to which of the following?
- thermal burns to the stomach
- flying debris and propelled objects*
- deceleration impact with a hard surface
- compression of air-containing organs

Compression of air-containing organs is common in the _____ ____ ____. Deceleration injuries _____ during the tertiary phase, and _____ _____ can occur during any phase of the blast, depending upon whether the _____ ____ is superheated, if flaming objects are striking the patient, or if the patient is thrown into a burning area. A _____, _____ abdomen indicates there are _____ _____ under the skin, and not surface injuries to the dermis from _____. This injury was most likely caused by flying debris or propelled objects _____ the patient.

internal injuries, primary blast phase, striking, occur, thermal burns, pressure wave, rigid, tender, burns,
Worsening, limited, extensive, airway compromise, hoarseness, on fire, explosion, Blast injury impact, thrown away, hit by debris, pressure wave, compression

17
This statement about the vital signs of a patient with an ___ is correct. Vital signs vary greatly since they are related to the area and extent of cardiac damage.*
Vital signs in MI patients depend on the _____ ___ _____ of underlying heart _____ and the patient's response to the insult.

damage, location and extent, AMI

Vocabulary 3
acid /'æs.ɪd/ kyselina
airway /'eə.weɪ/ dýchací cesty
alkali /'æl.kəl.aɪ/ alkálie, zásada
alkalosis /ˌælkə'ləu.sɪs/ alkalóza, zvýšený výskyt zásaditých látek v těle
antidote /æn.tɪ.dəut/ protijed, protilátka, protilék
aspiration /ˌæspɪ'reɪʃən/ aspirace, dýchání
auditory / 'ɔ:dɪtərɪ/ auditivní, sluchový
awake /ə'weɪk/ probudit se, probrat se, být vzhůru, bdělý

away /ə'weɪ/ pryč, daleko
Beck's triad /'traɪ.æd/ Beckova triáda, nízký arteriální tlak, vysoký venózní tlak, chybějící tep na srdečním hrotu při srdeční tamponádě spolu s oslabenými ozvami
blast /blɑ:st/ výbuch, výstřel, rána, poryv
burn / bɜ:n/ popálenina, hořet
bury /'ber.i/ zahrabat, pohřbít
canal /kə'næl/ kanálek
capillary /kə'pɪl.ər.i/ **refill** /'ri:.fɪl/ zpětné plnění kapilár
cell /sel/ buňka
charcoal /'tʃɑ:r.koʊl/ dřevěné uhlí, živočišné uhlí
chemistry /'kem.ɪ.stri/ chemické pochody složení, vlastnosti, procesy
clearly /'klɪə.li/ jasně
command /kə'mɑ:nd/ příkaz, ovládnutí, kontrola, velení
complete /kəm'pli:t/ dokončený, hotový, úplný, doplnit, dokončit, skončit
composed /kəm'pəuzd/ **of** složený z
compression /kəm'preʃən/ komprese, stlačení, stisknutí, slisování
concern /kən'sɜ:n/ zájem, starost, obavy, znepokojení
conduct /kən'dʌkt/ provádět, vést, řídit, chování, počínání
confused /kən'fju:zd/ zmatený, popletený
containment /kən'teɪn.mənt/ uzavření, omezení

contaminant /kənˈtæm.ɪ.nənt/ znečisťující látka

content /kənˈtent/ obsah, náplň

contusion /kənˈtjuː.ʒən/ pohmožděnina, zhmožděnina

cramp /kræmp/ křeč

crash /kræʃ/ havárie, nehoda, zhroucení, srážka, nabourat

critical /ˈkrɪt.ɪ.kəl/ kritický, zlomový, rozhodující, nebezpečný

crush /krʌʃ/ **syndrome** /ˈsɪn.drəʊm/ těžký stav vzniklý rozsáhlým rozdrcením kosterního svalstva např. při zavalení, následek dlouhého tlaku na svalstvo, zejm. paží a nohou

dead /ded/ mrtvý

debris /ˈdeb.riː/, /ˈdeɪ.briː/ trosky, úlomky, pozůstatky, poškozená tkáň, buněčný odpad, zbytky, nečistota

deceleration /diːˌseləˈreɪʃən/ zpomalení, zbrzdění

decontamination /ˌdiː.kən.tæm.ɪˈneɪ.ʃən/ dekontaminace, odmoření

deformity /dɪˈfɔː.mɪ.ti/ deformita, zdeformování, znetvoření

deny /dɪˈnaɪ/ odmítat, zapřít, popřít, popírat

dermis /ˈdɜː.mɪs/ dermis, škára, kožní vrstva

determine /dɪˈtɜː.mɪn/ určit, stanovit, zjistit, rozhodnout

diffuse /dɪˈfjuːz/ pronikat, rozšířit se, roztrousit (se)

disrupt /dɪsˈrʌpt/ narušit, zkomplikovat, přerušit, roztrhat

distant /ˈdɪs.tənt/ vzdálený, odměřený, nepřístupný

distension /dɪˈsten.tʃən/ roztažení

downwind /ˌdaʊnˈwɪnd/ po větru, ve směru větru

due /djuː/ **to** /tʊ/ kvůli, následkem, v důsledku, díky

dig /dɪg/ **out** /aʊt/ vykopat, vyhrabat

dyspnoea /dɪs.pniː.ə/ dyspnoe, dušnost, porucha dýchání

expansion /ɪkˈspæn.tʃən/ expanze, rozpínání, roztahování, rozrůstání

explosion /ɪkˈspləʊ.ʒən/ exploze, výbuch (též přen.)

extrication /ˌek.strɪˈkeɪ.ʃən/ vyproštění, vysvobodit, vyprostit

fireworks /ˈfaɪəˌwɜːk/ rachejtle, zábavní pyrotechnika

flaming /ˈfleɪ.mɪŋ/ planoucí, hořící

flash /flæʃ/ blesk, záblesk, blesknout, vznítit se, zapálit se

flying /ˈflaɪ.ɪŋ/ létající

force /fɔːs/ síla, účinnost, nutit, vyvíjet tlak, zatlačit, natlačit

foreign /ˈfɒr.ən/ **body** /ˈbɒd.i/ cizí tělísko

garbled /ˈgɑː.bl̩d/ zkomolený, překroucený

gradual /ˈgræd.jʊ.əl/ postupný, pozvolný

ground /graʊnd/ zem, území, dopadnout, přistát

haemodynamic /ˌhiː.mə.daɪˈnæm.ɪk/ hemodynamický, týkající se krevní cirkulace

hoarseness /hɔːsnɪs/ ochraptění, chrapot, chraplavost

illegal /ɪˈliː.gəl/ nezákonný

impact /'ɪm.pækt/ dopad, náraz, úder, účinek, vliv, výsledek, dopadat
incomprehensibly /ɪnˌkɒm.prɪ'hen.sɪ.b̩li/ nesrozumitelně
initially /ɪ'nɪʃ.əl.i/ nejprve, zpočátku, původně, na začátku
injury /'ɪndʒərɪ/ úraz
intestine /ɪn'tes.tɪn/ střevo, trakčník
judge /dʒʌdʒ/ posoudit
jugular /'dʒʌg.jə.lər/ jugulární, hrdelní, krční, týkající se hrdla
lactic /'læk.tɪk/ **acid** /'æs.ɪd/ kyselina mléčná
limited /'lɪm.ɪ.tɪd/ limitovaný, omezený, malý
liquefaction /ˌlɪkwɪ'fækʃən/ zkapalnění
localize /'ləʊ.kəl.aɪz/ lokalizovat, určit polohu
lung /lʌŋ/ plíce
major /'meɪ.dʒə/ hlavní, významný, větší, důležitý, závažný, převážný
mean /miːn/ znamenat
membrane /'mem.breɪn/ membrána, blána, blána kryjící tělesnou část, orgán ap.
METTAG, Medical /'med.ɪ.kəl/ **Emergency** /ɪ'mɜː.dʒənt .si/ **Triage** /'triː.ɑːʒ/ **Tag** /tæg/ označování pacientů dle závažnosti zdravotního stavu
mid /mɪd/ střední
middle /'mɪd.l̩/ **age** /eɪdʒ/ střední věk, 40-65 let
minor /'maɪ.nə/ menší, drobný, malý, nezletilý

motor /'məʊ.tər/ motorický, pohybový
nasopharynx /ˌneɪ.zə'fær.ɪŋks/ nosohltan
necrosis /ne'krəʊsɪs/ nekróza, odumření, místní odumírání tkáně
object /'ɒb.dʒɪkt/ objekt, věc
obstruction /əb'strʌk.ʃən/ překážka, ucpání
oedema /ɪ'diː.mə/ edém, otok
oropharynx /'ɔː.rə 'fær.ɪŋks/ orofarynx, ústní část hltanu
overpressure /ˌəʊ.və'preʃ.ər/ nadměrný tlak
paradoxus /'pær.ə.dɒk.səs/ paradoxní
pedestrian /pɪ'destrɪən/ chodec
peers /pɪərz/ vrstevníci
perfect /'pɜː.fekt/ perfektní, dokonalý, bezvadný
phase /feɪz/ fáze, stádium, etapa
pinch /pɪntʃ/ štípnout, stisknout
pinna /pin.ə/ aurikula, ušní boltec
point /pɔɪnt/ okamžik, bod, hrot, špička, pracovní konec nástroje
presentation /ˌprez.ən'teɪ.ʃən/ vzhled, projevení, představení, prezentace
profound /prə'faʊnd/ hluboký, silný
propelled /prə'peld/ poháněný, hnaný
properly /'prɒp.əl.i/ vhodně, náležitě, řádně
pull /pʊl/ táhnout, zatahat
radial /'reɪ.di.əl/ radiální, vřetenní
rarely /'reə.li/ vzácně, jen zřídka
referred /rɪ'fɜːd/ **pain** /peɪn/ přenesená bolest, bolest

pociťovaná v jiném místě než kde je její příčina

release /rɪ'li:s/ propustit, povolit, vypouštět, uvolňovat

renal /'ri:.nəl/ renální, ledvinový

response /rɪ'spɒns/ odpověď, reakce

revise /rɪ'vaɪz/ revidovat, opravit, přehodnotit

rigid /'rɪdʒ.ɪd/ rigidní, tvrdý, pevný, přísný, neohebný, tuhý, strnulý

rock /rɒk/ zatřást, otřást

rupture /'rʌp.tʃər/ ruptura, natržení, protržení, zlomení, kýla, výhřez

score /skɔ:/ docílit, skóre, dosažený výsledek

serious /'sɪə.ri.əs/ opravdový, vážný, závažný, těžký

singe /sɪndʒ/ ožehnutí, lehká popálenina

sinus /'saɪ.nəs/ sinus, dutina (nosní)

snore /snɔ:r/ chrápat, zachrápání

sodium bicarbonate /ˌsəʊ.di.əm.baɪ'kɑ:.bən.ət/ hydrouhličitan sodný, soda

sound /saʊnd/ zvuk, znít

speech /spi:tʃ/ řeč, mluvení

spill /spɪl/ rozlít, rozsypat, vysypat

spinal /'spaɪ.nəl/ páteřní, míšní

sputum /'spju:.təm/ sputum, hlen při vykašlávání

statement /'steɪt.mənt/ prohlášení, výpověď

stimulus /'stɪm.jʊ.ləs/ pl **stimuli** podnět, popud

stomach /'stʌm.ək/ žaludek, břicho

stridor /straɪd.ər/ stridor, pískavý zvuk při ztíženém dýchaní

strike /straɪk/ (struck, struck) zasáhnout, postihnout, udeřit

superheat /'su:.pəˌhi:t/ přehřát, přehřívat páru ap.

surface /'sɜ:.fɪs/ povrch, hladina, zevnějšek, vynořit se

sustain /sə'steɪn/ vydržet, snést, utrpět

swelling /'swelɪŋ/ otok, opuchlina

tag /tæg/ cedulka, visačka, označit jmenovkou, cedulkou

tender /'ten.dər/ měkký, citlivý

tertiary /'tɜ:.ʃər.i/ terciární, třetího stupně

thermal /'θɜ:.məl/ tepelný

thready /'θred.i/ nitkovitý

throughout /θru:'aʊt/ ve všech částech, po celou dobu

throw /θrəʊ/ (threw, thrown) mrštit, hodit

tissue /'tɪʃ.u:/, /'tɪs.ju:/ tkáň, papírový kapesník

trench /trentʃ/ zákop

triage /'traɪ.ɪdʒ/ rychlé třídění raněných a nemocných, stanovení priorit dle naléhavosti

tympanic /'tɪm.pə.nik/ **membrane** /mem.breɪn/ ušní bubínek

tympanic /'tɪm.pə.nik/ tympanický, bubínkový

upper /'ʌp.ər/ horní

venous /'vi:.nəs/ žilní

victim /'vɪk.tɪm/ oběť

voice /vɔɪs/ hlas, hlasový, vyslovit vyjádřit (názor, mínění)

wave /weɪv/ vlna, kývat, mávnout čím

withdraw /wɪðˈdrɔː/ stáhnout,
ustoupit, odejít
withdrawal /wɪðˈdrɔː.əl/ ukončení,
odstranění
witness /ˈwɪt.nəs/ svědek, svědčit,
potvrdit podpisem
zone /zəʊn/ zóna, oblast

Part 5
Gynaecology, obstetrics, paediatrics

Unit I

I

Supine hypotension syndrome occurs from the reduction of cardiac output due to compression of the inferior vena cava.*
_____ hypotension syndrome (or vena cava syndrome) occurs when the pregnant _____ compresses the _____ ____ ____ when the patient is in a supine position. This results in a _____ in blood return back to the heart and a reduction of _____ _____. This syndrome can occur as early as the third month of gestation.

Supine, cardiac output, inferior vena cava, decrease, uterus

2

You are caring for a female patient who is at thirty-five weeks' gestation. She was involved in a car accident and complains of neck pain. You suspect spinal injury and fully immobilize her on a long spine board.
You would then carefully ____ the board on its left side 10-15 degrees.*
The backboard must be tilted on its left side 10-15 degrees

to prevent supine _____
_____. Tilting the board will allow the _____ to displace to the left and prevent compression of the _____ vena cava.

hypotension syndrome, uterus, tilt, inferior

3

The major concern with a prolapsed cord is that it will be compressed and reduce blood flow to the infant, resulting in _____.*
The major concern with a prolapsed cord is _____ of the cord by the head of the infant. This can result in a reduced ____ ____ to the infant and can lead to foetal hypoxia.

compression, blood flow, hypoxia

4

Abdominal pain in the region of the ovary during ovulation is known as _____.
Mittelschmerz is German for '_____ pain' and is defined as abdominal pain in the region of the ovary during _____.*

middle, ovulation, Mittelschmerz

5

In obstetrics, a woman's parity refers to her number of _____ deliveries.*

'This is common obstetric medical terminology. The term *gravida* means number of _____.
_____ or gravidity refers to the number of times a woman has been _____.
A multigravida and _____ pregnancy history includes many pregnancies and no births.
_____ is when a woman has been pregnant more than once. A nullipara is a woman who has not yet delivered her first child.

viable, pregnant, nullipara, Multigravida, Gravida, pregnancies

6
Your patient is 26 years old and thirty weeks pregnant. She complains of sudden severe tearing abdominal pain with some minor vaginal bleeding. Upon careful _____, her abdomen is very tender, and her uterus seems to be tightly _____.
You suspect abruptio placentae.* Abruptio placentae is the premature separation of the placenta from the uterus. There are different _____ that can occur depending on the severity of the abruption.
Classic presentation includes a sudden, _____, tearing pain and the development of a _____ boardlike abdomen. Bleeding

can be severe or not present depending on many factors.

stiff, palpation, sharp, presentations, contracted

7
Placental abruption is a _____ _____ caused by:
• _____ of the fertilized ovum in a fallopian tube
• the uterus covering the _____ opening
• premature separation of the placenta from the uterine wall*
• spontaneous _____
It is a true medical emergency because it poses a life threat to the mother and _____.

foetus, medical emergency, abortion, implantation, cervical

8
The normal _____ changes to vital signs during the second trimester of pregnancy include the following: blood pressure _____, _____ _____ rises.*

physiological, pulse rate, falls

9
The next four questions are based on the following scenario:
You are called to the scene of a 26-year-old female patient who

is twenty-seven weeks pregnant and in active labour. The patient states the baby is coming. You perform a visual examination of the perineum and notice a prolapsed cord.

You would immediately place the patient in which position?
- hips _____ as much as possible*
- knee-chest position*

Position the mother with the hips elevated as much as possible or in the knee-chest position in an attempt to _____ pressure on the cord.

You would instruct the patient to:
- push with each contraction
- pant with each contraction*
- bear down
- hold her breath

You would instruct the patient to pant with each contraction to prevent _____ ____ and applying pressure on the cord. With a gloved hand, place two fingers into the vagina to elevate the presenting part to relieve pressure on the cord. Provide oxygen and rapid transport to a hospital that can perform a _____ _____.

Additional treatment would include, with a gloved hand, placing two fingers into the vagina to raise the foetus off the cord, providing oxygen and transport.*

Care for the prolapsed cord would include:
- application of a sterile dressing*
- attempting to reposition the cord
- packing in ice to prevent it from drying

Applying a sterile _____ to the exposed cord will minimize _____ change. If the cord is exposed to room temperature, the temperature of blood _____ to the infant will decrease. This can cause hypothermia.

Additionally, a temperature change of the blood may cause the umbilical vessels to _____ resulting in _____ blood flow to the infant.

relieve, caesarean delivery, elevated, bearing down, raise, spasm, dressing, flowing, decreased, temperature

10

The hormone secreted by the _____ _____ that stimulates the uterus to produce stronger _____ is called oxytocin.* The medication (oxytocin) is used to induce labour or control _____ haemorrhage.

> postpartum, pituitary gland, contractions

of the abdomen and nausea are also common with PID.

> chills, Guarding, suffering from, walking

11

The most common sexually _____ disease is called:

- chlamydia*
- gonorrhoea
- syphilis
- herpes

Gonorrhoea, syphilis, and _____ are also _____ transmitted diseases.

> herpesvirus, sexually, transmitted

12

You are treating a 20-year-old female complaining of abdominal pain that becomes more intense when walking. She states that if she shuffles her feet when she walks, the pain isn't as intense. Other signs and symptoms include fever, _____, and nausea. This patient is most likely _____ ____:

- endometritis
- pelvic inflammatory disease*
- ruptured ovarian cyst
- mittelschmerz
- cystitis

Pelvic inflammatory disease is often accompanied by increased pain when _____.
The patient will bend forward and take short, slow steps. _____

13

The next three questions are based on the following scenario: You are called to a 32-year-old female who is in her twenty-eighth week of pregnancy. She complains of dizziness, blurred vision, and a feeling that she is going to pass out. She is emotionally _____ and crying. At her doctor's _____ last week, her doctor scolded her for gaining too much weight. Her hands and ankles are oedematous, and her face is puffy. Vitals are as follows: BP, 178/108; pulse, 104; respirations, 24.

You suspect that this patient:

- is emotionally upset
- has preeclampsia*
- has borderline hypotension
- has postpartum depression

_____ signs and symptoms of preeclampsia include headache, dizziness, _____, blurred vision, nausea, vomiting, proteinuria, hypertension, and oedema.

Treatment for this patient would include:

- rapid transport with lights and siren
- administering nitroglycerin to lower the blood pressure
- transporting for psychiatric evaluation
- keeping the patient calm and transporting without lights and siren*

If you suspect preeclampsia, you should ____ _____ to prevent seizures, which include keeping the patient calm and transporting without lights and sirens.

You are en route to the hospital when the patient has a _____ ___ _____.

Treatment for this patient includes maintaining an airway, administering oxygen, administering magnesium sulphate 2-5 grams, and monitoring vital signs.* Treatment of seizure activity in eclampsia includes placing the patient in the left lateral _____ position, maintaining the airway, administering high-flow oxygen, _____ IV access, and administering 2-5 grams of magnesium sulphate IV. If seizures cannot be controlled, sedatives may be required.

establishing, Common, upset, confusion, take precautions, recumbent, grand mal seizure, appointment

14

The next two questions are based on the following scenario:
Your patient is a 38-year-old _____ in her thirtieth week of gestation. She presents with bright red vaginal bleeding but _____ abdominal pain. Her _____ is soft and feels out of place. Her problem began following sexual intercourse. You suspect:

- a uterine rupture
- placenta praevia*
- an ectopic pregnancy
- abruptio placentae

Placenta praevia is usually in a multigravida in her third trimester of pregnancy. A recent history of _____ _____ or vaginal examination just before the onset of vaginal bleeding is not uncommon. The onset of painless bright red vaginal bleeding or spotting is considered the _____ ____ of placenta praevia.
Management of this patient includes IV fluids, high-flow oxygen, and transport for evaluation.*
A vaginal exam should not be attempted when placenta praevia is suspected. The exam may

_____ the placenta and cause severe haemorrhage.

puncture, sexual intercourse, hallmark sign, denies, multigravida, uterus

15
APGAR assessment of a newborn should be performed at ___ ___ ____ minutes after birth.*
It is important to wait one full minute to perform the first _____ assessment. A second APGAR should be _____ at five minutes.

APGAR, one and five, performed

16
If the amniotic sac has not ruptured and the baby's head _____, you should use your fingers to _____ and puncture the sac, then push the sac away from the nose and mouth.*
If the _____ ___ is present around the baby's head, use your fingers to pinch the sac and then ____ __ ____ from the nose and mouth. Using a scalpel or scissors is not recommended.

amniotic sac, push it away, emerges, pinch

17
_____ _____ should be performed on any newborn with a

heart rate less than __ _____ per minute.*
If a newborn's heart rate is 60-80 and does not increase despite _____ and _____, it is necessary to start chest compressions.

60 beats, stimulation, ventilation, Chest compressions

18
Your 26-year-old female patient complains of nausea, dizziness, sudden onset of sharp left lower-quadrant pain, and shoulder pain. You suspect:
• a ruptured appendix
• an ectopic pregnancy*
• cholecystitis
• kidney stones
An ectopic pregnancy should be suspected when _____ ____ is present in women of childbearing age who are sexually active. An ectopic pregnancy can be difficult to _____ from other conditions. The classic _____ of symptoms includes abdominal pain, _____ bleeding, and amenorrhoea.
Other symptoms include _____ pain to the shoulder, nausea, vomiting, or syncope. Signs of shock may be present if the _____ ruptures.

distinguish, vaginal, abdominal pain, referred, triad, ectopic

19

The function of the placenta includes all of the following:

- the transfer of antibodies*
- the transfer of _____ ___
  _____*
- the excretion of CO_2 and waste products*

The placenta has many functions including the transport of oxygen, nutrients, and other substances to the foetus and the _____ of CO_2 and other _____ products.

excretion, waste, oxygen and nutrients

20

What is the most appropriate care for a suspected _____-_____ patient? Perform a limited _____ _____ and care for injuries requiring immediate treatment.*
EMS providers should limit the patient's history to the elements necessary to provide care. Patient contact should be ___-_____ and supportive.

non-judgemental, sexual-assault, physical examination

Vocabulary I

abortion /əˈbɔː.ʃən/ potrat, přerušení těhotenství

abruptio placentae /æbˈrʌp.ʃɪ.əʊ. pləˈsen.tiː/ předčasné odloučení placenty

abruption /əˈbrʌp.ʃən/ odtržení

amenorrhoea /ˌeɪ.men.əˈriː.ə/ amenorea, vynechávání menstruačního krvácení

amniotic /ˌæm.niˈɒt.ɪk/ **sac** /sæk/ plodový vak

antibody /ˈæn.tiˌbɒd.i/ protilátka, vlastní, v těle

appendix /əˈpen.dɪks/ apendix, červovitý přívěsek slepého střeva

apply /əˈplaɪ/ aplikovat, požádat, platit, použít

appointment /əˈpɔɪnt.mənt/ funkce, místo, schůzka, jednání

bear /beər/ **down** /daʊn/ tlačit, vyřítit se, ležet svou vahou na

bend /bend/ (bent, bent) ohnout, sklonit, pokrčit, oblouk, ohnutí, ohyb

blurred /blɜːd/ neostrý, nejasný, zastřený, rozmazaný

boardlike /bɔːd.laɪk/ podobný desce

borderline /ˈbɔː.də.laɪn/ hranice, mezní, hraniční

breath /breθ/ dech

caesarean section /sɪˌzeə.ri.ənˈsek. ʃən/ císařský řez

care /keə/ **for** /fɔː/ sb starat se, mít zájem, ošetřovat

careful /ˈkeə.fəl/ opatrný, pečlivý, důkladný

cervical /səˈvaɪ.kəl/ krční, krčkový

childbearing /ˈtʃaɪldˌbeə.rɪŋ/ rození dětí

chill /tʃɪl/ vychladit, zimnice

chlamydia /kləm.iˈde.ə/ Chlamydia, lat. rod mikroorganismů schopných množení jen v buňce, obligátní intracelulární paraziti

cholecystitis /ˌkəʊ.lɪ.sɪˈstaɪ.tɪs/ cholecystitida, zánět žlučníku

compress /kəmˈpres/ obklad, stlačit, zmáčknout

condition /kənˈdɪʃ.ən/ stav, fyzická kondice, potíže, onemocnění, podmínka

contract /kənˈtrækt/ stáhnout, zúžit se

cord /kɔːd/ šňůra, pupečník

cyst /sɪst/ cysta

cystitis /sɪˈstaɪ.tɪs/ cystitida, zánět močového měchýře

decrease /dɪˈkriːs/ snížit se, zmenšit, pokles

delivery /dɪˈlɪv.ər.i/ porod, narození

distinguish /dɪˈstɪŋ.gwɪʃ/ rozlišit, rozeznat, odlišit

eclampsia /ɪˈklæmp.si.ə/ eklampsie, pozdní gestóza, komplikace těhotenství

ectopic pregnancy /ekˌtɒp.ɪkˈpreg.nən.si/ mimoděložní těhotenství

emerge /ɪˈmɜːdʒ/ objevit se, vynořit se

emotionally /ɪˈməʊ.ʃən.əl.i/ emočně, citově

endometritis /ˌen.də.miˈtraɪ.tɪs/ endometritida, zánět děložní sliznice

establish /ɪˈstæb.lɪʃ/ navázat, založit, vytvořit, ustavit, vybudovat

evaluation /ɪˌvæl.juˈeɪ.ʃən/ ohodnocení, ocenění, zhodnocení, vyhodnocení

excretion /ɪkˈskriː.ʃən/ exkrece, vyměšování, vylučování

exposed /ɪkˈspəʊzd/ exponovaný, odhalený, obnažený, nechráněný, vystavený

fallopian tube /fəˌləʊ.pi.ənˈtjuːb/ vejcovod

fertilize /ˈfɜː.tɪ.laɪz/ oplodnit

flowing /ˈfləʊ.ɪŋ/ proudící, plynoucí, tekoucí

foetal /ˈfiː.təl/ fetální, plodový

forward /ˈfɔː.wəd/ dopředu

gonorrhoea /ˌgɒn.əˈriː.ə/ gonorea, kapavka

gravida /ˌgræv.ɪ.də/ gravidní

gravidity /grævˈɪd.ɪ.ti/ gravidita, těhotenství

gynaecology /ˌgaɪ.nəˈkɒl.ə.dʒi/ gynekologie

hallmark /ˈhɔːl.mɑːk/ typický znak, známka

herpes /ˈhɜː.piːz/ zoster /zɒ.stər/ pásový opar

herpes /ˈhɜː.piːz/ herpes opar

herpes /ˈhɜː.piːz/ simplex /ˈsɪm.pleks/ opar rtu

herpes-virus /ˈhɜː.piːzˈvaɪ.rəs/ skupina virů způsobující opary

hip /hɪp/ bok, kyčel

hold /həʊld/ pořádat, podržet, pojmout, obsahovat

implantation /ˌɪm.plænˈteɪ.ʃən/ implantace, uhnízdění vajíčka v děloze

instruct /ɪnˈstrʌkt/ instruovat, nařídít, dát pokyn
kidney /ˈkɪd.ni/ stones /stəʊnz/ ledvinové kameny
knee /niː/ -chest /tʃest/ position / pəˈzɪʃ.ən/ pacientka spočívá na kolenou a horní části hrudníku (při porodu)
labour /ˈleɪ.bər/ porodní stahy, začátek porodu
light /laɪt/ světlo
magnesium /mægˈniː.zi.əm/ sulphate /ˈsʌl.feɪt/ síran hořečnatý
minimise /ˈmɪn.ɪ.maɪz/ minimalizovat
minor /ˈmaɪ.nə/ menší, drobný, malý, nezletilý
mittelschmerz /mɪtl.ʃmərθ/ bolest v oblasti vaječníků uprostřed ovulačního cyklu
multigravida /mʌl.ti'græv.ɪ.də/ vícekrát těhotná
newborn /ˈnjuː.bɔːn/ novorozenec
non-judgemental /ˌnɒn.dʒʌdʒˈmen.təl/ neodsuzující
nullipara /nʌˈlɪp.ər.ə/ žena, která dosud nerodila
nutrient /ˈnjuː.tri.ənt/ výživná látka, živina
obstetrics /ɒbˈstetrɪks/ porodnictví
oedematous /ɪˈdiː.mə.təs/ edémový, oteklý
ovarian /əʊˈveə.ri.ən/ ovariální, týkající se vaječníků
ovary /ˈəʊ.vər.i/ vaječník
ovum /ˈəʊ.vəm/ pl ova vajíčko
oxytocin /ˌɒk.sɪˈtəʊ.sɪn/ hormon tvořený v hypothalamu a vylučovaný do krve v zadním

laloku hypofýzy, má význam pro stahy dělohy při porodu
pack /pæk/ zábal, obal
packing /ˈpæk.ɪŋ/ balení, balicí materiál
paediatrics /ˌpiː.diːˈæt.rɪks/ pediatrie
pant /pænt/ těžce oddechovat, supět, popadat dech
parity /ˈpær.ɪtɪ/ rovnost, rovnoprávnost
pass /pɑːs/ out /aʊt/ omdlít, ztratit vědomí
pelvic /ˈpel.vɪk/ inflammatory / ɪnˈflæm.ə.tər.i/ disease /dɪˈziːz/ zánětlivé onemocnění pánve
perform /pəˈfɔːm/ vykonat, provést, udělat, fungovat
perineum /ˌper.ɪˈniː.əm/ hráz, u muže úsek mezi análním otvorem a odstupem šourku, u ženy mezi análním otvorem a spojením stydkých pysků
pituitary gland /pɪˈtjuː.ɪ.tər. i.glænd/ hypofýza, podvěsek mozkový
placenta /pləˈsen.tə/ praevia/ priː. vi.ə/ vcestné lůžko, překrývá děložní otvor a brání normálnímu průběhu porodu
postpartum /ˌpəʊstˈpɑː.təm/ poporodní, následující po porodu
precaution /prɪˈkɔː.ʃən/ opatrnost, preventivní opatření, bezpečnostní opatření, předběžné opatření
preeclampsia /ˌpriː.ɪˈklæmp.si. ə/ preeklampsie, těhotenské

onemocnění s otoky, bílkovinou v
moči a vysokým krevním tlakem
premature /ˈprem.ə.tʃər/
předčasný, nedonošený,
předčasně narozený
presenting /prɪˈzent.ɪŋ/ **part** /pɑːt/
procházející část, při porodu
product /ˈprɒd.ʌkt/ produkt,
výsledek
prolapsed /prəʊˈlæpst/ vyhřezlý,
snížený trubicový orgán
proteinuria /ˈprəʊ.ti:n.jʊəˈriː.ə/
proteinurie, vylučování bílkovin
moči
puffy /ˈpʌf.i/ opuchlý, oteklý
puncture /ˈpʌŋk.tʃə/ punkce, vpich,
otvor propíchnutí, propíchnout
push /pʊʃ/ tlačit, posunout,
postrčit, strčit, prodrat se
recumbent /rɪˈkʌm.bənt/ ležící
reposition /ˌriː.pəˈzɪʃən/ přemístit,
přesunout, posunout
scalpel /ˈskæl.pəl/ skalpel
scissors /ˈsɪz.əz/ nůžky, sevření
scold /skəʊld/ vynadat
separation /ˌsepəˈreɪʃən/ separace,
oddělení, odloučení, rozdělení
severity /sɪˈver.ɪ.ti/ krutost,
vážnost, útrapy
sexual /ˈsek.sjʊəl/ **intercourse** /ˈɪn.
tə.kɔːs/ pohlavní styk
shuffle /ˈʃʌf.l̩/ šourat, vléci se
siren /ˈsaɪərən/ siréna
spot /spɒt/ skvrna, zpozorovat,
všimnout si
spotting /spɒt.ɪŋ/ krvavý výtok
z dělohy mezi menstruačními
obdobími

state /steɪt/ stav, uvádět,
prohlašovat
stiff /stɪf/ tvrdý, ztuhlý, neohebný
supportive /səˈpɔː.tɪv/ nápomocný,
podporující
suspected /səˈspek.tɪd/ suspektní,
domnělý podezřelý
syphilis /ˈsɪf.ɪ.lɪs/ syfilis
tender /ˈten.dər/ měkký, citlivý
tightly /ˈtaɪt.li/ těsně
umbilical /ʌmˈbɪl.ɪ.kəl/ pupeční
upset /ʌpˈset/ podráždění,
rozrušený, znepokojený, narušit
uterine /ˈjuː.tər.aɪn/ **wall** /wɔːl/
uterinní, děložní stěna
viable /ˈvaɪ.ə.bl̩/ životaschopný,
funkční
vision /ˈvɪʒ.ən/ vidění, zrak
waste /weɪst/ **product** /ˈprɒdʌkt/
odpadní produkt
weight /weɪt/ váha

Unit 2

I

The next two questions are based on the following scenario:
You arrive on the scene of a 25-year-old female who states she is nine months pregnant and is in _____ labour. The patient states she is gravida 3, para 2. She states that her _____ _____ about 15 minutes ago and the baby is coming. Vital signs are as follows: BP, 152/86; pulse, 96; respirations, 24.
The term *gravida* means number of pregnancies.*
Upon _____ examination, you notice that crowning is present. You should prepare for _____ because the birth of the baby is imminent.*

apparent, delivery, water broke, visual

2

The next two questions are based on the following scenario:
You arrive on the scene of a motor vehicle crash and notice that a car has struck a telephone pole. There is extensive damage to the vehicle.
You find a confused female in her mid twenties complaining of neck, chest, and abdominal pain. She keeps asking if her baby is going to be okay. You find out that she is eight months pregnant.

Assessment reveals a large laceration to the forehead with active bleeding. BP, 96/54; pulse, 142 with pale, cool skin; respirations, 24 and shallow. Treatment includes administering 100% oxygen, rapid _____ from the vehicle with C-spine immobilization onto a backboard, placing her on a _____ on the left side, starting two large-bore IVs while en route to the hospital.

During transport, she suddenly goes into cardiac arrest. The patient is apnoeic and _____, and the cardiac monitor shows ventricular fibrillation.
What should be your next action? Defibrillate, _____ ___, intubate, and administer epinephrine 1 mg IVP.*
Treatment for a pregnant patient in cardiac arrest would include defibrillation, CPR, intubation, and administration of appropriate _____.

medications, extrication, backboard, begin CPR, pulseless

3

You are treating a 22-year-old female _____ __ severe abdominal pain and left shoulder pain. Vital signs are as follows: BP, 88/64; pulse, 128 and regular; respirations of 22; skin, cool and wet. She states that

she has a small amount of pink vaginal _____. This patient is most likely experiencing:
- a ruptured ectopic pregnancy*
- endometriosis
- pelvic inflammatory disease
- amenorrhoea

An ectopic pregnancy should __ _____ when abdominal pain is present in women of childbearing age who are _____ active. An ectopic pregnancy can be difficult to distinguish from other _____. The classic triad of symptoms includes abdominal pain, vaginal bleeding, and _____.

conditions, discharge, be suspected, complaining of, amenorrhoea, sexually

4
You are providing positive-pressure _____ to a newborn.
Regarding oxygen administration to a newborn, this statement is correct: never _____ a newborn of oxygen for fear of oxygen toxicity.*
If central cyanosis is present or you are unsure about the _____ of ventilation, the administration of _____ oxygen is necessary.

deprive, supplemental, ventilation, adequacy

5
To prevent over- or undertransfusion of blood from the umbilical cord to the _____, the correct _____ of the newborn until the umbilical cord __ _____ should be at the level of the vagina.*
Keep the newborn at the ____ level of the vagina with the head slightly _____ than the rest of the body.
This will prevent over- or undertransfusion of blood from the umbilical cord to the newborn and facilitate _____ of secretions from the nose and mouth to help to prevent _____.

aspiration, positioning, same, drainage, newborn, lower, is clamped

6
The umbilical vein carries oxygenated blood from the placenta to the foetus.
The umbilical cord consists of one ____ and two _____.*
The umbilical vein carries oxygenated blood from the _____ to the foetus. The umbilical arteries transport _____ products from the foetus to the placenta.

waste, arteries, vein, placenta

7

Contraction intervals are correctly _____ from the beginning of one contraction to the _____ of the next.*
Many health-care providers _____ measure intervals from the end of one contraction to the beginning of the next.
Contraction length is correctly measured from the beginning of one contraction to ___ ___ of that contraction.*

beginning, measured, incorrectly, the end

8

You have a female patient at thirty-nine weeks' gestation. She has _____ contractions _____ 45-60 seconds at 1- to 2-minute intervals and is crowning. Treatment for this patient should include preparing for delivery.*
Regular contractions lasting 45-60 seconds at 1- to 2-minute intervals and _____ indicate that delivery is imminent.

regular, crowning, lasting

9

Four assessment manoeuvres used to _____ foetal position is called the Leopold manoeuvre.*

The Leopold manoeuvre is _____ of the abdomen in four different assessment steps. This is used to identify the _____ of foetuses and the foetal presentation, presenting ____, degree of descent, point of maximum intensity of foetal heart tones, and internal _____ of the foetus.

palpation, determine, part, number, rotation

10

You are delivering a child when you observe the umbilical cord _____ around the neck.
Your first action should be to gently _____ the cord from around the neck.*
Initial care for _____ ____ (cord around the neck) is to first try to gently remove the cord from around the neck. If this is not successful and the cord is so tight that it is _____ labour, it will be necessary __ _____ the cord in two places and ___ between the clamps.

wrapped, to clamp, nuchal cord, remove, inhibiting, cut

11

You are delivering a child in a breech presentation. You have delivered the feet and chest. You note that the _____ of the child is

moving and suspect that the child is attempting to breathe. You should insert two fingers in the vagina to form an airway around the infant's ____ ___ _____.*
If the infant starts to breathe with its face pressed against the vaginal wall, it is necessary __ _____ two fingers in the vagina to form __ _____ around the infant's nose and mouth.

> an airway, nose and mouth, chest, to insert

12
Applying gentle _____ to the infant's head to prevent explosive delivery is essential because this will allow the _____ to stretch and reduce the chance of tearing.*
Applying gentle countertraction to the infant's head to prevent _____ delivery is essential to decrease the likelihood of tearing of the perineum and decrease the potential for rapid _____ of the baby's skull through the birth canal, which may cause _____ injury.

> countertraction, intracranial, expulsion, explosive, perineum

13
Meconium-stained _____ _____ indicates a foetal hypoxic incident.*

Hypoxia causes an increase in _____ activity along with the relaxation of the ____ _____, which allows meconium to pass into the amniotic fluid.

> digestive, anal sphincter, amniotic fluid

14
The next two questions are based on the following scenario:
You are sent to a private residence for a 13-month-old child with a barky cough. He is awake, slow to respond, and visibly uncomfortable. The _____ cough is audible without a stethoscope, but lung sounds reveal inspiratory stridor at rest. There is use of _____ muscles, and you note nasal flaring.

You would suspect the child to be suffering from:
• epiglottitis
• croup*
• bronchiolitis
• a common cold
_____ is a viral infection of the upper airway that causes inflammation of the _____ region that can lead to airway _____. Inspiratory stridor is often present. Other assessment findings include nasal flaring, tracheal tugging or retractions. The vital signs of this patient

are compensatory to the airway obstruction.

This child can be categorized as a child who is experiencing:
- respiratory arrest
- respiratory insufficiency
- prerespiratory arrest
- respiratory failure*

Respiratory failure is _____ for the following reasons: tachypnoea, tachycardia, nasal flaring, _____, audible airway noises, (stridor/barky) cough, and slowness to respond, which indicates a decreased level of _____.

> barky, Croup, retractions, accessory, obstruction, consciousness, subglottic, evident

15
You have been called to treat a 5-year-old child previously diagnosed with an upper respiratory infection. She now presents with increased work of breathing, fever, and increased cough. The child appears pale, is lying on the couch, and slow __ _____. She has obvious nasal flaring with a respiratory rate of 8 per minute.
This child is most likely in respiratory distress with _____ respiratory failure.*
Respiratory distress is defined as the inability to maintain _____ _____ sufficient to meet the needs of the body. Evidence of abnormal respirations (tachypnoea or bradypnoea) or increased work of breathing, use of accessory muscles, nasal flaring, _____, and decreased _____ can also signal respiratory distress in the paediatric patient.

> to respond, gaseous exchange, mentation, grunting, impending

16
Signs and symptoms associated with shaken baby syndrome might include an intracranial haemorrhage, resulting from ____ _____ between the brain and skull in children under the age of 24 months.*
The result of _____ _____ in a baby less than 24 months old may include damage to nerve tissues deep _____ ___ _____ and torn veins between the brain and the skull, which can cause severe bleeding.

> violent shaking, within the brain, torn veins

17
You respond to a call for a 2-month-old female who is reported by the mother to be seizing. Upon arrival, you find the infant lying in a crib motionless;

no _____ _____ is evident. The mother reports that the episode began approximately 10 minutes ago. Your assessment reveals a flaccid infant with slow respiration of 10 per minute, bulging anterior fontanelle, and several areas of bruising on the extremities __ _____ _____ of healing.

From the information given and the general appearance of the infant, you suspect child abuse, most probably shaken baby syndrome.*

You may suspect _____ ____ _____ based on the _____ __ the anterior fontanelle without fever or overhydration as a cause. In addition, the multiple areas of bruising provide information that may indicate _____ _____.

in various stages, shaken baby syndrome, child abuse, bulging of, seizure activity

18

Intraosseous access allows for the administration of fluids, medications, and blood products into the ____ _____.

Possible complications of intraosseous infusion include all of the following: osteomyelitis, fractures, and compartment syndrome.*

IO infusions will generally improve the patient's condition or improve his or her vascular volume, thereby increasing the BP and cardiac output.

_____ can occur if the needle is left in place for longer than twenty-four hours.

_____ can occur when the extremity is not well stabilized or an attempt was made at an improper site where the bone is weaker.

_____ _____ occurs when extravasation is not detected.

Fractures, bone marrow, Compartment syndrome, Osteomyelitis

19

The MOST appropriate _____ manoeuvre for an infant in SVT involves holding ice packs firmly to the face.

Apply ice to the ____ of the infant, being careful not to obstruct the nose and mouth. If the child is old enough to follow _____, have the child hold his or her _____ and blow into an occluded straw or _____ the child to bear down.

encourage, face, breath, directions, vagal

20

You are dispatched to a private residence for an 8-year-old boy complaining of trouble breathing.

On arrival, you find the patient _____, with blue lips and rapid, laboured respirations. He is able to answer questions with only one- or two-word _____. Physical examination reveals a respiratory rate of 50 per minute and diminished breath sounds, and _____ are heard over the right lung field with dullness to percussion. He also has a temperature of 104 °F (40 °C). Based on your assessment, this patient may be experiencing respiratory _____, most probably due to pneumonia.* The patient may be experiencing respiratory failure, most probably due to _____ based on tachypnoea, increased work of breathing, diminished breath sounds, dullness to _____, and elevated temperature.

pneumonia, sentences, percussion, crackles, lethargic, failure

21
Answer the next four questions on the basis of the following information.
You respond to the residence of a 4-year-old male who was found in his backyard head down in a 5-gallon (19 l) bucket of water. The child, according to the mother, was in the water _____ 4 minutes.

The child is cyanotic, pulseless, and apnoeic. The ECG shows he is in asystole. The child weights approximately 40 pounds (18 kg).

A physician at the scene of an accident instructs you to provide care for a patient that you know to be inappropriate given the patient's present condition. Your best course of action will be to contact the medical control physician and ask him to speak with the on-scene physician.* The medical control physician should be able to engage with the on-scene physician in discussion with the patient's condition, the level of care that will be provided by the EMS _____, and the transportation and destination decisions.
What would be the most reliable method for determining the proper medication dosing for this paediatric patient? Use the Broselow Tape or another length-weight _____ system.*
All of the following medications can be given through the endotracheal tube to the paediatric patient: lidocaine, epinephrine, and atropine.*
Valium is usually given orally or rectally.
After endotracheal intubation of this patient, what step should be done first? Confirm the ETT placement.*

Your first step following
placement of the ET tube is
to confirm its placement in the
trachea. After _____ of
its placement, secure the tube
with tape or using a commercial
device to help _____ dislodging
of the tube. Pay especially close
_____ to these tubes as they
are easily displaced, even when
secured.
Depending upon which size of
tube you use, it may or may not
be a cuffed tube. Medication
administration will follow after
confirmation of _____ and
securing the tube.

---

attention, placement,
approximately, prevent, personnel,
measuring, confirmation

Vocabulary 2
accessory /ək'ses.ər.i/ akcesorní,
přídatný
activity /æk'tɪv.ɪ.ti/ aktivita,
činnost
adequacy /'æd.ə.kwə.si/
přiměřenost
amenorrhoea /ˌeɪ.men.ə'riː.ə/
amenorea, vynechávání
menstruačního krvácení
anal /'eɪ.nəl/ anální, řitní
apnoeic /æp'niː.ɪk/ apnoický, bez
dechu
apparent /ə'pær.ənt/ zřejmý,
patrný, jasný
asystole /ə.sɪs.tə.lɪ/ asystola,
asystolie, uvolnění srdeční

svaloviny, zástava srdeční
činnosti
at /ət/ **rest** /rest/ v klidu, bez
pohybu
attempt /ə'tempt/ pokus,
pokoušet se, snažit
audible /'ɔː.dɪ.b|/ slyšitelný
backyard /ˌbæk'jɑːd/ dvorek,
zahrada za domem
barky /'bɑː.ki/ štěkavý
bear /beər/ **down** /daʊn/ tlačit,
rodit
birth /'bɜːθ/ **canal** /kə'næl/ porodní
cesta
bone /bəʊn/ **marrow** /'mær.əʊ/
kostní dřeň
break /breɪk/ (broke broken)
prasknout, zlomit, rozbít
breech /briːtʃ/ **presentation** /
ˌprez.ən'teɪ.ʃən/ poloha koncem
pánevním
bucket /bʌkɪt/ kbelík, vědro
bulge / bʌldʒ/ naběhnout, zduřet,
vyboulit se, vyklenutí, vydutí,
vyboulenina
clamp /klæmp/ svorka, upevnit
svorkou, spona, sepnout
cold /kəʊld/ nachlazení, rýma
commercial /kə'mɜːʃəl/ obchodní,
komerční, průmyslově vyráběný
compartment /kəm'pɑːt.
mənt/ **syndrome** /'sɪn.drəʊm/
kompartmentový syndrom,
imobilizace nervu nebo šlachy v
určitém prostoru
confirmation /ˌkɒn.fə'meɪ.ʃən/
potvrzení, schválení
contraction /kən'træk.ʃən/ stah,
stažení, smrštění

countertraction /ˌkaʊn.tərˈtræk.ʃən/ protitah, repozice zlomeniny tahem ze dvou opačných stran

course /kɔːs/ průběh, kúra (léčebná), postup

crackle /ˈkræk.ļ/ praskot, praskání, šustění

crash /kræʃ/ havárie, nehoda, zhroucení, srážka, nabourat

crib /krɪb/ (dětská) postýlka

croup /kruːp/ difterický krup, dětský zánět hrtanu, štěkavý kašel, hrtanová křeč

crowning /ˈkraʊ.nɪŋ/ stadium porodu, kdy se hlava plodu objeví v rodidlech

defibrillate /ˌdiːˈfɪb.rɪ.leɪt/ defibrilovat

deprive /dɪˈpraɪv/ zbavit, sebrat, připravit o co

descent /dɪˈsent/ klesání

destination /ˌdes.tɪˈneɪ.ʃən/ destinace, místo určení, cílová stanice cíl cesty

detect /dɪˈtekt/ zjistit, objevit, určit

discharge /dɪsˈtʃɑːdʒ/ výtok, odtok, sekret, výměšek, propustit, vyměšovat, vylučovat

dislodge /dɪˈslɒdʒ/ uvolnit, vytlačit, vypudit

distinguish /dɪˈstɪŋ.gwɪʃ/ rozlišit, rozeznat, odlišit

drainage /ˈdreɪ.nɪdʒ/ odvodnění, odtok

dullness /ˈdʌl.nəs/ tupost, netečnost, hloupost

endometriosis /ˌen.dəʊˌmiː.triˈəʊ.sɪs/ endometrióza, ložiska tkáně podobná děložní sliznici na neobvyklých místech

engage /ɪnˈgeɪdʒ/ obsadit, zaměstnávat, zapadat, zajistit

epiglottitis /ˌep.ɪ.gləˈtaɪ.tɪs/ epiglotitida, zánět příklopky hrtanové

essential /ɪˈsen.tʃəl/ základní, důležitý, hlavní

explosive /ɪkˈspləʊ.sɪv/ **delivery** /dɪˈlɪv.ər.i/ překotný porod

expulsion /ɪkˈspʌl.ʃən/ expulze, vypuzení z těla, vykašlávání, vypuzení

extravasation /eksˌtræ.vəˈseɪ.ʃən/ extravazát, výron, únik tekutiny do okolní tkáně

facilitate /fəˈsɪl.ɪ.teɪt/ usnadnit, ulehčit

fear /fɪə/ strach, obava, úzkost

flaccid /ˈflæksɪd/ ochablý, povadlý

fontanelle /ˌfɒn.təˈnel/ fontanela, neosifikované místo v lebce novorozeněte

gallon /ˈgæl.ən/ galon, v Británii 4,546 l, v USA 3,785 l

gaseous /ˈgeɪ.si.əs/ plynný

gently /ˈdʒent.li/ jemně, mírně

grunt /grʌnt/ chrčet, chrochtat

heal /hiːl/ hojit, léčit, vyléčit se, zahojit

ice /aɪs/ **pack** /pæk/ sáček s ledem, ledový obklad

imminent /ˈɪm.ɪ.nənt/ bezprostřední, hrozící, blízký, nadcházející

impending /ɪmˈpen.dɪŋ/ blížící se, bezprostředně hrozící, nastávající

improper /ɪmˈprɒp.ər/ nesprávný, nestandardní, nezákonný

improve /ɪmˈpruːv/ zlepšit, zotavit se, uzdravit se

inability /ˌɪn.əˈbɪl.ɪ.ti/ neschopnost, nemožnost, nezpůsobilost

incident /ˈɪnt.sɪ.dənt/ incident, mimořádná událost, případ

indicate /ˈɪn.dɪ.keɪt/ indikovat, označit, ukazovat

infusion /ɪnˈfjuː.ʒən/ infuze, nalévání, nálev

inhibit /ɪnˈhɪb.ɪt/ zabránit, tlumit, zpomalovat, znemožnit

insuffiency /ˌɪn.səˈfɪʃ.ənt.si/ nedostatečnost

intraosseous /ˌɪn.trəˈɒs.i.əs/ intraoseální, nitrokostní

intubate /ɪnˈtjuː.beɪt/ intubovat, zavést rourku do průdušnice

likelihood /ˈlaɪ.kli.hʊd/ pravděpodobnost

measure /ˈmeʒ.ər/ měřit, opatření

meconium /mɪˈkəʊ.nɪ.əm/ mekonium, smolka, první stolice novorozeněte

mentation /menˈteɪ.ʃən/ duševní pochody

motionless /ˈməʊ.ʃən.ləs/ nehybný, bez hnutí

nuchal /nuː.kəl/ šíjový

osteomyelitis /ˌɒs.ti.əʊ.maɪ.əlˈaɪ.tɪs/ osteomyelitida, zánět kosti a kostní dřeně

overhydration /ˌəʊvə.haɪˈdreɪ.ʃən/ nadměrná hydratace, zavodnění

pain /peɪn/ bolest, bolet, trápit

pelvic /ˈpel.vɪk/ **inflammatory** / ɪnˈflæm.ə.tər.i/ **disease** /dɪˈziːz/ zánětlivé onemocnění pánve

potential /pəˈten.ʃəl/ potenciál, možnost, schopnost, potenciální schopnost, možnost že se něco stane

prerespiratory /ˌpriːˈres.pər.əˌtor.i/ předrespirační

presentation /ˌprez.ənˈteɪ.ʃən/ vzhled, projevení představení, prezentace

regarding /rɪˈgaː.dɪŋ/ ohledně, pokud jde o

relaxation /ˌriː.lækˈseɪ.ʃən/ relaxace, odpočinek, zmírnění

remove /rɪˈmuːv/ odstranit, vyjmout

residence /ˈrez.ɪ.dəns/ rezidence, obydlí

retraction /rɪˈtræk.ʃən/ retrakce, stažení, odtažení, zatažení

rotation /rəʊ ˈteɪ.ʃən/ rotace, otáčení, obíhání

seize /siːz/ chytit, ovládnout, mít záchvat

seizure / ˈsiː.ʒə/ křečový stav, záchvat (nemoci), záchvatový

sentence /ˈsen.təns/ věta

shake /ʃeɪk/ (shook, shaken) třást, otřást, chvět

shaken /ˈʃeɪkən/ **baby** /ˈbeɪ.bi/ **syndrome** /ˈsɪn.drəʊm/ syndrom třeseného dítěte, zdravotní poškození malého dítěte nešetrným třesením a cloumáním (zejména hlavičky a krku)

sphincter /ˈsfɪŋk.tər/ svěrač

stage /steɪdʒ/ stádium, etapa

stethoscope /'steθ.ə.skəʊp/
stetoskop, přístroj zesilující zvuky
v tělních dutinách
subglottic /sʌb'glɒt.ɪk/ subglotický,
pod hlasivkami
suddenly /'sʌd.ən.li/ náhle,
najednou
thereby /ˌðeə'baɪ/ tímto, a tím
tight /taɪt/ těsný, pevný
torn /tɔːn/ roztržený, roztrhaný
tracheal / trə'kiː.əl/ tracheální,
průdušnicový
tug /tʌg/ trhnutí, cuknutí

umbilical cord /ʌm'bɪl.ɪ.kəlˌkɔːd/
pupeční šňůra
uncomfortable /ʌn'kʌmp f.tə.b|/
nesvůj, necítící se dobře
unsure /ʌn'ʃɔːr/ nejistý, nesmělý
ventricular /ven'trɪk.jə.lər/
fibrillation /ˌfaɪ.brɪ'leɪ.ʃən/, /ˌfɪb.
rɪ'leɪ.ʃən/ fibrilace srdečních
komor
violent /'vaɪələnt/ agresivní,
prudký, silný, násilný
wrap /ræp/ zabalit, obal

Unit 3

1

Defibrillation in an infant or child is _____ every 2 minutes as indicated.*

After five cycles of CPR (2 minutes), _____ the rhythm and pulse and defibrillate again if a _____ rhythm is present.

shockable, reassess, repeated

2

You have just delivered a ____-____ baby in your ambulance. The initial APGAR score is 5.

Treatment should consist of effective ventilation.*

Most newborn infants respond quite favourably to _____, drying, suctioning, and _____. Occasionally, administration of oxygen with assisted ventilations may be necessary. Vascular access and ___ are utilized only after the infant fails to _____ effectively to ventilatory assistance.

stimulation, full-term, warming, respond, CPR

3

Which of the following clinical _____ is MOST consistent with _____ ingestion in a child?

- diaphoresis, miosis, tachycardia, and bronchospasm
- hypertension, tachycardia, diaphoresis, and mydriasis.*
- miosis, bradycardia, hypoventilation, and hypotension
- mydriasis, diarrhoea, hypothermia, and hallucinations

Hypertension, tachycardia, diaphoresis, and _____ (dilated pupils) are consistent with cocaine or _____ use.

presentations, amphetamine, mydriasis, cocaine

4

Which of the following assessment finding would indicate that a paediatric patient is progressing from respiratory distress to respiratory failure?

- nasal flaring
- _____ rate over 32
- poor muscle tone*
- grunting/head bobbing

Nasal _____, elevated respiratory rate, and grunting and head bobbing all indicate respiratory distress. The development of poor _____ ____ indicates the patient is tiring and is an _____ sign of respiratory failure.

respiratory, muscle tone, flaring, ominous

5

While enjoying an off day from work, you hear your neighbour screaming. You rush outside to see her _____ her 4-year-old child from the swimming pool. The child is limp, blue, and ___ _____ to any stimulus. What should you do? Send the mother to call 112, open an airway, and initiate _____ _____.*
The ____ rescuer should initially provide rescue breathing to the child while someone is sent to call 112.

pulling, lone, rescue breathing, not responsive

6

Identify the anatomical differences in the paediatric airway compared to the _____ _____. The airway diameter is smaller, the larynx is more anterior, and the tongue is proportionally larger.*
The airway _____ in children is smaller than an adult airway. The larynx is more _____, making visualization difficult. The _____ is proportionally larger to the jaw.

anterior, tongue, diameter, adult airway

7

Beta blocker ingestion in small children would ____ likely cause:
- acute hypoglycaemia*
- agitation or irritability
- marked hypertension
- ventricular fibrillation

Ingestion of beta blockers, ethanol or other _____, _____, or oral hypoglycaemic agent can lead to hypoglycaemia.

insulin, MOST, alcohols

8

It is important to compare central and _____ pulses in the paediatric patient to determine:
- the presence of shock*
- skin colour
- mental status
- airway patency

The presence or absence of shock may be indicated by a difference between the _____ and peripheral pulses. Pulse _____ or deficit may be a sign of poor peripheral _____.

perfusion, central, peripheral, differences

9

A child wearing a helmet strikes a large rock with his bicycle and flies over the _____. The patient would MOST likely suffer:
- associated head injury

- stretching or tearing injuries to the kidneys
- open or closed fractures to the lower extremities
- compression injuries to the intraabdominal organs*

Injury from bicycle handlebars typically includes _____ injuries to the intraabdominal organs and _____ injuries. Upper _____ injuries are also common.

> pancreatic, extremity, compression, handlebars

10
You have administered lidocaine to an 8-year-old. _____, decreased mental status, muscle twitching, and seizures are side effects that may result from its administration.*
Lidocaine has central nervous system properties that cause drowsiness, decreased _____ _____, muscle _____, and the possibility of _____.

> Drowsiness, seizures, twitching, mental status

11
Of the following _____ below, which is most likely to _____ ____ shaken baby syndrome?
- hypoglycaemia

- abdominal bruising
- subdural haematoma*
- lower-extremity fracture
___ _____ (including the possibility of a subdural haematoma) is a _____ _____ in shaken baby syndrome.

> common finding, Head injury, choices, result from

12
Your squad is dispatched to the scene of a 6-year-old child with an elevated temperature. The mother tells you that the child was fine last night and got up this morning complaining of a sore throat and trouble swallowing.
The initial assessment reveals a sick-looking child who is leaning forward in the _____ _____. He is obviously drooling. From this information you suspect:
- bronchiolitis
- croup
- epiglottitis*
- meningitis

_____ is a bacterial infection causing acute _____ of the epiglottis and the soft tissues above the glottic opening. Clinical findings include but are not limited to sudden onset of high fever 102-104 °F (38-40 °C), pain on _____, typically sitting in tripod position, and _____.

Epiglottitis, swallowing, drooling, tripod position, swelling

13

During transport of a child with epiglottitis, he becomes _____ and apnoeic. You are still able to _____ a weak pulse at a rate of 64 per minute. Your immediate action should be to position the child's head and provide bag-valve mask ventilation with 100% oxygen.* Any external _____ of the epiglottis (i.e. intubation or OPA _____) can cause complete airway obstruction in the child with epiglottitis. Carefully _____ the child's head and provide positive pressure ventilation with 100% oxygen.

palpate, unresponsive, manipulation, position, insertion

14

Your patient is an ill-appearing 4-month-old lying in his mother's arms. The mother tells you that the infant won't take a bottle and cries whenever she moves. Your exam reveals a lethargic infant, warm to touch, with fine pinpoint _____ on the abdomen, chest, and face. The infant's _____ appears to be bulging.

The information gained on exam should lead you to suspect meningitis.*
Recognize the syndrome of fever and petechia as a medical emergency. Inflammation of the _____ will cause the fontanelle __ _____ and appear full. _____ should be suspected in this patient.

to bulge, petechia, meninges, fontanelle, Meningitis

15

This statement correctly relates to paediatric seizures: febrile seizures correlate to the speed in which the temperature rises, not to the _____ of the fever. How fast the _____ of the child rises will increase a child's risk for developing a _____.

seizure, degree, temperature

16

The next two questions are based on the following scenario:
You are dispatched to a local department store when a concerned customer notices an infant left unattended in a car. It is bitterly cold outside. Once you gain entry into the car, you find the infant to be dusky in colour with no activity or _____. The respiratory rate is

12 per minute and irregular with _____ and short sighs.
The heart rate is 64 per minute with weak central pulses. The infant's hands are cold to touch. Capillary refill is 5 seconds. Your immediate action should be to ventilate with a bag-valve mask device and 100% oxygen.* Recognize that the infant has inadequate oxygenation (_____ colour) and immediately begin bag-valve mask ventilation with 100% oxygen.

After obtaining _____ _____ and delivering the pharmacological intervention, the patient's heart rate increases to 130 per minute with strong central pulses but no peripheral pulses.
To further stabilize the infant, the next course of action should be to begin rewarming the patient.* Considering the _____ temperature to be very cold, hypothermia is a significant cause of the patient's presentation.
Begin _____ the patient.

> movement, ambient, rewarming, venous access, dusky, grunting

17
A 7-year-old child has been _____ by a car and is lying _____ on the street. He has _____ head trauma.

Identify the signs of Cushing's triad: increased BP, bradycardia, and abnormal respirations.*
_____ _____ (sometimes referred to as Cushing's reflex or response) characteristically presents with an _____ blood pressure, bradycardia, and abnormal (usually ____) respirations.

> elevated, slow, struck, motionless, obvious, Cushing's triad

18
Seizure-like activity triggered by stimuli other than cerebral electrical discharges, such as major mood disorders or severe environmental stress, is defined as:
- partial seizure
- partial complex seizure
- generalized seizure
- pseudoseizure*

_____ _____ (neurogenic) is a distributive shock, producing hypotension relative to an increase in the vascular space in the absence of a loss of body fluids.
A _____ ____ injury results in a lack of communication between the _____ and the ____ so there is no response to catecholamine release, resulting in bradycardia and hypotension.

spinal cord, Spinal shock, brain, body

19
To ensure that an infant's head is in a neutral position during _____ _____, you should:
- provide slight flexion of the head
- place padding under the infant's shoulders*
- _____ a towel roll behind the infant's neck
- use _____ rolls for lateral head stabilization

An infant has a large head in comparison to the rest of the body. To maintain the infant's head in a neutral position, place padding under the infant's _____.

shoulders, spinal immobilization, place, towel

20
You respond to a MVC involving a young child. The child is found apnoeic but still has a _____ pulse. You immediately begin positive-pressure ventilation with a bag-valve mask device. You note that the left side of the chest moves but the right does not. _____ _____ are absent on the right side, and the _____ is deviated to the left.

Your immediate action is to perform a needle decompression on the right side.*
The signs and symptoms are consistent with a _____ _____ (absent breath sounds, tracheal _____, little or no chest movement on the affected side). Immediate needle decompression is warranted.

tension pneumothorax, trachea, palpable, Lung sounds, deviation

21
Your patient is a 5-year-old girl who presents with breathing difficulty of rapid _____. She is sitting upright and _____. Her temperature is 104.6 °F (40.3 °C). What should you suspect? Epiglotitis.*
What does the appropriate management of a child with _____ consist of? Airway maintenance and administration of humidified oxygen.*
Management of epiglottitis consists of airway _____, oxygen, and prompt transport.

drooling, maintenance, epiglottitis, onset

Vocabulary 3

agitation /ˌædʒ.ɪˈteɪ.ʃən/ nervozita, rozrušení, vzrušení, znepokojení

ambient /ˈæm.bi.ənt/ okolní, prostředí se týkající

bitterly /ˈbɪt.ə.li/ prudce, ostře

bob /bɒb/ pohodit hlavou, pohupovat se, poskakovat

catecholamine /kat.ə.kəl.am.in/ katecholamin, nejběžnější jsou epinefrin (adrenaline), norepinefrin (noradrenalin) a dopamin

compare /kəmˈpeər/ porovnat, srovnat

comparison /kəmˈpærɪsən/ srovnání, porovnání

complex /kɒm.pleks/ složitý

correlate /ˈkɒrɪˌleɪt/ souviset, být ve vzájemném vztahu

deviate /ˈdiː.vi.eɪt/ odchýlit se

discharge /dɪsˈtʃɑːdʒ/ výtok, odtok, sekret, výměšek,

dispatch /dɪˈspætʃ/ vyslat, poslat, odeslat, odeslání

drool /druːl/ slintat, sliny tekoucí z úst

drowsiness /ˈdraʊ.zɪ.nəs/ ospalost, mátožnost

dusky /ˈdʌs.ki/ tmavý, tlumený o barvě

favourably /ˈfeɪ.vər.ə.bli/ příznivě

fly /flaɪ/ (flew, flown) letět

full-term (infant) /fʊlˈtɜːm/ plně donošené dítě, kojenec narozený mezi 38. a 41. týdnem

generalized /ˈdʒen.ə r.ə.laɪzd/ všeobecný

handlebar /ˌhæn.dl̩.bɑː/ řídítka jízdního kola

humidified /hjuːˈmɪd.ɪ.faɪd/ zvlhčený

identify /aɪˈden.tɪ.faɪ/ identifikovat, určit, rozeznat, rozpoznat, ztotožňovat se

ingestion /ɪnˈdʒes.tʃən/ přijímání potravy, trávení

intraabdominal /ɪn.trə.æbˈdɒm.ɪ.nəl/ intraabdominální, nitrobřišní

irritability /ˌɪr.ɪ.təˈbɪl.ɪ.ti/ iritabilita, dráždivost, podráždění, podrážděnost

kidney ˈkɪd.ni/ ledvina

lean /liːn/ **forward** /ˈfɔː.wəd/ naklonit se dopředu

limp /lɪmp/ ochablý, skleslý

lone /ləʊn/ osamocený, samotný

maintenance /ˈmeɪntɪnəns/ údržba, péče, zachování, udržování

miosis /maɪˈəʊ.sɪs/ mióza, abnormální kontrakce zornice

mood /muːd/ **disorder** /dɪˈsɔː.dər/ porucha nálady, nejčastější je deprese a bipolární porucha

muscle /ˈmʌsəl/ **tone** /təʊn/ tonus svalové napětí

mydriasis /maɪˈdraɪ.ə.sɪs/ mydriáza, rozšíření zornice

occasionally /əˈkeɪ.ʒən.əl.ɪ/ příležitostně, občas

ominous /ˈɒmɪnəs/ zlověstný, hrozivý

onset /ˈɒnˌset/ propuknutí, začátek

padding /ˈpæd.ɪŋ/ vycpávka, vatování

pancreatic /ˌpæŋ.krɪˈæ.tɪk/ pankreatický, týkající se slinivky břišní

partial /ˈpɑː.ʃəl/ částečný, dílčí

patency /ˈpeɪ.tənt .si/ průchodnost

perfuse /pəˈfjuːz/ perfundovat, promývat

petechia /piˈtiː.ki.ə/ pl **petechiae** petechie, tečkovité krvácení z kapilár

pin-point, **pinpoint** / ˈpɪn.pɔɪnt/ velmi přesný, špička špendlíku

prompt /prɒmp t/ promptní, okamžitý

property /ˈprɒp.ə.ti/ vlastnost

proportionally /prəˈpɔː.ʃən.əli/ úměrně, přiměřeně

pseudoseizure /ˈsjuː.dəʊ.ˈsiː.ʒər/ falešný, nepravý záchvat

pull /pʊl/ táhnout, zatahat

reassess /ˌriː.əˈses/ přehodnotit, znovu posoudit

responsive /rɪˈspɒnt.sɪv/ vnímavý, reagující, citlivý na co

result /rɪˈzʌlt/ výsledek, mít za následek

rewarm /ˌriːˌwɔːm/ znovu zahřát

rock /rɒk/ kámen, skála

roll /rəʊl/ stočit, svinout, rulička

rush /rʌʃ/ spěchat, udělat ve spěchu, příval, nával

sick-looking /sɪkˈlʊk.ɪŋ/ vypadající jako nemocný

sigh /saɪ/ povzdech, vzdechnutí, zavzdychat

slight /slaɪt/ nepatrný, mírný, drobný

sore /sɔː/ **throat** /θrəʊt/ bolest v krku

spinal /ˈspaɪ.nəl/ **cord** /kɔːd/ mícha

squad /skwɒd/ oddíl, tým

stretch /stretʃ/ protáhnout, protažení

swallow /ˈswɒl.əʊ/ polykat, spolknout, hlt

tiring /ˈtaɪə.rɪŋ/ vyčerpávající

towel /taʊəl/ ručník

trigger /ˈtrɪg.ər/ spustit, vyvolat, vzbudit, spoušť zbraně

tripod /ˈtraɪ.pɒd/ trojnožka

twitch /twɪtʃ/ škubat, trhat, záškuby částí svalů

unattended /ˌʌn.əˈten.dɪd/ bez dozoru, nehlídaný

warrant /ˈwɒr.ənt/ oprávnit, opravňovat, vyžádat si, zasluhovat

Unit 4

1

Your assessment of an unresponsive 7-year-old child reveals that he is _____ and _____. After performing a 2-minute period of ___, you assess his cardiac rhythm, which reveals _____ _____.
You should defibrillate and immediately resume CPR.*

> ventricular fibrillation, CPR, apnoeic, pulseless

2

A small child has fallen through the ice while skating. After 30 minutes, the child is pulled from the icy water, apnoeic and pulseless.
Your first action in the management of this child should be to secure the child's airway and control the cervical spine.* Since it is unknown if there are any C-spine injuries from the ____ through the ice, you must _____ ___ _____ and control the cervical spine during _____.

> secure the airway, fall, resuscitation

3

You have intubated a 6-week-old infant found in respiratory arrest.

While performing ventilation, the child becomes blue, and the pulse rate drops into the lower 50s. Your next step should be to auscultate the chest.* _____ of the chest for proper endotracheal tube _____ is necessary. If lung sounds are diminished or absent, it may be necessary to _____, ventilate, _____, and then reintubate.

> extubate, placement, reassess, Auscultation

4

A child has suffered multisystem trauma, and IV access cannot be obtained. You determine the best _____ of action would be establish an IO.
A _____ for intraosseous insertion is _ _____ of the lower extremity.*

> a fracture, course, contraindication

5

An injury to which abdominal organ is most likely to cause death in the paediatric patient?
- pancreas
- liver*
- spleen
- kidney

The liver is a _____, vascular organ in the right upper quadrant.

_____ or _____ of the liver can cause severe _____. Injury to the liver is the most common abdominal injury that leads to death in paediatrics.

> haemorrhage, solid, laceration, Rupture

6

You have performed a _____ _____ _____ on a child and are prepared to transport. In which situation is it appropriate to perform the detailed exam en route to the hospital?

- fracture of the humerus
- amputated thumb
- mottled skin with tachycardia*
- fractured tibia with numbness in the foot

A sign of poor perfusion includes _____ ____ and tachycardia. This is indicative of _____, and a detailed exam should be performed en route to the hospital. Other indicators of shock include weak peripheral pulses and prolonged _____ _____ time.

> shock, capillary refill, mottled skin, Rapid Trauma Survey

7

You are treating a child with a tension pneumothorax. Needle decompression is needed.

The correct site for insertion of needle is the top of the third rib in the midclavicular line.* _____ the needle over (on top of) the second or third rib avoids _____ puncturing or laceration of the adjoining _____ and _____ located at the inferior border of the ribs.

> Inserting, inadvertent, nerves, vessels

8

Concerning paediatric airway management, this statement is true: bradycardia can result from suctioning a child.* _____ may result in bradycardia from stimulation of the _____ _____, particularly in children less than 6 months old. Do not use _____ suction attempts.

> Suctioning, prolonged, vagus nerve

9

Which of the following is most likely to cause shock in a child?

- laceration to the face
- a fractured radius
- cerebral oedema
- a splenic injury*

The _____ is a blood-filled organ located in the left upper quadrant. _____ _____ can cause injury to the spleen, resulting in _____

____ and shock. The spleen is the most injured organ resulting in shock, while the ____ is the most injured organ resulting in death of a paediatric patient.

> Blunt trauma, spleen, liver, blood loss

10

Which action is most important when _____ an unresponsive child?

- performing chest compression
- checking for a pulse
- administering supplemental oxygen
- manually opening the airway*

Establishing a _____ _____ is the most important treatment ____ in providing care for an _____ patient.

> unresponsive, patent airway, treating, step

11

You respond to the local high school football practice field for a sports injury. The coach tells you that the patient made a tackle and, after the play, did not ___ __. Your patient is _____ on the ground with all of his equipment on. He is _____ but slow to answer questions.

You should remove the football _____ if you do not have an easy access to the airway.*
Unless special circumstances exist such as respiratory distress or airway _____, the helmet should not be _____ by EMS.

> get up, awake, compromise, supine, helmet, removed

12

Cuffed endotracheal tubes are usually not _____ in children under the age of 8.*
In a child less than 8, the normal anatomic _____ at the level of the _____ _____ provides a functional cuff and eliminates the need for a cuffed tracheal tube under most _____.

> narrowing, circumstances, cricoid cartilage, indicated

13

Suctioning of the infant's mouth and nose should be performed after:

- ___ ____ is clamped and cut
- the infant _____ to cry
- the chest ___ ____ _____
- the head has been delivered*

> begins, the cord, has been delivered

14

You are assessing a newborn infant who presents with respiratory distress. Physical _____ reveal that the patient has a low birth weight, a small head, and small eye openings. Besides the obvious respiratory distress, you might suspect the infant to be suffering from:

- a heroin _____
- crack cocaine ingestion
- foetal alcohol syndrome*
- apnoea of _____

Characteristics of a newborn with foetal _____ _____ include low birth weight, a small head, and small eye openings.

alcohol syndrome, overdose, infancy, findings

15

You are assessing an 18-month-old male who presents with obvious _____ _____. Inspiratory stridor is heard with evident use of all _____ _____. The trouble breathing is worse at night. No other significant findings are visible. The child is not on medications and has otherwise been well. You suspect:

- epiglottitis
- asthma
- bronchiolitis
- croup*

_____ _____, absence of drooling, trouble swallowing, and symptoms persistently worse at night leads to the conclusion of ___ _____.

the croup, Inspiratory stridor, breathing difficulty, accessory muscles

16

External signs that may indicate an intraabdominal injury in a paediatric patient may include:

- pale skin, abdominal contusion, seat belt abrasions across the abdomen*
- dilated pupils, bradycardia, poor peripheral pulses
- tracheal deviation, JVD

____ ____, abdominal contusion, ____ ____ abrasions, or unexplained _____ may suggest the possibility of intraabdominal injury with a probability of abdominal _____.

haemorrhage, seat belt, Pale skin, shock

17

From the following list, identify an example of distributive shock:

- hypovolaemic shock
- anaphylactic shock*
- cardiogenic shock
- psychogenic shock

_____ _____ is a shock state that exists when there is no loss of ____ _____ but the fluid distribution is altered from an increase in the vascular space or leaking of fluid from the _____ _____. This results in an _____ of fluid relative to the vascular space. Types of distributive shock include anaphylactic, septic, and neurogenic.

vascular space, insufficiency, body fluid, Distributive shock

18
You are _____ ___ a child with respiratory distress. You note a _____, high-pitched sound with each breath. You suspect this is indicative of:
- stridor*
- wheezing
- crackles
- rhonchi

_____ is a harsh, high- or low-pitched sound caused by breathing through a partially blocked airway; wheezing is a high- or low-pitched _____ sound. Crackles/rhonchi represent _____ in the larger bronchial airways.

Stridor, fluid, whistling, caring for, harsh

19
A priority in evaluating a 2-year-old with diarrhoea and vomiting includes determining:
- temperature _____
- a viral infection
- a respiratory _____
- adequate hydration*

Of the choices listed, evaluating the patient for adequate hydration is the ___ _____. Evaluating the patient's _____ and the presence of infection are necessary, but secondary to determining adequate hydration.

top priority, temperature, elevation, infection

20
You have initiated an IO line in a paediatric patient suffering from severe _____. What is the most reliable indicator of the successful placement of the IO needle?
- take an X-ray
- the ability to draw arterial blood through the IO
- aspiration of bone marrow*
- no evidence of fractures after insertion

One of the ways to determine _____ _____ of the IO needle is by aspiration of the ____ _____. Additionally, an unobstructed infusion of fluid without evidence of infiltration can also be used. _-____ are not needed to confirm placement. You should not be able to aspirate _____ _____ from a properly placed IO needle.

arterial blood, bone marrow, successful placement, X-rays, dehydration

21
Answer the next five questions on the basis of the following information.
You arrive to find a 6-year-old on the floor of his classroom, unconscious, incontinent, and responsive to pain only.
The school nurse states that the child shook _____ for approximately 2 minutes and has been _____ ever since. She knows that he takes phenobarbital because she gave him one at lunch, but she is unable to provide further medical history.
This child most likely suffers from seizure disorder.*
The clinical presentation is one of seizures that could occur for a variety of _____, including diabetes. However, the use of the drug phenobarbital is commonly associated with _____ _____.
Phenobarbital is an example of a sedative or anticonvulsant.*

If this child is on medication, why did he have this episode at school? Medications only limit the number of seizures a person has; they do not always eliminate the seizures.*
Anticonvulsants serve to limit the number of seizures a patient has, but they do not stop them from occurring altogether.
Treatment for this patient should include oxygen and monitoring.*
This patient should be transported to a hospital because medication levels need to be determined by laboratory analysis.*
This patient needs to be _____ to a hospital because medication levels should be assessed by laboratory methods. Seizures may or may not continue to occur.

reasons, transported, unconscious, seizure disorders, violently

Vocabulary 4
abrasion /əˈbreɪ.ʒən/ odřenina, oděrka
adjoining /əˈdʒɔɪ.nɪŋ/ sousední, vedlejší
alter /ˈɒl.tər/ změnit
amputate /ˈæm.pju.teɪt/ amputovat
anticonvulsant /ˌæn.tɪ.kən.ˈvʌl.sənt/ antikonvulzivní, protikřečový
aspirate /ˈæs.pɪ.rət/ aspirovat, vdechnout, odsát, odsávat
blood /blʌd/ **loss** /lɒs/ krevní ztráta

175

bone /bəʊn/ **marrow** /ˈmær.əʊ/ kostní dřeň

border /bɔː.dər/ okraj, hranice

cardiogenic /ˈkɑː.di.ə.ˈdʒen.ɪk/ **shock** /ʃɒk/ kardiogenní šok, způsobený těžkou poruchou srdeční funkce, komplikace rozsáhlého či opakovaného infarktu myokardu

coach /kəʊtʃ/ vést, učit, trenér

compromise /ˈkɒmprə͵maɪz/ oslabit, ohrozit, vydat v nebezpečí, zhoršit, kompromis

conclusion /kənˈkluː.ʒən/ závěr, úsudek

crack /kræk/ čistý kokain (hovor. název)

cricoid /ˈkraɪ.kɔɪd/ **cartilage** /ˈkɑː.təl.ɪdʒ/ chrupavka prstencová, nejspodnější chrupavka hltanová

croup /kruːp/ difterický krup, dětský zánět hrtanu, štěkavý kašel, hrtanová křeč

cuff /kʌf/ manžeta, záložka

distributive /dɪˈstrɪbjʊtɪv/ distributivní, rozdělený

draw /drɔː/ pohybovat se, táhnout, natáhnout, načerpat

equipment /ɪˈkwɪp.mənt/ vybavení, zařízení, výstroj

foetal /ˈfiː.təl/ fetální, plodový

get up /get.ʌp/ vstát, být vzhůru

harsh /hɑːʃ/ drsný, výrazný

helmet /ˈhel.mət/ helma

humerus pl -ri /ˈhjuː.mə.rəs/ humerus, kost pažní

hydration /haɪˈdreɪ.ʃən/ hydratace, zavodnění

inadvertent /͵ɪn.ədˈvɜː.tənt/ neúmyslný, nepozorný, nedbalý

incontinent /ɪnˈkɒn.tɪ.nənt/ inkontinentní, neschopný udržet moč, stolici

indicator /ˈɪn.dɪ.keɪ.tər/ indikátor, ukazatel

infancy /ˈɪn.fənt.si/ dětství (útlé)

inferior /ɪnˈfɪə.ri.ər/ dolní

infiltration /͵ɪn.fɪlˈtreɪ.ʃən/ infiltrace, prosakování, prostoupení orgánů zánětlivými či nádorovými buňkami či jinými látkami

laceration /͵læsəˈreɪʃən/ lacerace, tržná rána

leaking /liː.k.ɪŋ/ výtok, vytékání

list /lɪst/ seznam, soupis

liver /ˈlɪv.ər/ játra

mottled /ˈmɒt.|d/ skvrnitý, flekatý, žilkovaný

narrow /ˈnær.əʊ/ úzký, těsný, omezený, zúžit

numbness /ˈnʌm.nəs/ necitlivost, znecitlivění, ochromení, pocit necitlivosti

nurse /nɜːs/ zdravotní sestra, ošetřovat

obvious /ˈɒb.vi.əs/ zjevný, jasný, samozřejmý, nápadný

overdose /ˈəʊ.və.dəʊs/ nadměrná dávka, předávkování

pancreas /ˈpæŋ.kri.əs/ pankreas, slinivka břišní

partially /ˈpɑː.ʃəl.i/ částečně, zčásti

patent /ˈpeɪ.tənt/ průchodný

pitch /pɪtʃ/ výška, poloha (tónu)

priority /praɪˈɒr.ɪ.ti/ priorita, přednost

psychogenic /ˌsaɪ.kəʊˈdʒɛ.nɪk/ psychogenní, mentálního původu
puncture /ˈpʌŋk.tʃər/ punkce, vpich, otvor propíchnutí, propíchnout
radius /ˈreɪ.di.əs/ vřetenní kost
responsive /rɪˈspɒnt.sɪv/ vnímavý, reagující, citlivý na co
resume /rɪˈzjuːm/ pokračovat, zvovu začít
seat /siːt/ **belt** /belt/ bezpečnostní pás
sedative /ˈsed.ə.tɪv/ sedativum, utišující lék
seizure / ˈsiː.ʒər/ **disorder** /dɪˌsɔː. dər/ epilepsie
skate /ˈskeɪ.t/ bruslit
space /speɪs/ prostor, mezera, vzdálenost
spleen /spliːn/ slezina
splenic /spliːn.ɪk/ splenický, slezinný
survey /ˈsɜː.veɪ/ průzkum, přehled, vyšetření, prohlídka, posoudit

tackle /ˈtæk.l/ zákrok, napadat hráče, obrat o míč
thumb /θʌm/ palec na ruce
tibia /ˈtɪb.i.ə/ pl -ae holeň, kost holenní
vagus /veɪ.gəs/ pl -gi bloudivý nerv, X. hlavový nerv
weight /weɪt/ váha, hmotnost
whistle /ˈwɪs.l/ pískat, hvízdat, pískání
X-ray /ˈeks.reɪ/ rentgen, vyšetřit rentgenem

Unit 5

I

You are performing _____ _____ with a bag-mask device for an _____ child.
- How often should you _____ rescue breaths? Once every 6 seconds.*

> provide, apnoeic, rescue breathing

2

A small child has been struck by a car travelling approximately 25 ___. The child is unresponsive. The airway manoeuvre of choice for this patient is:
- jaw thrust with C-spine stabilization*
- head tilt/chin lift
- _____ with jaw thrust
- hyperflexion of the head to the _____ position

With the probability of significant trauma and C-spine injury, the child's airway should be assessed using a ___-_____ manoeuvre while stabilizing the _____ _____. Head tilt/chin lift, hyperextension, and hyperflexion cause manipulation of the cervical spine and are not indicated when cervical spine injury is suspected.

> jaw-thrust, cervical spine, sniffing, MPH, hyperextension

3

Which of the following findings or factors would make you ___ ___ immediate transport of a pregnant woman rather than _____ delivery in the field?

a) the mother's urge to push
b) the presence of crowning
c) meconium-stained amniotic fluid*
d) multiparity with explosive births

Because meconium staining in the amniotic fluid can indicate _____ _____, it may mean that the best thing to do is to transport the mother immediately. Choices a, b, and d suggest that birth is imminent and transport is ___ _____. If you must deliver the infant when _____ staining is present, you should be prepared to provide immediate _____ of the trachea and to _____ the child prior to stimulation, drying, warming, or positioning.

> not advisable, meconium, foetal distress, intubate, attempt, suctioning, opt for

4

During delivery you notice that the _____ _____ is discoloured and has a foul odour.
What should you do first?
Suction the upper airway using a meconium aspirator.*

Suction the newborn before stimulating it so it can _____. Endotracheal suctioning may be _____ if meconium is noted in the _____ _____.

> breathe, amniotic fluid, upper airway, warranted

5
How should you _____ bleeding after the normal _____ of an infant? Perform fundal massage.* Massaging the top of the uterus _____ it to contract and _____ control of normal postpartum bleeding.

> promotes, control, stimulates, delivery

6
In the prehospital management of a very ill neonate, interventions should be reassessed at 30-second intervals.* Interventions during a neonatal _____ should be assessed often so that _____ are noted as soon as they _____.

> changes, occur, resuscitation

7
You must perform chest compressions on a newborn infant if, after oxygenation and ventilation, the heart rate persists in being less than 80/min.*

The threshold for _____ in a newborn infant is 80 beats per minute, and the range where you would consider the ____ ___ compressions along with other _____ is between 60 and 80 bpm.
Any infant with a heart rate less than 60 bpm should immediately receive _____, but if the rate remains between 60 and 80 and is not rapidly increasing despite positive-pressure _____ with 100% oxygen, you should perform chest compressions for 30 seconds, reassess, and repeat as needed.

> ventilation, bradycardia, treatments, need for, compressions

8
Which is the correct method to stimulate _____ in a neonate?
- Hold it by the feet while you slap the buttocks.
- Slap the soles of the feet and rub the back.*
- Let the cool air cause it to shiver a little.
- Rub the head but avoid touching the fontanelle.

Stimulate a neonate by slapping the soles of the feet and rubbing the back. The infant should not be allowed to lose any ____ ___, and you should avoid _____ the head to keep from putting any pressure on the _____.

> fontanelle, body heat, touching, respirations

9
How should you control bleeding after the normal delivery of an infant?
- Pack the vagina with _____ _____.
- Apply _____ pressure on the genitalia.
- _____ the pelvis.
- Perform fundal massage.*
Massaging the top of the _____ stimulates it to contract and promotes control of normal _____ bleeding.

> Elevate, direct, uterus, postpartum, sterile gauze

10
The minimum-size bag-valve mask device used for neonates, infants, and children should be 450 ml.*
Although it is likely that the ___-_____ ____ will not deliver 450 ml of volume, it is important to have a device _____ __ delivering excessive volumes because, as the bag __ _____, there is dead space from which air cannot be _____ expelled.

> is compressed, fully, bag-valve mask, capable of

11
An isotonic solution is one that has an electrolyte composition like that of blood plasma.*
_____ _____ such as Ringer's lactate or normal _____ have electrolyte compositions similar to that of _____ _____ although they lack the large protein molecules found within blood.

> blood plasma, Isotonic solutions, saline

12
One way to determine the size of the endotracheal tube to use in a child is to use the following equation: 16 plus the child's age divided by 4.
Another consideration is the size of the child's cricoid ring.*
__ _____ to the child's age, the size of the _____ ____ should be based on the size of the cricoid ring, which is ___ _____ part of a child's airway.

> the narrowest, endotracheal tube, In addition

13
Cardiac arrest in young children is most commonly associated with respiratory problems or diseases.*

Most _____ cardiac arrests are the result of _____ accidents that result in respiratory _____.

preventable, compromise, childhood

14

A late sign of _____ in children is called bradycardia.*
Bradycardia in a child is an _____ sign of a _____ brain.

hypoxic, ominous, hypoxia

15

Why is _____ of the paediatric patient with a bag-valve mask more difficult than ventilation of an adult? It is more difficult to create a ____ ____ in an infant.*
The bridge of the nose in a paediatric patient may make a mask seal more difficult to _____. Additionally, the mask size needed to fit in paediatric patient's face may not be available.

achieve, good seal, ventilation

16

Which of the following statements regarding _____ _____ in the paediatric patient is correct?

• The curved _____ is preferred in infants and children.
• The narrowest _____ of the airway in infants and children is just below the glottic opening.*
• Cuffed _____ tubes should be used in children under the age of 8.

Straight laryngoscope blades are preferred in children. Uncuffed tubes are needed in order to be firmly seated at the narrowing of the _____.

trachea, airway management, blade, diameter, endotracheal

17

An 18-month-old female presents with lethargy. The parent states that the patient began looking _____ a few hours ago and has become increasingly _____ to arouse. The patient had exhibited ____ feeding and vomited once prior to your arrival. She presents with ____, cool skin, a pulse rate of 200, and a respiratory rate of 40. She responds to _____ stimuli with a weak cry. The EKG shows a rapid narrow complex tachydysrhythmia.
What is the patient's primary problem? Dysrhythmia.*
The relatively _____ ____ of this condition and lack of dehydration

history points to a primary dysrhythmia as the _____ _____ of her presentation.

underlying cause, difficult, poor, pale, painful, irritable, sudden onset

18
Answer the next three questions on the basis of the following information.
You respond to the home of a 2-year-old girl who is experiencing _____ and difficult breathing. The child's mother states that she has had a cold for the past several days and a seal-like bark for the past 20 minutes. Physical exam reveals she has a fever of 102 °F (38.9 °C) and ___, ___ skin. Inspiratory _____ is heard upon auscultation of lung sounds. Vital signs are as follows: blood pressure, 100/70; pulse rate of 100; and respiratory rate of 40 that is laboured and with sternal retractions noted. This patient is most likely _____ _____ croup.*
This patient is exhibiting the classic signs and symptoms of croup.
What is the _____ treatment for this child? Saline given by nebulizer treatment and oxygen.*
A _____ saline mist is the appropriate treatment of croup.

Do not interfere with the airway in case there is any tissue swelling present.
A related disease or condition that can result in rapid and total airway obstruction is called epiglottitis.*
Epiglottitis, a condition whereby the patient's airway can become _____ obstructed, is related to croup.

stridor, suffering from, appropriate, laboured, nebulized, totally, hot, dry

19
Your patient is 2 years old. How can you reassure her before listening to her chest with your stethoscope? Gain her trust by letting her listen to your chest first.*
_____ can often be reassured by being allowed to handle _____ objects. They will not understand detailed _____ and should not be _____ to disassemble equipment.

Toddlers, allowed, explanations, unfamiliar

20
You respond to a 2-year-old female who is postictal following seizure activity. The patient's parents report that the child was sleeping when she began to shake and turn blue. She has had

a runny nose, but she has had no medications lately. There is no history of seizures.
This patient is most likely suffering from which condition? A febrile seizure.*
Fever-induced _____ are common in young children with only minor illnesses. Once a child has a febrile seizure, he or she is _____ _ repeat episodes, which can occur at _____ temperatures than the first seizure.
What vital signs would you expect this patient to have? Increased body temperature, tachycardia, and tachypnoea.*
_____ body temperature, tachycardia, and tachypnoea are common in a child who is recently postictal from febrile seizures.
What would be the appropriate treatment if this patient continues in a prolonged _____ state? Remove the child's excess clothing, administer oxygen and an IV, and transport.*
Oxygen, an IV, and transport is an appropriate treatment for this patient. Remove excess clothing from the patient to passively cool him or her, but do not allow the patient to get chilled. _____ the child with room-temperature water if the temperature is excessively high.
Never use _____ on the skin as a cooling agent. Alcohol can

be absorbed directly through the skin.

alcohol, prone to, Increased, postictal, lower, seizures, Sponge

21
Your patient is 10 months old. He has tachypnoea and wheezing and a fever of 100.6 °F (38.1 °C). What do you suspect is wrong with your patient? Bronchiolitis.*
_____ and tachypnoea in a child younger than age 1 is most often due to bronchiolitis brought on by the RSV virus. Asthma in children this young often presents as _____.
Epiglottitis will often have a fever _____ ____ 100.6 °F (38.1 °C), and the epiglottitis patient will be drooling as respiratory distress _____.
Croup will present with junky-sounding airways and the classic ____-_____ cough.

worsens, seal-barking, higher than, Wheezing, coughing

Vocabulary 5

absorb /əb'zɔːb/ absorbovat, vstřebat

achieve /ə'tʃiːv/ dosáhnout, docílit, uspět

advisable /əd'vaɪ.zə.bḷ/ vhodný, záhodný

amniotic fluid /ˌæm.ni.ɒt.ɪk'fluː.ɪd/ plodová voda

arouse /ə'raʊz/ vzbudit, probudit

aspirator /æs.pə.reɪ.tər/ aspirátor, přístroj na odsávání

bark /bɑːk/ štěkat

buttock /'bʌt.ək/ hýždě, zadek

chill /tʃɪl/ vychladit, zimnice

chin /tʃɪn/ brada

composition /ˌkɒm.pə'zɪʃ.ən/ skladba, složená

cooling /'kuː.lɪŋ/ ochlazování

cuff /kʌf/ manžeta, záložka

curved /kɜːvd/ zahnutý, zakřivený

disassemble /ˌdɪs.ə'sem.bḷ/ rozmontovat, rozložit

equation /ɪ'kweɪ.ʒən/ rovnice, srovnání

expel /ɪk'spel/ být vyloučen, vypudit, vyhnat

febrile /'fiː.braɪl/ febrilní, horečnatý

feeding /ˌfiː.dɪŋ/ krmení, výživa, stravování

firmly /'fɜːm.li/ pevně

fit /fɪt/ odpovídat, pasovat, slučovat se, zapadat, odpovídat, v dobré kondici

foul /faʊl/ odporný

fundal /'fʌn.dəl/ týkající se fundu, dna

fundus /'fʌn.dəs/ pl. -di fundus, dno f. uteri dno dělohy

handle /'hæn.dḷ/ zvládnout, poradit si, ovládat, brát do ruky, manipulovat

hyperflexion /ˌhaɪ.pə'flæk.ʃən/ hyperflexe, násilné ohnutí

irritable /'ɪr.ɪ.tə.bḷ/ iritabilní, dráždivý, podrážděný

isotonic /aɪ.səʊ'tɒn.ɪk/ izotonický, se stejným osmotickým tlakem

jaw /dʒɔː/ čelist

junky- /'dʒʌŋ.ki/ **sounding** / 'saʊndɪŋ/ rachotivý

keep from /kiːp/ (kept, kept) ubránit, ubránit se, uchovat

lack /læk/ nedostatek, postrádat, chybět

lactate /læk'teɪt/ laktát, mléčnan, sůl nebo ester mléčné kyseliny, tvorba l. ve velkém rozsahu způsobuje okyselení vnitřního prostředí, metabolickou acidózu

lift /lɪft/ pozvednout, zdvih

massage /'mæs.ɑːʒ/ masáž, masírovat

mist /mɪst/ mlha, aerosol

MPH, Miles /maɪlz/ **Per** /pə/ **Hour** / aʊə/ mil za hodinu (1 pozemní míle 1609 m)

multiparity /mʌl.ti'pær.ɪt.ɪ/ vícečetný porod

need /niːd/ potřeba, nutnost

neonate /ˌniː.əʊ'neɪt/ neonatus, novorozenec

odour /'əʊ.dər/ odér, pach, zápach

opt /ɒpt/ vybrat si, zvolit

oxygenation /'ɒk.sɪ.dʒə.neɪ.ʃən/ oxygenace, okysličení

point /pɔɪnt/ **to** /tʊ/ ukázat, namířit, upozornit

postictal /ˈpəʊstˈɪkt.əl/ následně po prodělaném záchvatu, po mrtvici, po epileptickém záchvatu

preventable /prɪˈven.tə.bļ/ jemuž lze předejít, ne nevyhnutelný

prior /ˈpraɪə/ **to** /tʊ/ před, přede

put /pʊt/ **pressure** /ˈpreʃ.ər/ vyvinout tlak na

range /reɪndʒ/ rozmezí, rozsah, pohybovat se, být v rozmezí

reassure /ˌriː.əˈʃɔːr/ uklidnit, utěšit

retraction /rɪˈtræk.ʃən/ retrakce, stažení, odtažení, zatažení

room /ruːm/ prostor, místo, pokoj

RSV, Human /hjuːmən/ **Respiratory** /rɪˈspɪr.ə.tər.i/ **Syncytial** /sɪnˈsɪ.ʃi.əl/ **Virus** /ˈvaɪrəs/ lidský respirační syncyciální virus, je častým původcem těžkých respiračních infekcí v pediatrii

rub /rʌb/ mnout, masírovat, potřít, namazat, drhnout, otřít

runny /ˈrʌn.i/ slzící oči z rýmy

seal /siːl/ tuleň, lachtan

seated /ˈsiː.tɪd/ posazený, uložený

shiver /ˈʃɪv.ər/ chvění, třes, třást se, chvět se

slap /slæp/ poklepat

sniffing /snɪf.ɪŋ/ čichání

sole /səʊl/ chodidlo, ploska

solution /səˈluː.ʃən/ řešení, roztok, rozpuštění

sponge /spʌndʒ/ mycí houba, omývat

stain /steɪn/ skvrna, zašpinit

straight /streɪt/ přímo, přímý, rovný

swelling /ˈswelɪŋ/ otok, opuchlina

tachydysrhythmia /ˌtæk.ɪ.dɪsˈrɪθ.mɪə/ tachyarytmie, nepravidelná a urychlená srdeční akce

threshold /ˈθreʃ.həʊld/ práh, hranice

thrust /θrʌst/ úder, vražení, tah

tilt /tɪlt/ naklonit, sklon, sklopit

toddler /ˈtɒd.lər/ batole, dítě učící se chodit

turn /tɜːn/ **blue** /bluː/ zmodrat

underlying /ˌʌndəˈlaɪ.ɪŋ/ skrytý, pod povrchem, základní, spodní

unfamiliar /ʌn.fəˈmɪl.i.ər/ cizí, neznámý

urge /ɜːdʒ/ naléhat, nutkání, naléhavá potřeba

ventilation /ˌven.tɪˈleɪ.ʃən/ dýchání, ventilace

Part 6
Operations

Scene safety; legal considerations; vehicle operations; communications; documentation; infection controlling; quality improvement; DNR; basic patient assessment; basic physiology; hazardous materials; mass-casualty incidents; scene management

Unit I

I

You arrive on the scene of a two-car MVC. The driver of the first vehicle is _____.
Consent for this patient is said to be:
- informed
- implied*
- expressed
- involuntary

_____ is assumed from any patient requiring emergency _____ who is physically, mentally, or emotionally unable to provide expressed consent.

intervention, Consent, unconscious

2

A properly written _____ ____ _____ (PCR) is important because the PCR may be the only _____ for pertinent information for receiving _____

_____ as well as other people interested in the event.*

health-care professionals, patient-care report, source

3

Which of the following patients would _____ most from the application of the PASG/MAST?
- a 10-year-old male, suspected spinal _____, no blood loss
- 72-year-old female, suspected _____ shock, no blood loss
- 40-year-old male, suspected lower-extremity fracture, low blood pressure*
- 67-year-old female, suspected _____ sprain, high blood pressure

Indications for the use of the PASG are to control bleeding, stabilize fractures, and _____ blood pressure.

raise, benefit, cardiogenic, fracture, ankle

4

The PCR is a legal document, making it necessary to record accurate incident times.*
All _____ _____ are to be recorded accurately for legal purposes, including time of _____, time of _____, time

of arrival, time of medication _____, etc.

administration, incident times, dispatch, call

5
Findings that require no _____ _____ but require documentation as evidence of a thorough history and exam are termed pertinent negatives.* _____ _____ are findings that require no medical treatment but help to show the completeness of the paramedic's _____ ___ ____ on the PCR.

Pertinent negatives, history and exam, medical intervention

6
The proper way to correct a written error on the PCR is to draw a single line through the error, initial, and date the area.* To _____ an error on a PCR,_ _____ ____ should be struck through the error, with the EMT/ paramedic's _____ next to the error and dated.

a single line, initials, correct

7
An incomplete or _____ patient-care report may cause subsequent caregivers to provide inappropriate treatment based on the report.*
The _____ and completeness of the patient-care report may have a significant _____ on ongoing care and treatment of the patient.

accuracy, illegible, impact

8
Revisions to the original patient-care report are done on a separate _____ ____ and then attached to the original.* Revisions are acceptable and must be done on a _____ report form and then _____ to the original document.

attached, separate, report form

9
Appropriate _____ language on a PCR includes:
• medical terminology*
• slang
• personal opinion
• personally acceptable abbreviations
Medical _____ is an integral part of good _____ on a PCR.

documentation, terminology, professional

10
A telephone is an example of:
• simplex
• duplex*
• multiplex
• trunked
A duplex communication system allows the user to both _____
___ _____ at the same time. A _____ _____ allows a person to listen or speak at one time. A multiplex system allows a person to listen and speak, as well as _____ ___. A trunked system pools all frequencies and routes transmissions to the next available frequency.

listen and speak, transmit data, simplex system

11
For communication to be effective, the _____ must give appropriate:
• ideas
• encodings
• decodings
• feedback to the sender*
_____ is a vital part of communication, allowing the sender to know that the receiver understands the _____.

Feedback, message, receiver

12
When communicating medical information, using _____

_____ can shorten transmission and provide an _____ form of communication.*
Proper terminology helps to make communication clear, _____, and unambiguous.

concise, unambiguous, proper terminology

13
Disadvantages of a simplex system may include the process being slower and more formal.*
In a simplex system the user is able _____ to listen or speak. The major _____ include the fact that the process is slower, more formal, and ___ _____ discussion.

not facilitating, only, disadvantages

14
A disadvantage of using a cellular telephone for EMS communications is that geography can _____ ___ the system or signs.*
An advantage of _____ _____ includes promoting a less formal, _____ discussion of EMS events. Disadvantages include ____ __ _____ signals due to geographical area or cell sites.

shorter, lost or broken, cellular telephones, interfere with

15

Functions of an EMS dispatcher include all of the following:
- call taking*
- alerting and directing the EMS response*
- giving prearrival instructions to the caller*

EMS _____ serve by receiving the call, taking information regarding the _____ of the event, and providing prearrival _____ to assist prior to the EMS unit's arrival.

nature, instructions, dispatchers

16

Communication from the EMS dispatcher that provides the caller with _____ _____, may be life-sustaining to the patient during a critical event and provides immediate _____ to the caller as well as ongoing information to responding units is called:
- incident data collection
- predispatch education
- prearrival instructions*
- incident referral data

_____ instructions provide immediate instructions and assistance to patients prior to the arrival of EMS units.

Prearrival, emotional support, assistance

17

Bacteria, viruses, and fungi are _____ of:
- pathogenic hosts
- non-specific inflammatory _____
- disease processes
- infectious agents*

_____ _____ have the potential of causing an infection.

infectious agents, examples, agents

18

The body's first line of _____ against infection is:
- the skin*
- the _____ system
- the gastrointestinal _____
- the humoral response

The skin is the body's first line of defence against _____ _____.

infectious agents, system, defence, respiratory

19

You respond to the home of a patient with an unknown illness for two days. You approach the call, suspecting an infectious or _____ disease. What action is not appropriate for the patient's care?

189

- Gloves and protective eye goggles are worn.*
- A full history and detailed physical exam is obtained.*
- Make the patient a 'load and go' due to the potential for paramedic exposure.
- Dispose of supplies and sharps appropriately on disposition of the patient.*

Making this patient a ___ ___ ___ patient based on the information provided is an _____ action.

communicable, 'load and go', inappropriate

20

Proper care of the patient with known HIV includes all of the following:

- effective hand washing*
- use of eye protection and gowns where exposure to _____ _____ in large quantities is possible*
- BSI based on task performed*

Isolation of the HIV patient is an inappropriate action. Care includes being supportive, using appropriate BSI based on the task being performed, effective hand washing, _____ of equipment, and care in the use of equipment, especially _____.

sharps, disinfection, bodily fluids

Vocabulary I

abbreviation /əˌbriː.viˈeɪ.ʃən/ zkratka

accuracy /ˈæk.jʊ.rə.si/ přesnost, správnost

accurate /ˈæk.jʊ.rət/ pečlivý, přesný

alert /əˈlɜːt/ bdělý, čilý, zvýšená ostražitost, stav pohotovosti, varovat

assistance /əˈsɪs.tənt s/ asistence, pomoc, podpora

assume /əˈsjuːm/ domnívat se, převzít, vzít na sebe odpovědnost, zaujmout

bodily /ˈbɒd.ɪ.li/ tělesný

care /keər/ pečovat, starat se, péče

cell, cellular /ˈsel.jʊ.lər/ telephone / ˈtelɪˌfəʊn/ mobilní telefon

communicable /kəˈmjuː.nɪ.kə.b|/ nakažlivý, přenosný

completeness /kəmˈpliːt.nəs/ úplnost, kompletnost

concise /kənˈsaɪs/ stručný, výstižný, zkrácený

consideration /kənˌsɪd.əˈreɪ.ʃən/ úvaha, zřetel, kritérium, faktor, který je třeba brát v úvahu

decode /diːˈkəʊd/ dekódovat, rozluštit

direct /daɪˈrekt/ nasměrovat, zamířit, řídit, dohlížet

disadvantage /ˌdɪs.ədˈvɑː.n.tɪdʒ/ nevýhoda

dispatcher /dɪˈspætʃər/ dispečer

dispose of /dɪˈspəʊz/ odklidit, odstranit, zbavit se něčeho

disposition /ˌdɪs.pəˈzɪʃ.ən/ rozmístění, umístění

duplex /ˈdjuː.pleks/ dvojitý, zdvojený

encode /ɪnˈkəʊd/ zakódovat, zašifrovat

express /ɪkˈspres/ vyjádřit, projevit, vyslovit

feedback /ˈfiːd.bæk/ zpětná vazba

fluid /ˈfluː.ɪd/ tekutina, kapalina

form /fɔːm/ formulář

fungus /ˈfʌŋ.gəs/ (pl **fungi**) houba, plíseň:

goggle /ˈgɒg.l̩/ ochrané brýle

gown /gaʊn/ plášť

handwash /ˈhændˌwɒʃ/ mýt ruce

health /helθ/ **care** /keə/ zdravotní péče

healthcare /helθ.keə/ zdravotní péče

host /həʊst/ hostitel

humoral /ˈhjuː.mər.əl/ humorální, týkající se tělesných tekutin

illegible /ɪˈledʒ.ə.bl̩/ nečitelný

implied /ɪmˈplaɪd/ implicitní, nepřímo vyjádřený

inappropriate /ˌɪn.əˈprəʊ.pri.ət/ nepatřičný, nevhodný, neúčelný

infectious /ɪnˈfek.ʃəs/ nakažlivý, infekční

inflammatory /ɪnˈflæm.ə.tər.i/ zánětlivý

initial /ɪˈnɪʃ.əl/ iniciála, šifra

integral /ˈɪn.tɪ.grəl/ nedílný, celý

involuntary /ɪnˈvɒləntərɪ/ bezděčný, mimovolný, vůlí neovladatelný, nedobrovolný

isolation /ˌaɪ.səl.eɪ.ʃən/ izolace, osamění, odloučení

legal /ˈliːgəl/ právní

line /laɪn/ linka, čára

mass /mæs/ hmotnost, hmota, objem, hromadění velké množství

multiplex /ˈmʌl.tɪ.pleks/ mnohonásobný

ongoing /ˈɒŋˌgəʊ.ɪŋ/ trvající, pokračující, přetrvávající, dále probíhající

opinion /əˈpɪn.jən/ názor, mínění

paramedic /ˌpær.əˈmed.ɪk/ zdravotnický záchranář

pathogenic /ˌpæθ.əˈdʒen.ɪk/ patogenní, choroboplodný

pertinent /ˈpɜː.tɪnənt/ týkající se, související, případný

pool /puːl/ nahromadit se

prearrival /ˌpriː.əˈraɪ.vəl/ před příjezdem

promote /prəˈməʊt/ podporovat, prosazovat

protection /prəˈtek.ʃən/ ochrana, zabezpečení

quantity /ˈkwɒn.tɪ.ti/ kvantita, počet, množství

record /ˈrekɔːd/ záznam, nahrát, zapsat

referral /rɪˈfɜː.rəl/ doporučení kam, odkázání ke specialistovi, předání do péče

report /rɪˈpɔːt/ oznámit, podat zprávu, informovat

revision /rɪˈvɪʒ.ən/ revize, pozměnění, přepracování

sender /ˈsen.dər/ odesilatel

separate /ˈsep.ər.ət/ oddělený, samostatný

shorten /ˈʃɔː.tən/ zkrátit

simplex /ˈsɪm.pleks/ jednosměrný přenos (tech.)

single /ˈsɪŋgəl/ jeden, jediný, jednoduchý

slang /slæŋ/ slang, hantýrka, nadávat

sprain /spreɪn/ podvrtnout, vymknout, vyvrtnutí, výron

subsequent /ˈsʌb.sɪ.kwənt/ pozdější, následující

take /teɪk/ **care** /keər/ pečovat, starat se

task /tɑːsk/ úkol, úloha

trunking /ˈtrʌŋkɪŋ/ systém sdílených telefonních linek, umožňuje služby pro velký počet lidí současně

unambiguous /ˌʌnæmˈbɪgjuəs/ jednoznačný, zcela jasný

Unit 2

I

Which of the following hepatitis groups is NOT transmitted via _____?
- Hepatitis A*
- Hepatitis B
- Hepatitis C
- Hepatitis D

Hepatitis A is transmitted via the ___/_____ route.

blood, oral/faecal

2

The next two questions are based on the following scenario:
You are called to a local _____ _____ for a gentleman with complaints of a cough for two or three weeks, night sweats, and weight loss. You suspect:
- hepatitis A
- HIV
- TB (tuberculosis)*
- meningitis

_____ presents with a chronic cough _____ for two to three weeks, low-grade fever, and night sweats. Certain populations are at a higher risk of developing TB, including children less than 3 years old and _____ patients.

You diagnose the above illness and know the disease is spread through:
- exposure to blood
- exposure through airborne droplets*
- exposure to body fluids
- direct physical contact

Tuberculosis, geriatric, homeless shelter, persistent

3

You respond to a home of a patient with complaints of a sudden onset of fever/chills, joint pain, neck stiffness, and severe headache. Upon examination the medics note a petechial rash. You suspect:
- rabies
- influenza
- hepatitis A
- meningitis*

Meningitis signs and symptoms include a _____ _____, vomiting, fever, and _____ of sudden onset. The patient may have a petechial rash and usually has _____ _____.

muscle rigidity, chills, severe headache

4

The causative organism of _____ ___ is the varicella zoster virus, which is a member of the:
- varicella virus group
- zoster virus group
- herpesvirus group*
- rubivirus group

The _____ group also contains a virus responsible for genital herpes and the common ____ ____.

chicken pox, cold sore, herpesvirus

5
Reportable infectious/communicable disease exposures _____:
- contact of infectious materials with eye, mouth, or mucous membrane*
- working with a partner with a URI
- contact with blood and body fluids on intact gloves
- spill of infectious material in the EMS unit with no contact

_____ includes contact of infectious material with eyes, mouth, exposed mucous membrane, or _____ skin.

include, nonintact, Exposure

6
Exercising the degree of care, skill, and judgement that would be expected under like or similar _____ by a similarly trained, reasonable paramedic in a similar _____or location is the _____ __:
- duty to act

- standard of care*
- malfeasance
- proximate cause

community, definition of, circumstances

7
The four _____ of a negligence claim include:
- the duty __ ___*
- breach of duty*
- proximate cause*
- _____ damages*

elements, to act, actual

8
You arrive on the scene of a two-car MVC (motor vehicle collision). The driver of the first vehicle is _____. Consent for this patient is said to be:
- informed
- implied*
- expressed
- involuntary

Consent is assumed _____ from any patient requiring emergency intervention who is physically, mentally, or emotionally unable to provide expressed _____.

implied, unconscious, consent

9
You and your partner are treating a 16-year-old female with lower-abdominal pain. The

patient's husband arrives and informs you his wife may be _____.
You can treat this patient without parental consent based on the fact that an emancipated minor is considered an adult.*
Care for this patient would not require _____ _____ because the patient is married and therefore an _____ minor.

pregnant, emancipated, parental consent

10
You are called to the middle of a bridge to transport a violent patient who is suicidal. Per local police, the patient threatened to jump from the bridge and needs a psychiatric evaluation. The patient refuses transport, threatening to sue anyone who touches him. You transport this patient against his ____ based on involuntary consent.*
This patient can be treated and transported against his will under _____ _____. Law enforcement personnel can direct transport and treatment of a patient who is _ _____ to himself or others.

involuntary consent, a threat, will

11
You and your partner are treating a patient who needs to be transported to the hospital for chest pain. You have established an IV, placed the patient on the monitor, and administered oxygen and aspirin. Your partner checks his watch and notes that his _____ __ ____. You remove the monitor and politely tell the patient that the oncoming crew will come and _____ him to the hospital shortly. Leaving this patient is an example of:
- false imprisonment
- assault
- battery
- abandonment*

_____ is the termination of the paramedic-patient relationship without ensuring appropriate ____ ___ the patient.

Abandonment, care for, shift is over, transport

12
Unlawful _____ of an individual without his or her consent could lead the paramedic open to _____ __ battery.*
Battery is an unlawful touching of someone without his or her _____.

consent, touching, allegations of

13

_____ directives are documents that express the patient's wishes in the event that he or she is _____ or otherwise unable to _____ his or her choice for care.
These include living wills and do not resuscitate orders and durable power of attorney for health care.*
Durable power of attorney for _____ ____ or health care proxy, once signed and witnessed, are effective until the patient revokes them.

health care, express, unconscious, Advance

14

The paramedic's primary responsibility at a crime scene or _____ scene is:
- quality patient care
- _____ documentation
- thorough knowledge of the event
- to protect self and other EMS personnel*

The primary responsibility of the paramedic at all scenes is the _____ of himself or herself and other ___ _____.

EMS personnel, protection, accident, quality

15

Laws that protect a paramedic if he or she acts __ ____ _____, is not negligent, acts within his or her scope of _____, and does not accept _____ for service constitutes the Good Samaritan laws.*

payment, in good faith, practice

16

You and your partner are overheard in the elevator discussing a patient's injuries from a motor vehicle crash. Your conversation included pertinent personal and medical information about the patient.
A call was placed to your _____ because you failed to keep patient confidentiality.*
Breach of _____ – any medical or personal information about a patient should not be discussed __ _____ or released without the patient's consent.

in public, confidentiality, supervisor

17

Commonly mandated injuries that are reportable to local authorities include all of the following:
- child abuse or neglect*
- animal bites*
- gunshot/stab wounds*

Injuries reportable to local authorities include spousal abuse, child _____ __ _____, elder abuse, sexual _____, gunshot/ stab wounds, animal bites, and _____ diseases.

> assault, communicable, abuse or neglect

18
Intentional false communication that injures another person's _____ or good name is a definition of:
- invasion of privacy
- breach of confidentiality
- informed slander
- defamation*

Defamation includes _____, which is verbal, and libel, which is _____.

> slander, written, reputation

19
Personal protective equipment used to operate safely in the rescue environment includes all of the following:
- head _____*
- eye protection*
- ____ protection*
- personal flotation devices*
- _____ protection*
- high visibility clothing*
- specialized _____*

> protection, footwear, thermal, hand

20
It is generally considered _____ to walk in fast-moving water:
- ankle
- knee-deep*
- waist
- chest

Walking in fast-moving water places the person at risk of having an _____ pinned and then being pulled under by ___ _____.

> extremity, the current, unsafe

Vocabulary 2
abuse /ə'bjuːz/ zneužívání, týrání, zneužívat
act /ækt/ akt, zákon
airborne /'eə,bɔːn/ přenášený vzduchem
allegation /ˌæl.ə'geɪ.ʃən/ nařčení, obvinění (nepodložené)
assault /ə'sɒlt/ útok, napadení, přepadnout
authority /ɔː'θɒr.ɪ.ti/ oprávnění, pravomoc, úřad, správní orgán, úřední činitelé
battery /'bæt.ər.i/ útok, ublížení na zdraví
be /biː/ **over** /'əʊ.vər/ být skončený
bite /baɪt/ kousnout, uštknout, kousnutí
breach /briːtʃ/ porušení, nedodržení

causative /ˈkɔ:.zə.tɪv/ kauzativní, příčinný, způsobující

chickenpox /ˈtʃɪk.ɪn.pɒks/ varicela, plané neštovice

claim /kleɪm/ požadavek, nárok

cold /kəʊld/ sore /sɔ:r/ opar na rtu, v nose

confidentiality /ˌkɒn.fɪ.den.tʃiˈæl.ɪ.ti/ důvěrnost informací, mlčenlivost

consent /kənˈsent/ souhlas, svolení

constitute /ˈkɒn.stɪ.tju:t/ znamenat, představovat

crew /kru:/ posádka

crime /kraɪm/ zločin, trestný čin

current /ˈkʌr.ənt/ proud

damage /ˈdæm.ɪdʒ/ poškodit, poškození, škoda

defamation /ˌdefəˈmeɪʃən/ pomluva, hanobení

directive /daɪˈrek.tɪv/ směrnice

Do Not Resuscitate /rɪˈsʌs.ɪ.teɪt/ order /ˈɔ:.dər/ pokyn neoživovat

droplet /ˈdrɒp.lət/ kapka, kapička

durable /ˈdjʊərəbəl/ trvalý

duty /ˈdju:tɪ/ povinnost, úkol

elder /ˈeldə/ starší člověk

element /ˈelɪmənt/ element, prvek, součást

emancipated /ɪˈmæn.sɪ.peɪ.tɪd/ emancipovaný, zletilý

enforcement /ɪnˈfɔ:.smənt/ prosazování, prosazení, vymáhání, vynucení

expressed /ɪkˈspresd/ vyjádřený, projevený, vyslovený

faecal /ˈfi:.kəl/ fekální, týkající se stolice

faith /feɪθ/ víra, důvěra, náboženské vyznání

false /fɒls/ imprisonment /ɪmˈprɪz.ən.mənt/ neoprávněné zadržení

fast-moving /fɑ:stˈmu:.vɪŋ/ rychle se pohybující

flotation /fləʊˈteɪ.ʃən/ equipment /ɪˈkwɪp.mənt/ plovací vybavení

footwear /ˈfʊt.weər/ obuv

genital /ˈdʒen.ɪ.təl/ genitálie, pohlavní

grade /greɪd/ stupeň, kvalita

gunshot /ˈgʌn.ʃɒt/ střela, výstřel

hepatitis /ˌhep.əˈtaɪ.tɪs/ hepatitida, zánět jater

herpes-virus /ˈhɜ:.pi:zˈvaɪ.rəs/ skupina virů způsobující opary

homeless /ˈhəʊm.ləs/ bez domova, bezdomovec

implied /ɪmˈplaɪd/ implicitní, nepřímo vyjádřený

influenza /ˌɪn.fluˈen.zə/ chřipka

informed /ɪnˈfɔ:md/ informovaný, poučený

intentional /ɪnˈtenʃənəl/ úmyslný, záměrný

invasion /ɪnˈveɪ.ʒən/ narušení, vpád

involuntary /ɪnˈvɒləntərɪ/ nedobrovolný

judgment /ˈdʒʌdʒ.mənt/ úsudek, názor, soudnost, posouzení, soud, odsouzení

law /lɔ:/ právo, zákon

libel /ˈlaɪ.bəl/ pomluva, křivé nařčení

living /ˈlɪvɪŋ/ will /wɪl/ poslední vůle

malfeasance /mæl'fi:.zəns/ trestný čin

mandate /'mæn.deɪt/ nařizovat

minor /'maɪ.nə/ malý, nezletilý

mucous membrane /ˌmjuː. kəs'mem.breɪn/ sliznice

neglect /nɪ'glekt/ zanedbání, zanedbávat

negligence /'neglɪdʒəns/ nedbalost

negligent /'neg.lɪ.dʒənt/ nedbalý

nonintact /ˌnɒn.ɪn'tækt/ neintaktní, nikoli nedotčený

oncoming /'ɒnˌkʌmɪŋ/ blížící se, protijedoucí

overhear /ˌəʊvə'hɪə/ vyslechnout (náhodou)

parental /pə'ren.təl/ rodičovský

personnel /ˌpɜːsə'nel/ personál

petechial /pi'tiː.ki.əl/ petechiální, týkající se petechie

pin /pɪn/ špendlík, spona

polite /pə'laɪt/ slušný, zdvořilý

power /paʊər/ of attorney /ə'tɜː.ni/ plná moc, oprávnění advokáta

privacy /'praɪvəsɪ/ soukromí

proximate /'prɒk.sɪ.mət/ nejbližší, bezprostřední

proxy /'prɒk.sɪ/ zástupce, zmocněnec

rabies /'reɪ.bi:z/ vzteklina

reportable /rɪ'pɔː'tebəl/ podléhající hlášení

responsibility /rɪˌspɒn.sə'bɪ. lɪ.tɪ/ zodpovědnost, povinnosti, závazky pracovní

resuscitate /rɪ'sʌs.ɪ.teɪt/ oživovat

revolve /rɪ'vɒlv/ rotovat, otáčet se, točit se

rigidity /rɪ'dʒɪd.ɪ.ti/ rigidita, tuhost, ztuhlost, pevnost, tvrdost

rubivirus /ruː.bɪ'vaɪ.rəs/ rubivirus, virus způsobující rubeolu (zarděnky)

scope /skəʊp/ prostor, příležitost, rozsah

shelter /'ʃel.tər/ přístřeší, úkryt

shift /ʃɪft/ posunovat, přemístit

sign /saɪn/ znak, známka, znamení, podepsat

skill /skɪl/ dovednost, schopnost, zkušenost

slander /'slɑːndə/ pomluva, hanobení

spousal /'spaʊzəl/ manželský

standard /'stæn.dəd/ standard, zásada, obvyklý, běžný

stiffness /'stɪf.nəs/ strnulost, ztuhlost, ztuhnutí

sue /sjuː/ zažalovat, podat žalobu

supervisor /'suː.pə.vaɪ.zər/ dozor, nadřízený

sweat /swet/ pot, potit se

termination /ˌtɜː.mɪ'neɪ.ʃən/ ukončení

thorough /'θʌr.ə/ důkladný, podrobný

threat /θret/ hrozba, ohrožení, výhrůžka

threaten /'θret.ən/ hrozit, vyhrožovat

touch /tʌtʃ/ dotknout se, dotek

transmit /trænz'mɪt/ přenášet, rozšířit

treat /triːt/ zacházet, jednat, léčit

unlawful /ʌn'lɔː.fʊl/ nezákonný, protizákonný

unsafe /ʌnˈseɪf/ nebezpečný,
zdravotně závadný
varicella /ˌvær.ɪˈsel.ə/ varicela,
plané neštovice
visibility /ˌvɪz.ɪˈbɪl.ɪ.ti/ viditelnost
waist /weɪst/ pas
will /wɪl/ vůle
wish /wɪʃ/ přát, přání
witness /ˈwɪt.nəs/ svědek, svědčit,
potvrdit podpisem
zoster /zɒ.stər/ pásový opar

Unit 3

I

Low-head dams are considered drowning machines due to recirculating currents created by water moving over a uniform obstruction.*

Low-head dams create a recirculating current, which can repeatedly ____ the victim under the water, making _____ difficult. These dams also make _____ _____ hazardous.

> rescue operations, escape, pull

2

The body responds to cold water by rapidly losing heat. Protective measures exist within the body, which stimulates a parasympathetic response, decreasing heart rate, causing peripheral vasoconstriction, and shunting blood to the core. This cold protective response is known as the mammalian dive reflex.*

The _____ ____ _____ is a protective physiologic response which increases _____ by shunting blood to the core, _____ heart rate, and dropping ____ _____. These factors are affected by the person's age and ____ _____ and the water temperature.

> decreasing, survivability, health status, mammalian dive reflex, blood pressure

3

The following are considered oxygen-deficient environments or _____ spaces:
- storage tanks*
- grain bins or _____*
- _____ vaults*
- wells*
- manholes*

> confined, underground, silos

4

You are the first unit on the scene of a multiple-vehicle crash. Upon arrival, each of the following actions would be appropriate:
- establish scene command*
- the scene size-up*
- control scene hazards*

The first unit to arrive on the scene should begin the scene size-up, which includes _____ _____, calling for backup units, controlling any _____, and locating any _____ _____. It would not be appropriate for the primary unit to locate and transport the ____ _____ injured patient.

> hazards, most critically, establishing command, triage patients

5

Which of the following definitions best describes a disaster?

- motor vehicle collision with two to three patients
- an everyday incident that generates three or more patients
- a bus or train collision with 25-30 injured
- an incident that overwhelms resources and may damage the infrastructure of a region*

_ _____ is an incident that may generate hundreds of patients, ___ _____ the existing resources, and may damage the _____ of the region, shutting down railroads, hospitals, and other normal operations.

may overwhelm, A disaster, infrastructure

6

You are assigned the duties of a safety officer under the incident command of a local mass-casualty _____. You understand the _____ of this position to:

- monitor all on-scene actions to ensure no potentially harmful situations are created
- coordinate all operations of this incident that involve outside agencies
- collect data regarding the incident and relay information to the press or media
- act as an officer who supervises a specific safety unit or area*

The safety officer monitors all on-scene actions to ensure that no potentially _____ _____ are created.

harmful situations, responsibilities, incident

7

The S in the acronym START is for:

- suitable
- simple*
- salvageable
- sorting

_____ stands for simple triage and rapid transport. This system focuses on four easily identifiable _____: (1) ability to walk, (2) respiratory _____, (3) pulses/perfusion, (4) _____ status.

findings, START, effort, neurological

8

You are the _____ _____ at a car-versus-bus collision. Your first victim is approximately 30 years old, awake, alert, and oriented.

He is the driver of the car that collided with the bus head-on. He complains of lower-abdominal pain and has obvious _____ to both femurs. Respirations, 24; pulse, 140; BP, 80/ palpated; capillary refill, >2 sec. How would you triage the following patient?
- green
- yellow
- red*
- black

This patient should be tagged Red with immediate life threats, including the possibility of bilateral _____ _____ and intraabdominal bleeding.

femur fractures, triage officer, deformity

9
You are treating a patient with diabetic ketoacidosis. The patient is tachycardic and has deep, rapid respirations.
The most likely cause for the ____, _____ respirations is that the body is compensating for a low pH by increasing respirations.*
The _____ recognizes a decrease in pH or an excess of H+ ions and attempts to compensate by _____ the respiratory effort.

brain, increasing, deep, rapid

10
You are treating a patient with hyperventilation syndrome due to an anxiety attack.
What acid-base derangement will hyperventilation produce? Respiratory alkalosis.*
_____ _____ results from an _____ in respirations and an excessive _____ of CO_2.

Respiratory alkalosis, elimination, increase

11
Hyperventilation resulting from pure anxiety leads to:
- _____ acidosis
- respiratory alkalosis*
- a decreasing blood pH
- hepatic failure

_____ can result in an excess elimination of _____ _____ leading to respiratory alkalosis.

Hyperventilation, respiratory, carbon dioxide

12
Parenteral routes of drug administration include all of the following:
- intravenous*
- intramuscular*
- topical*

_____ _____ for the delivery of medication include all those areas _____ the gastrointestinal tract. Parenteral routes include _____, _____, intramuscular, subcutaneous, topical, and _____. The sublingual route administers the drug through the enteral route, or through the gastrointestinal tract.

> intravenous, inhalations, Parenteral routes, outside, endotracheal

13

The six rights of medication administration include:
- right _____*
- right dose*
- right time*
- right _____*
- right patient*
- right _____*

> medication, route, documentation

14

A 53-year-old female who is being treated for chronic pain with morphine sulphate continues to complain of pain despite taking her medications __ _____. The patient is most likely experiencing what _____ to this medication?
- _____ reaction
- tolerance*
- dependence
- antagonism

Tolerance is a decreased response to the ____ _____ of a drug after taking the drug over a period of time.

> as prescribed, response, same amount, allergic

15

At the scene of an MVC your ambulance should __ _____ at least 100 feet (30.5 metres) from the accident, uphill, and upwind to ensure:
- ___ _____ of the vehicle
- the safety of your crew*
- that the crime scene is not violated
- clear distance for secondary units to arrive

The number one _____ of every EMS call is assurance of your personal safety.

> priority, the safety, be parked

16

The following statements regarding scene safety with regard to helicopter and air medical transport are all true:
- Generally, a helicopter requires a _____ ____ of approximately 100 feet (30.5 metres) by 100 feet (30.5 metres).*
- Ensure that the landing zone is _____ __ wires,

loose debris, towers, or vehicles.*
- Mark the landing zone with a single flare and do not shine lights directly into the pilot's eyes.*

The helicopter should _____ be approached in a crouched position away from the tail rotor. Approach a helicopter that is on a slight incline from the _____ side.

downhill, landing zone, cautiously, clear of

17

Promptly recognizing the need for _____ management, assessing the scene for _____, contacting dispatch to mobilize other units for care and _____ of the patient, and establishing rapport with the patient and other paramedics on the scene represent the paramedic's:
- ethical responsibility
- roles*
- triage criteria
- care responsibility

Recognizing an emergency exists, assessing the situation, managing the emergency care, _____ efforts of your team as well as other agencies involved in the care and transportation of the patient, and establishing _____ with the patient and other

EMS crew are all examples of a paramedic's roles.

transportation, coordinating, rapport, danger, emergency

18

In the _____ C-FLOP, when describing the practices of the Incident Management System, the O _____ ___:
- operations*
- ongoing assessments
- order of command
- officer in charge

The mnemonic C-FLOP stands for C - command, F -_____/ administration, L - logistics, O - operations, P - planning.

stands for, finance, mnemonic

19

The next questions are based on the following scenario:
You are assigned to triage patients at the scene of an explosion in a park. You are using the METTAG system of triage.

The first victim you come in contact with has no palpable pulse and no respiratory effort. The patient has a major laceration on the scalp with an open skull fracture.
You would tag this person as Black.*

The designation of this patient would be _____ due to the _____ of signs of life and injuries that were possibly _____ with life. The morgue area should be a triage area away from other treatment areas.

The next patient with whom you come into contact is a 34-year-old female who is wandering around the incident, looking for her 3-year-old daughter. The patient has multiple abrasions to her face and arms.
You would most likely triage this patient as Green.*
This patient can be triaged to the _____ treatment area. The green treatment area is the area where patients require _____ __ __ care in preparation for transport.

The third patient you find is awake, alert, and oriented. The patient has tachypnoea with shallow respirations. Your assessment reveals a sucking chest wound on the right side of the chest, a fracture of the right femur, and a large laceration on the forehead.
You will most likely _____ this patient as Red.*
This patient has _____ injuries that require immediate attention. The ___ treatment area has the equipment and skilled providers

to best care for, stabilize, and transport this patient.

incompatible, absence, little or no, green, critical, triage, red, black

20
You and your partner are the first EMS unit to arrive on the scene of a single-car MVC, car versus pole. Electrical lines are down across the car. One victim is trapped inside the vehicle. What action would be most correct? Contact dispatch and have the _____ _____ turn the power off to the lines prior to attempting rescue of this patient.*
The rescuer's ___ _____ is the safety of himself or herself and other rescuers. Attempting any rescue prior to cutting power to the downed lines would _____ the safety of rescuers and the patient.

power company, jeopardize, top priority

Vocabulary 3
antagonism /ænˈtæg.ə.nɪ.zəm/ antagonismus, protiklad, rozpor
assign /əˈsaɪn/ zadat, přidělit
assurance /əˈʃɔː.rəns/ jistota, zajištění, pojištění
back-up /ˈbæk.ʌp/ podpořit, podložit, záloha

be /biː/ **in charge** /tʃɑːdʒ/ **of** být zodpovědný za, mít na starost

bin /bɪn/ zásobník, nádoba

carbon /ˈkɑː.bən/ **dioxide** /daɪˈɒk.saɪd/ oxid uhličitý

cautiously /ˈkɔː.ʃəs.li/ opatrně, ostražitě

command /kəˈmɑːnd/ příkaz, ovládnutí, kontrola, velení

company /ˈkʌm.pə.ni/ společnost, firma

confined /kənˈfaɪnd/ stísněný, omezený, být omezen na

core /kɔːr/ střed těla

crouch /kraʊtʃ/ skrčit se, přikrčit se

dam /dæm/ hráz, přehrada

dependence /dɪˈpen.dənt s/ závislost

derangement /dɪˈreɪndʒd.mənt/ vyšinutí, pomatenost, porucha

diabetic /ˌdaɪəˈbet.ɪk/ diabetický

disaster /dɪˈzɑː.stər/ pohroma, neštěstí, katastrofa

distance /ˈdɪs.tənt s/ vzdálenost

dive /daɪv/ potápět se v moři ap.

down /daʊn/ dole, spadnout, srazit

downhill /ˌdaʊnˈhɪl/ dolů z kopce, pod kopcem

drop /drɒp/ klesnout, spadnout, pokles, kapka, upustit na zem

electrical /ɪˈlek.trɪ.kəl/ **line** /laɪn/ elektrické vedení

elimination /ɪˌlɪm.ɪˈneɪ.ʃən/ eliminace, vylučování, odstranění, vypouštění

escape /ɪˈskeɪp/ únikový, utéct, uniknout, uprchnout

flare /fleər/ zarudnutí, vzplanout

forehead /ˈfɒrɪd/, /ˈfɔːˌhed/ čelo hlavy

generate /ˈdʒen.ər.eɪt/ generovat, shromáždit, vytvořit, vyvolat

grain /greɪn/ obilí, zrní

harmful /ˈhɑːm.fəl/ škodlivý, zhoubný, zdravotně závadný

hazard /ˈhæz.əd/ hazard, riziko, nebezpečí

head-on /ˌhedˈɒn/ čelně, zepředu

health /helθ/ **status** /ˈsteɪ.təs/ zdravotní stav

identifiable /aɪˈden.tɪ.faɪ.ə.bl̩/ identifikovatelný, rozpoznatelný

incline /ɪnˈklaɪn/ sklánět se, tíhnout, mít sklon

incompatible /ˌɪn.kəmˈpæt.ɪ.bl̩/ inkompatibilní, neslučitelný

infrastructure /ˈɪn.frəˌstrʌk.tʃər/ infrastruktura

intramuscular /ˌɪn.trəˈmʌs.kjʊ.lər/ intramuskulární, nitrosvalový

intravenous /ˌɪn.trəˈviː.nəs/ nitrožilní

jeopardize /ˈdʒep.ə.daɪz/ ohrozit

landing /ˈlændɪŋ/ **zone** /zəʊn/ místo přistání, přistávací plocha

locate /ləʊˈkeɪt/ najít, vypátrat

loose /luːs/ volný, uvolněný, nepřivázaný

mammalian /məˈmeɪ.li.ən/ týkající se savců

manhole /ˈmænˌhəʊl/ otvor, průlez, kanalizace

morgue /mɔːg/ márnice

operation /ˌɒp.ərˈeɪ.ʃən/ operace, zásah, akce

order /ˈɔːdə/ příkaz

overwhelm /ˌəʊ.vəˈwelm/ přemoci, zdolat
parenteral /pəˈren.tə.rəl/ mimostřevní
peripheral /pəˈrɪf.ər.əl/ periferní, okrajový, obvodový
power /paʊər/ elektrický, elektřina
prescribe /prɪˈskraɪb/ předepsat, naordinovat lék
press /pres/ tlačit, tisknout
promptly /ˈprɒmptlɪ/ ihned, okamžitě
railroad /ˈreɪl.rəʊd/ železniční trať
rapport /ræˈpɔːr/ vzájemné porozumění, souznění
recirculate /riːˈsɜː.kjʊ.leɪt/ recirkulovat
relay /ˈriː.leɪ/ přenos, vysílání
repeatedly /rɪˈpiː.tɪd.li/ opakovaně, opětovně
rotor /ˈrəʊtə/ rotor, pohyblivá část motoru
safety /ˈseɪftɪ/ bezpečnost, ochranný
salvageable /ˈsæl.vɪdʒə.bl̩/ zachranitelný
scalp /skælp/ vlasová pokožka, kůže pokrývající lebeční kosti, kůže na temeni hlavy
shine /ʃaɪn/ svítit, zářit, lesk
silo /ˈsaɪ.ləʊ/ silo, nádoba na skladování obilí
simple /ˈsɪm.pl̩/ prostý, jednoduchý
sorting /ˈsɔːt.ɪŋ/ třídění, roztřídění, řazení
stand /stænd/ **for** /fə/ znamenat, značit

storage /ˈstɔː.rɪdʒ/ ukládání, uchovávání, uschování
sublingual /sʌbˈlɪŋ.gwəl/ sublingvální, podjazykový
suitable /ˈsjuː.tə.bl̩/ vhodný
supervise /ˈsuː.pəˌvaɪz/ dohlížet, mít na starost
survivability /səˈvaɪv.əˈbɪl.ə.ti/ schopnost přežít, přetrvat
tail /teɪl/ zadní část, ocas
tank /tæŋk/ cisterna, nádrž
tolerance /ˈtɒl.ər.əns/ tolerance, snášenlivost
topical /ˈtɒp.ɪ.kəl/ místní
underground /ˌʌn.dəˈgraʊnd/ podzemní
uphill /ˌʌpˈhɪl/ nahoru
upwind /ˌʌpˈwɪnd/ proti větru
vault /vɔːlt/ klenba
violate /ˈvaɪəˌleɪt/ narušit, porušit, přestoupit
wander /ˈwɒn.dər/ toulat se, bloudit
well /wel/ studna, šachta výtahová, schodišťová ap.
wire /waɪər/ drát

Unit 4

1

You are the paramedic in charge of a single patient entrapped in a vehicle that was involved in a head-on crash. The extrication of this patient will require a lengthy period of time.

Your _____ during the time of disentanglement will be that management of this patient will remain the same as for other emergency patients. Initiation of assessment and care should be started as soon as possible.* Keep in mind that rapid

_____ ___ _____ may not be possible. Management of this patient should remain the same as similar emergency patients. You must _____ assessment and care as soon as possible.

> initiate, extrication and transport, responsibility

2

You are transporting a patient who has been exposed to a hazardous material. You have come into contact with this patient with Level D hazmat protection equipment on.

You have most likely experienced a secondary exposure.* For a secondary contamination, Level D _____ protection equipment is the lowest level of protection. Level D equipment consists of structural fire-fighting, or turnout, gear. _____

_____ occurs when an uncontaminated person comes ____ _____ with a contaminated person.

> into contact, Secondary contamination, hazmat

3

The paramedic faces many stress-inducing situations. All of the following are phases of the stress response:
- alarm reaction*
- resistance*
- exhaustion*

The three phases of the body's _____ to stress are alarm reactions (of the _____ __ _____ response), resistance, and exhaustion. As the body sustains increasing stress, the level of resistance to stress rises, and higher levels of stress must occur for the _____ _____ to occur. _____ follows as stress continues and coping mechanisms begin to fail.

> fight-or-flight, alarm reaction, response, Exhaustion

4

While eating lunch at a local eatery, you and your partner are _____ a call you had just completed. The patient's relative who is sitting at the next table _____ your partner talking about the patient's condition. Your partner has violated the patient's:

- right to consent
- right to confidentiality*
- _____ of refusal of treatment
- character by defamation

Information related to the patient's condition or treatment is considered _____ information.

> confidential, overhears, discussing, right

5

While assessing a patient complaining of abdominal pain, you should first:

- palpate/auscultate
- inspect/percuss
- inspect, then auscultate the abdomen.*
- palpate/percuss

Inspection is the visual assessment of the patient. Inspection can reveal many important aspects of the patient. _____ of abdominal sounds should _____ palpation and _____.

> Auscultation, precede, percussion

6

A 50-year-old male is experiencing an acute _____ of asthma. Your partner establishes an IV, and you prepare to administer albuterol via a handheld _____. Your actions are in direct accordance with your local protocol. This type of standing order is considered off-line medical direction.*

__-____ medical direction includes the authority of a medical director or advisory group to establish treatment protocols or standing orders.

> nebulizer, exacerbation, Off-line

7

You and your partner respond to the home of an elderly gentleman who is unresponsive. Your assessment reveals no respiratory effort, skin that is cool and mottled with obvious pooling, and no palpable pulse. The patient's wife presents a valid Do Not Resuscitate order. All of the actions below would be correct:

- Address the wife using gentle eye contact and choose appropriate words.*
- Explain to the wife that her loved one has died; do not use terms that can be misinterpreted.*

- Offer assistance to the survivor(s) if necessary.* This patient has a valid ___ (Do Not Resuscitate) order and no obvious _____ __ ____. The correct actions would be to address the survivor in terms that leave no doubt about the outcome of the _____. Use gentle, reassuring eye contact and offer any _____ that may be needed to the survivor.

assistance, DNR, signs of life, deceased

8

You are one of the many EMS workers who just completed working the scene of a _____ plane crash that left several hundred people ____ __ _____. You and your crew are called in for CISD (Critical Incident Stress Debriefing). You understand this to be:

- a technique for reducing stress on the scene that includes fluid replacement, food services, and change of assignments
- a formal, structured, planned intervention done by a trained team within 24-72 hours of a posttraumatic event. ____ ____ includes mental

health workers and peers.*

- a spontaneous post-call discussion of the events
- a short informal meeting that gives the crew a chance to vent and verbalize their feelings about this _____

incident, devastating, dead or injured, The team

9

Your crew is dispatched to the home of an obese woman who has fallen. The general rules for lifting and moving this patient include all of the following:

- Position the load as close to your body as possible.*
- Bend your knees; let the _____ _____ of the legs do the work of lifting.*
- Take your time, do not hurry, and maintain a wide base of support.*

Proper _____ _____ should be utilized during all patient encounters. Ask for assistance if needed. Do not _____ the rescuer's or the patient's safety.

jeopardize, lifting techniques, large muscles

10
Documentation of a patient's
_____ for care or transport
should include all of the following:
- the paramedic's advice to the patient*
- online medical control's _____*
- a complete narrative of the _____*

advice, event, refusal

11
Legislation that governs the
_____ of medicine and may
prescribe a physician's ability
to delegate authority to perform
medical acts by the paramedic is
called:
- licensure
- _____ direction
- _____ of care
- medical practice act*

standard, medical, practice

12
You ___ _____ the patient
involved in a two-car MVC with
severe blunt trauma to the
abdomen. You suspect internal
haemorrhage. The patient's BP is
100/52 with a pulse rate of 130.
You know the _____ in the
heart rate is the body's attempt to
maintain:
- metabolism
- system integration
- homeostasis*
- end-organ damage

_____ is the natural
tendency of the body to maintain
a steady state of _____ within
the body's internal environment.

Homeostasis, equilibrium,
elevation, are assessing

13
The _____ of water across a
cell membrane is known as:
- oncotic pressure
- osmosis*
- diffusion
- osmolarity

_____ is the movement of any
solvent (usually water) across a

____ _____.

Osmosis, cell membrane,
movement

14
The set of _____ ___ _____
that a paramedic is permitted to
perform during a medical situation
is called:
- primary practice
- consent to _____
- scope of practice*
- regional practice

_____ of practice is generally
defined by state statute and defines
what an EMS provider can _____.

Scope, duties and skills,
perform, practice

15

When is the use of reasonable force or use of restraints permissible for a patient?

- The patient is alert, cooperative, but _____.
- The patient has an altered level of consciousness caused by injury, substance abuse, or illness.*
- It is never appropriate to use any _____ on a patient.
- This is at the _____ of the paramedic or the crew's officer.

If the patient is altered and is placing himself or others in harm's way, the EMS provider should use any method within reason to _____ the patient's actions.

control, force, anxious, force

16

Drawing a patient's blood without her _____ may be an example of:

- battery*
- slander
- false imprisonment
- assault

In most situations, unpermitted _____ _____ is a form of battery. _____ is the threat of bodily harm.

physical contact, Assault, permission

17

In which of the following situations is an EMS provider required to make a report to law enforcement?

- suspected sexual assault*
- alcohol-related _____
- motor vehicle collision with _____
- illegal ____ possession

Most states require the reporting of _____ or neglect of children, spouses, or older adults; ____ and sexual assault; _____ and stab wounds; animal bites; and certain _____ diseases.

gunshot, communicable, trauma, rape, abuse, entrapment, drug

18

A patient is in respiratory distress. She has a _____ DNR order. Which of the following treatments is correct? _____ oxygen and a nebulized albuterol treatment.* 'Do not resuscitate' is not the same as '__ ___ _____'. Under these conditions, management of the condition is warranted.

valid, Provide, do not treat

19

The two primary goals of prehospital care of a

sexual-assault victim are to preserve the victim's privacy and dignity and to preserve all physical evidence for the police.* In order to preserve _____ _____ of the assault, avoid cleaning wounds and do not allow the victim to bathe or _____ her clothing. If clothing is removed during _____ _____, it should be placed in a brown paper bag and _____ ____ to police officers. Maintain the chain of custody carefully to _____ the evidence.

> change, patient care, handed over, physical evidence, preserve

20
You are dispatched to the home of a _____ patient who has signed a Do Not Resuscitate order. What should you do? Contact medical control before providing any patient care.*
Contact _____ _____ about the specific situation before providing care; this will allow you to provide the type of care that is _____ only. Some states have specific _____ to follow with DNR patients and may even provide various levels of care in a variety of circumstances.

> palliative, medical control, protocols, dying

21
The term *ethics* refers to:
- professional _____ of care
- rules, standards, and morals*
- upgrading standards __ ____
- moral code of _____
_____ refers to rules, standards, and morals that govern actions in a _____.

> Ethics, profession, standards, of care, conduct

Vocabulary 4
accordance /əˈkɔː.dənt s/ v souladu, ve shodě
address /əˈdres/ oslovit
advice /ədˈvaɪs/ rada, doporučení
advisory /ədˈvaɪ.zər.i/ poradenský, poradní
alarm /əˈlɑːm/ poplach, znepokojení
appropriate /əˈprəʊ.pri.ət/ náležitý, patřičný, odpovídající, přiměřený, příslušný, vhodný
authority /ɔːˈθɒr.ɪ.ti/ oprávnění, pravomoc, úřad, správní orgán
confidential /ˌkɒn.fɪˈden.t ʃəl/ důvěrný, tajný
confidentiality /ˌkɒn. fɪ.den.t ʃiˈæl.ɪ.ti/ důvěrnost informací, mlčenlivost

cope /kəʊp/ with /wɪð/ zvládnout, poradit si, vypořádat se, snášet, vyrovnat se, vydržet

custody /ˈkʌs.tə.di/ zadržení, vazba

debrief /ˌdiːˈbriːf/ vyslechnout hlášení o průběhu mise apod.

debriefing /ˌdiːˈbriːf.ɪŋ/ skupinový rozbor traumatické události, druh krizové intervence a pomoci, řízená diskuse spojená s edukací

deceased /dɪˈsiːst/ zemřelý

defamation /ˌdefəˈmeɪʃən/ pomluva, hanobení

delegate /ˈdel.ɪ.gət/ delegát, zástupce, pověřit

devastating /ˈdev.ə.steɪ.tɪŋ/ devastující, zničující, katastrofální

dignity /ˈdɪg.nɪ.ti/ důstojnost (v chování)

direction /daɪˈrek.ʃən/ směr, vedení, řízení, pokyn, instrukce

disentanglement /ˌdɪs.ɪnˈtæŋ.gl.mənt/ rozpletení, vyproštění

drawing /ˈdrɔː.ɪŋ/ natáhnutí

eatery /ˈiːtərɪ/ veřejná jídelna

encounter /ɪnˈkaʊntə/ setkat se, setkání, zkušenost

entrap /ɪnˈtræp/ chytit do pasti, polapit

entrapment /ɪnˈtræp.mənt/ uvíznutí, chycení do pasti

equilibrium /ˌiːkwɪˈlɪbrɪəm/ rovnováha, vyrovnanost, vyváženost

ethics /ˈeθɪk/ etika, morálka

evidence /ˈevɪdəns/ důkaz, známka čeho, svědčit

exacerbation /ɪgˌzæsəˈbeɪʃən/ zhoršení, ztížení

exhaustion /ɪgˈzɔː.s.tʃən/ vyčerpání

fight or flight /ˌfaɪt.ɔː.ˈflaɪt/ reakce na nebezpečí, zůstat a čelit situaci nebo uprchnout

fire-fighting /ˈfaɪəˌfaɪ.tɪŋ/ protipožární zásahy

gear /gɪə/ rychlostní stupeň (u auta), výstroj, výzbroj, vybavení

govern /ˈgʌv.ən/ řídit, ovládat

gunshot /ˈgʌnʃɒt/ střela, výstřel

hand /hænd/ over /ˈəʊ.vər/ předat, odevzdat

hazmat /ˈhæz.mæt/ nebezpečný materiál

homeostasis /ˌhəʊ.mi.əʊˈsteɪ.sɪs/ homeostáza, dynamická rovnováha

integration /ˌɪn.tɪˈgreɪ.ʃən/ integrace, začlenění, včlenění

law /lɔː/ -enforcement /ɪnˈfɔːs.mənt/ agency /ˈeɪ.dʒən.si/ policie a bezpečnostní složky

lengthy /ˈleŋ.θi/ vleklý, zdlouhavý

licensure /ˈlaɪ.sən.ʃər/ udělení licence

lifting /lɪft.ɪŋ/ zdvihání, zvedání

load /ləʊd/ naložit, náklad, zátěž, zatížení, nálož

misinterpret /ˌmɪs.ɪnˈtɜː.prɪt/ nesprávně interpretovat, mylně vyložit

moral /ˈmɒrəl/ morálka, mravy

narrative /ˈnærətɪv/ vyprávění, příběh

oncotic /ɒŋ.kɒ.tɪk/ pressure /ˈpreʃ.ər/ onkotický tlak – osmotický tlak koloidu na membráně

pro koloid nepropustné. O. t.
nitrobuněčných bílkovin zajišťuje
objem intracelulární tekutiny. O. t.
plasmatických bílkovin přispívá k
udržení dostatečného cirkulujícího
objemu krve
online /ˈɒn.laɪn/ online, přímo
spojený
osmolarity /ɒz.məˈlær.ə.ti/
osmolarita, celkové množství
osmoticky aktivních částic
rozpuštěných v litru rozpouštědla,
obv. vody
osmosis /ɒzˈməʊ.sɪs/ osmóza,
samovolné pronikání molekul
rozpouštědla z méně
koncentrovaného roztoku do
roztoku koncentrovanějšího
outcome /ˈaʊtˌkʌm/ výsledek,
výsledek čeho, jak věc dopadne,
závěr
palliative /ˈpæl.i.ə.tɪv/ paliativní,
utišující, bolest zmírňující
peers /pɪərz/ vrstevníci
permissible /pəˈmɪs.ə.bļ/
přípustný, dovolený
permit /pəˈmɪt/ povolit, dovolit
pooling /puːl.ɪŋ/ nahromadění krve
nebo jiné tekutiny, nahromadění
krve je následkem dilatace a
zastavení oběhu v kapilárách a
žilách v oblasti
possession /pəˈzeʃ.ən/ majetek,
vlastnictví
posttraumatic /ˌpəʊst.trɔːˌmæt.ɪk/
posttraumatický, poúrazový
precede /prɪˈsiːd/ předcházet
časově

preserve /prɪˈzɜːv/ zachovat,
uchovat
rape /reɪp/ znásilnit, znásilnění
reasonable /ˈriː.zən.ə.bļ/ přijatelný,
rozumný
refusal /rɪˈfjuːzəl/ odmítnutí
regional /ˈriː.dʒən.əl/ regionální,
týkající se dané oblasti
right /raɪt/ právo
scope /skəʊp/ rozsah
solvent /ˈsɒl.vənt/ ředidlo,
rozpouštědlo
spouse /spaʊs/ choť, manžel/ka
standing /stænd.ɪŋ/ **order** /ˈɔːdə/
trvalý příkaz
statute /ˈstætjuːt/ zákon, předpis
steady /ˈsted.i/ stálý
survivor /səˈvaɪ.vər/ přeživší,
pozůstalý
take /teɪk/ **time** /taɪm/ trvat,
věnovat čas
turn out /ˈtɜːnˌaʊt/ zahnout ven,
naruby, projevit se
upgrade /ʌpˈgreɪd/ zlepšit,
stoupnout, zvýšení
valid /ˈvælɪd/ platný, oprávněný
vent /vent/ ventilovat, otvor,
průduch

VOLUME 2

Unit I

I

You are called for a 55-year-old man who suddenly collapsed. He is _____ ___ _____.
Initial management of this patient's airway should include the insertion of an oropharyngeal airway and ventilation with bag-valve mask.*
An apnoeic and pulseless patient is unlikely to have an intact gag reflex, _____ an OPA to help control the _____ _____.
A BVM will need at least 10 LPM of oxygen flow in order to adequately _____the patient during ventilations.

```
oxygenate, apnoeic and
pulseless, upper airway,
necessitating
```

2

You respond to a college fraternity where you encounter a 19-year-old male with a partially obstructed airway. According to witnesses, he was eating pizza and drinking beer when he began to _____ ___ ____ his throat.
The patient is able to speak in a _____ _____ only, and he has been coughing repeatedly for about 20 minutes.

What is the best treatment for this patient? Remove the _____ with forceps.*
A conscious patient with a partial obstructed airway should be dealt with by _____ _____ and continuous monitoring of patient status. Interventions like Heimlich manoeuvre are considered counterproductive as they may actually _____ the obstruction.
To perform a needle cricothyrotomy, you should place the patient supine with the head and neck hyperextended.*
A _____ _____ will place the anatomical structure.

```
hoarse whisper, hyperextended
position, worsen, identified,
obstruction, cough and grab,
encouraging coughing
```

3

Your patient is a 26-year-old male with a midshaft _____ _____ and no other apparent injuries. The patient is _____ and oriented, and all vital signs are normal. The best way to _____ this fracture is to use:

- the PASG/MAST
- a long spine board
- a traction splint*
- a softly padded board

In a stable patient, the PASG is unnecessary. The long board will not adequately immobilize this injury because the muscles of the leg will _____ and _____ the leg. A padded board may not provide adequate traction to prevent muscle spasms either, so the _____ _____ is the best choice.

---

shorten, immobilize, femur fracture, spasm, alert, transion splint

---

4

A 16-year-old male complains of a fever, sore neck, nausea, vomiting, and headache. During transport, he begins to have a _____. Which of the following would most likely be your field impression?

- _____ abscess
- cerebral _____
- meningitis*
- sepsis

While the other answers are possible, based upon the fever, vomiting, and headache complaints, this is most likely

_____.

---

seizure, neoplasm, meningitis, brain

5

Your patient is a 24-year-old female who shows signs and symptoms of pelvic _____ _____.

What is the goal of _____ _____ for this patient? Make the patient as comfortable as possible and transport to the hospital.*

The goal of prehospital care for patients with PID is to _____ _____. There is no need to perform a _____ _____ or ask any questions regarding sexual contacts.

---

provide comfort, inflammatory disease, vaginal exam, prehospital care

---

6

You respond to a 22-year-old male who is complaining of _____ _____ of chest pain. The patient states that the pain __ _____ and sharp and that it started when he surfaced from a _____ _____ from 60 feet (18.2 metres) down. The patient's diving partner states that the patient _____ too rapidly. What is this patient most likely suffering from? Pulmonary embolism.*
A too-rapid ascent from a scuba dive may result in a pulmonary embolism due to lung

_____.

What does the treatment for this patient consist of? IV, high-flow oxygen, and rapid transport to a recompression chamber.*
An IV, 100% oxygen via a nonrebreather mask, and transport to a _____ _____ are essential for this patient.
Due to his rapid ascent, this patient may also be suffering from

another diving-related emergency: decompression sickness.*
Due to the _____ of the dive and the rapid ascent, this patient may also be suffering from

_____ _____.

What is an additional possible problem associated with this injury? Nitrogen bubbles entering tissue spaces and smaller blood vessels.*

scuba dive, rapid onset, is tearing, decompression sickness, depth, surfaced, overinflation, recompression chamber

7

Your patient is a 28-year-old diver who has been using scuba equipment. His diving partner states that he was unconscious when he surfaced after _ ____.
You should suspect air embolism.*

___ _____ presents as _____ _____ (including unconsciousness) during or after _____ from a dive or as a sharp pain in the chest.
Due to his rapid ascent, this patient may also be _____ ____ another diving related emergency: decompression sickness.*
Due to the depth of the dive and the rapid ascent, this patient

may also be suffering from decompression sickness.
What is an additional possible problem associated with this injury? Nitrogen bubbles entering _____ _____ and smaller blood vessels.*
In this patient, nitrogen ___ _____ may have entered tissue spaces and blood vessels.

a dive, tissue spaces, Air embolism, ascent, suffering from, gas bubbles, neurological deficit

8

This statement about care of a near-drowning _____ is correct: the patient should be admitted to the hospital for observation.*
Due to the chance of post-event pulmonary oedema, all ___-_____ victims should be admitted to the hospital for _____.

victim, near-drowning, observation

9

Your patient is a 23-year-old man who complains of abdominal pain. The patient states that the pain began _____ and was originally located only in the area around the _____.
Now, however, it has moved to the _____ _____ quadrant. The

patient also complains of nausea and vomiting, and he has a fever of 102 °F (38.8 °C). Examination displays rebound _____.
What would you suspect? Apendicitis.*

> tenderness, right lower, suddenly, umbilicus

10

A patient suspected of having an _____ aortic aneurysm will receive oxygen, an IV, ECG monitoring, and rapid transport as part of his or her treatment. What else should you do when treating such a patient? _____ the PASG/MAST garment.*
Treat the patient for shock and transport rapidly. Do not _____ the abdomen. This is one of the few medical conditions that may still benefit from the use of PASG/MAST as the garment may tamponade any _____ that may be occurring. _____, which stimulate the cardiovascular system, should be avoided.

> Medications, bleeding, palpate, Apply, abdominal

11

A 42-year-old male complains of sudden, intense pain that is centred in his _____ _____. He is ____, ____, and diaphoretic,

especially _____ the level of his umbilicus. He is tachycardic and hypotensive.

- What condition best describes the patient presentation? Abdominal aortic aneurysm.*

The abdominal aorta is located in the _____-_____ space. A sudden _____ of pressure due to an aortic aneurysm will result in loss of perfusion below the site of injury.

> lower back, below, pale, cool, retro-peritoneal, loss

12

You are called to the home of a 36-year-old man who is having a seizure. His wife reports that he has not taken his _____ _____ lately and that he has now had three seizures in a row without _____ _____. You have _____ the airway and are now ventilating with the ____ _____ ____.

What should you do next? Begin an IV, monitor cardiac rhythm, and administer diazepam.*
For a patient in _____ _____, treatment consists of establishing an IV, monitoring cardiac rhythm, and administering diazepam to stop the seizures.

> status epilepticus, seizure pills, regaining consciousness, bag-valve mask, secured

13

What is the primary reason that diazepam is given to a seizure patient? To suppress the spread of electrical activity in the brain and relax muscles.*
Although diazepam (Valium) does reduce _____, it is given to seizure patients to suppress the spread of _____ _____ through the brain as well as to _____ _____.

> anxiety, relax muscles, electrical activity

14

A 52-year-old male has been ejected from a car. He is apnoeic, with a slow pulse palpated at the _____ _____.

What procedure would best manage this patient's airway? Ventilate with the bag-valve mask and attach to high-flow oxygen.* This patient needs immediate _____ ___ _____.

Using a bag-valve mask will _____ this task most effectively.

> accomplish, oxygenation and ventilation, femoral artery

15

Your patient is a 27-year-old male who is found unconscious on a bathroom floor. He is not breathing, has _____ _____,

and has a fresh _____ wound to his right forearm. He has _____ _____ that form a bluish streak over the veins on the backs on both hands. This patient is most likely suffering from which of the following?

- a seizure disorder
- multiple spider bites
- a narcotic overdose*
- anaphylactic shock

Common signs of a _____ _____ are described: pinpoint pupils are characteristic of heroin and narcotic use, a fresh puncture wound over a vein indicates a recent _____ ____, and _____ _____ over the veins is consistent with the presence of track marks.

> bluish scarring, multiple scars, puncture, narcotic overdose, injection site, pinpoint pupils

16

A 24-year-old female is complaining of chest pain and difficulty breathing. She has been up for three days studying for finals and has been taking ephedrine supplements to help her _____ _____ and alert. She also admits to drinking twelve _____ soft drinks in the past day. Vitals are as follows: BP, 80/40; P, 180 carotid; and R, 42. She is ____ _____ and lethargic.

The best treatment for this patient would include cardioversion at 100 joules.*
This patient presents in unstable supraventricular _____.
Her condition may _____ quickly; therefore, immediate synchronized _____ is indicated.

cardioversion, caffeinated, stay awake, tachycardia, very pale, deteriorate

17
Your patient is a 19-year-old female who has been stung by a stingray while swimming. What should you do after _____ that airway, breathing and circulation are intact? Apply heat or warm water to reduce pain and _____ the poison.* Heat will cause the _____ to break down and _____ the harm to the patient.

detoxify, poison, ensuring, lessen

18
Your patient is a comatose 56-year-old male. His breath smells fruity and sweet, and his respirations are very deep and rapid.
After the initial assessment, you should provide the following treatments: draw blood, start an

IV of 0.9% NaCl, and give a 500 ml fluid bolus.*
This patient is showing signs and symptoms of diabetic _____. Avoid the use of _____ _____ if at all possible.
At the minimum, you should obtain a _____ _____ before administering any glucose-containing solutions. The fluid bolus will help _____ the glucose contained within his blood.

glucose administration, glucometer reading, ketoacidosis, dilute

19
Your patient is a 30-year-old female who is complaining of a generalized rash and a dyspnoea after eating shellfish. The patient has small itchy red welts all over her body and says her tongue feels like it is swollen. She complains of difficulty moving air in and difficulty _____ _ ____ _____. This patient's vital signs show a blood pressure of 110/60; a pulse of 100, strong and regular; and a respiratory rate of 36. Her breathing is somewhat shallow and _____.
This patient is exhibiting the signs and symptoms of an allergic reaction.*

This patient's blood pressure is still _____ ___ the allergic reaction; therefore, the patient is not in anaphylactic shock.
This patient needs close monitoring because she could _____ ____ anaphylactic shock.*

compensating for, catching a full breath, progress into, laboured

20
You respond to a 17-year-old female found unconscious in her backyard by her parents. She has a newly developing skin rash on her right arm and is having difficulty breathing. You note that she is wheezing. Her parents state that she has no history of respiratory problems or other medical disorders.
Which of the following is a possible cause of her condition?
- anaphylaxis*
- febrile seizures
- status asthmaticus
- epiglottitis

The environment she is in and previously unseen ____, _____, difficulty breathing and negative past history are keys to this being a case of possible anaphylactic shock.
What is the first step in managing this patient? Aggressively manage the airway.*

You should aggressively manage the airway. It may be necessary to _____ _____ this patient, and you may get only one attempt. Once the tube contacts the larynx, the _____ _____ can spasm and completely shut off the airway.
The next step in treating this patient is to start a normal saline or Ringer's lactate IV and to give epinephrine*
Epinephrine is a potent _____ and can reverse many of the effects of histamine _____. This patient is __ _____ and should first be treated with epinephrine. If respiratory _____ continues once the epinephrine has entered the patient's system, you may try using diphenhydramine (another antihistamine) or albuterol to bring about _____.

antihistamine, distress, bronchodilation, carefully intubate, rash, vocal cords, in extremis, overload, wheezing

Vocabulary I

abdominal /æbˈdɒm.ɪ.nəl/ **thrust** / θrʌst/ břišní úder, první pomoc při dušení

abscess /ˈæb.ses/ absces

accomplish /əˈkʌm.plɪʃ/ dosáhnout, provést, uskutečnit

admit /ədˈmɪt/ připustit, uznat, hospitalizovat

aggressively /əˈgres.ɪv.li/ agresivně, útočně

air /ˈeər/ **embolism** /ˈem.bə.lɪ.zəm/ vzduchová embolie

anaphylaxis /ˌæn.ə.fɪˈlæk. sɪs/ anafylaxe, druh alergie, přecitlivělosti na cizorodou bílkovinu

ascent /əˈsent/ stoupání, výstup

bag /bæg/ **mask** /mɑːsk/ dýchací maska, ambuvak, resuscitační vak, samorozpínatelný vak s maskou

bolus /ˈbəʊ.ləs/ jednorázově podaná dávka léku

break /breɪk/ **down** /daʊn/ porucha, porušení, havárie, defekt, zhroutit se, nevydržet

bring /brɪŋ/ **about** /əˈbaʊt/ způsobit, vyvolat

bronchodilation /ˌbrɒŋ.kəʊ. ˈdɪleɪʃən/ dilatace, rozšíření průdušek

caffeinated /ˈkæf.ɪ.neɪ.tɪd/ s kofeinem (nápoj)

cardioversion /ˌkɑː.di.əˈvɜː.ʃən/ kardioverze, elektrický výboj použitý při léčbě srdečních arytmií

catching /ˈkætʃ.ɪŋ/ nakažlivý, přenosný

center /ˈsen.tər/ střed, centrum, středisko

comfortable /ˈkʌmf.tər.bəl/ pohodlný, příjemný

consciousness /ˈkɒn.ʃəs.nəs/ vědomí, povědomí

counterproductive /ˌkaʊn. tə.prəˈdʌk.tɪv/ kontraproduktivní, mající opačný účinek

cricothyreotomy /ˈkraɪ.kə.θaɪəˈrɒ. tə.mɪ/ krikotyreotomie, chirurg. rozdělení chrupavky prstencové a štítné

decompression /ˌdiː.kəmˈpreʃ.ən/ **sickness** /ˈsɪk.nəs/ dekompresní nemoc

deficit /ˈdef.ɪ.sɪt/ deficit, nedostatek

detoxify /diːˈtɒk.sɪ.faɪ/ detoxikovat

dilute /daɪˈluːt/ zředit, oslabit

diphenhydramine /di.fenˈhɪ. drə.mɪːn/ difenylhydramin, antihistaminikum, užívané v léčbě alergických poruch

diving /ˈdaɪ.vɪŋ/ **reflex** /ˈriː.fleks/ reflex zahrnující kardiovaskulární a metabolické adaptace pro uchování kyslíku vyskytující se u živočichů během potápění do vody

drowning /ˈdraʊn.ɪŋ/ tonutí, utopení

encourage /ɪnˈkʌr.ɪdʒ/ povzbudit, vést

femoral /ˈfemərəl/ femorální, stehenní

final /ˈfaɪ.nəl/ závěrečná zkouška

forceps /ˈfɔː.seps/ chirurgické, lékařské kleště

fraternity /frəˈtɜː.nə.ti/ bratrstvo, jednota
fruity /ˈfruː.ti/ ovocný
gag /gæg/ **reflex** /ˈriːfleks/ reflex zvracení
garment /ˈgɑːmənt/ oděv, oblek
glucose /ˈgluː.kəʊs/ glukóza, hroznový cukr
goal /gəʊl/ cíl
grab /græb/ snažit se popadnout
haemostasis /ˌhiː.məˈsteɪ.sɪs/ hemostáza, zástava krvácení, zástava krevní cirkulace
Heimlich maneuver /ˈhaɪm.lɪk.məˌnu.vər/ Heimlichův manévr je určený k vypuzení předmětu, který ucpal dýchací cesty
in extremis /ˌɪn.ɪkˈstriː.mɪs/ krajní, v krajním případě
itchy /ˈɪtʃ.i/ svědivý
MAST, **Military Anti-Shock Trousers** vojenské protišokové pneumatické kalhoty viz také PASG
mid /mɪd/ střední
NaCl, **sodium** /ˈsəʊ.di.əm/ **chloride** /ˈklɔː.raɪd/ chlorid sodný, kuchyňská sůl
near /nɪər/ téměř, blízko
necessitate /nəˈses.ɪ.teɪt/ vyžadovat, vynutit si
neoplasm /ˌniː.əʊˈplæz.əm/ zhoubný nádor
neurological /ˌnjʊə.rəˈlɒdʒ.ɪ.kəl/ neurologický
nitrogen /ˈnaɪ.trə.dʒən/ dusík, dusíkatý
nonrebreather /ˌnɒn.rəbrə.ðər/ **mask** / mɑːsk/ dýchací

maska jednocestnou klapkou, vydechnutý oxid uhličitý je vyloučen a není znovu vdechován
oropharyngeal /ˈɔː.rə.fəˈrɪn.dʒi.əl/ orofaryngeální, týkající se úst a hltanu
overinflation /ˌəʊvə.ɪnˈfleɪʃ.ən/ nadměrné naplnění vzduchem, nahuštění
overload /ˌəʊ.vəˈləʊd/ přetížit, přetížení
oxygenate /ˈɒk.sɪ.dʒə.neɪt/ okysličovat
padded /ˈpæd.ɪd/ vycpaný, s vycpávkou
PASG, **Pneumatic** /njʊˈmætɪk/ **Antishock** /ˈæn.tɪ.ʃɒk / **Garment** / ˈgɑːmənt/ nafukovací oblek, používaný k potlačení šoku, stabilizaci zlomenin, podporování hemostázy a zvýšení periferní cévní rezistence, viz také MAST
pneumatic /njʊˈmætɪk/ vzduchový, na stlačený vzduch
poison /ˈpɔɪ.zən/ jed, otrávit
pulseless /pʌls.ləs/ bez pulzu
recompression /ˌriː.kəmˈpreʃ.ən/ **chamber** /ˈtʃeɪm.bər/ rekompresní komora
regain /rɪˈgeɪn/ znovu získat, vrátit
retroperitoneal /ˌret.rəʊˌper.ɪ.təʊ.ˈniː.əl/ ležící za pobřišnicí
reverse /rɪˈvɜːs/ zvrátit, změnit, otočit, opačně, pozpátku
Ringer's lactate /lækˈteɪt/ Ringerův roztok, infuzní roztok, podobně jako fyziologický roztok je izotonický a obsahuje ionty sodíku a chloru, navíc pak obsahuje ionty

draslíku a vápníku, čímž je bližší
složení krevní plasmy
scar /skɑːr/ jizva, zjizvit
scuba diving /ˈskuː.bəˌdaɪ.vɪŋ/
potápění s dýchacím přístrojem,
sportovní potápění
shaft /ʃɑːft/ diafýza, střední část
dlouhé kosti
shellfish /ˈʃel.fɪʃ/ měkkýši, korýši
shut /ʃʌt/ **off** /ɒf/ vypnout, zastavit,
odtáhnout
softly /ˈsɒft.li/ jemně, tlumeně
sore /sɔːr/ bolavý, bolestivý
spasm /ˈspæz.əm/ křeč, záchvat
spider /ˈspaɪ.dər/ pavouk
spine /spaɪn/ **board** /bɔːd/ páteřní
deska
splint /splɪnt/ dlaha, zpevnit
dlahou
status /ˈsteɪ.təs/ status, stav
stingray /ˈstɪŋ.reɪ/ trnucha, rejnok
s jedovým bodcem na ocase
streak /striːk/ stopa, proužek
suddenly /ˈsʌd.ən.li/ náhle,
najednou
suffering /ˈsʌf.ər.ɪŋ/ from trpící čím
suit /sjuːt/ oblek
supplement /ˈsʌp.lɪ.mənt/ doplnit,
dodatek
suppress /səˈpres/ potlačit, zastavit
track /træk/ dráha, cesta, sledovat
traction /ˈtræk.ʃən/ trakce, tah
tube /tjuːb/ trubice, trubička

umbilicus /ʌmˈbɪl.ɪ.kəs/ pupek
unconsciousness /ʌnˈkɒn.ʃəs.nəs/
bezvědomí
unlikely /ʌnˈlaɪ.kli/
nepravděpodobný
unseen /ʌnˈsiːn/ neviditelný,
nevídaný
valve /vælv/ klapka, ventil
welt /welt/ šrám, podlitina
whisper /ˈwɪs.pər/ šeptat, šepot
worsen /ˈwɜː.sən/ zhoršit (se)

Unit 2

1

What is the reason for giving _____ beta agonists to patients with severe allergic reactions? To reverse bronchospasm and relax airways.*

____ _____ such as albuterol help in the treatment of severe allergic reactions by relaxing the _____ and thus relieving _____.

> Beta agonists, airway, bronchospasm, inhaled

2

Your patient is a 27-year-old male who has fallen from a 24-foot (7.3 m) ladder. As you are approaching and forming your general impression, you note that he is conscious and talking. What should you do first?

_____ stabilize his neck in a neutral position.*

The _____ is always given first priority, but in this case, since the patient __ _____, the first step in his assessment and care would be to stabilize the _____ _____ as you begin your ___ _____.

> ABC assessment, is talking, cervical spine, Manually, airway

3

When using the OPQRST _____ to assess a patient's pain, you would assess the R portion of the mnemonic by asking, 'Does the pain move anywhere?'*

R stands for _____. You should determine if the pain is radiating, _____, or causing any _____ _____.

> radiation, referred, associated problem, mnemonic

4

The focused history and physical examination of a patient begins after you have controlled the immediate threats to the patient's life.*

The purpose of the focused history and physical examination is to detect additional problems after you have controlled _____ _____ to the patient's life. The _____ _____ is typically performed during transport. _____ _____ may be consulted anytime during the call when you feel it is _____ or whenever your protocols and standing orders require it.

> appropriate, Medical control, ongoing assessment, immediate threats

5

Using your sense of touch during a physical examination is called palpation.*
The technique of _____ is using touch during a _____ _____ to gather information.
_____ is listening with a stethoscope;
_____ is using gentle tapping in order to identify the presence of air or fluid in body tissues.

Percussion, Auscultation, physical examination, palpation

6

What are the components of the focused history and physical exam? SAMPLE history and focused examination.*
The _____ _____ and physical exam, undertaken only after _____ _____ to life have been corrected, consists of ascertaining the nature of _____ __ _____, previous history (via SAMPLE), _____ _____, and focused exam.

focused history, illness or injury, immediate threats, vital signs

7

What is the purpose of the OPQRST mnemonic? To define the major complaint.*

The OPQRST mnemonic is used to define the ____ _____ associated with _____ _____ such as pain, dyspnoea, dizziness, and vague sensations. It is not usually used in trauma or _____ _____.

medical conditions, actual unconsciousness, chief complaint

8

What is a major concern when dealing with a patient with organophosphate poisoning? Exposure of rescuers to the poison.*
_____ to organophosphate is a major concern. Proper _____ _____ are _____ to rescuer safety.
_____ __ all patient clothing according to Environmental Protection Agency guidelines.

Dispose of, Exposure, paramount, isolation procedures

9

Your patient is a farmer who has employed a crop cluster to spray his fields. The fields were sprayed earlier today, and now, the farmer has teary eyes, nausea and vomiting, diarrhoea, and excessive salivation.

What was he most likely poisoned with? Organophosphates.*
The symptoms of organophosphate _____ are described by the acronym SLUDGE (excessive _____, _____, _____, diarrhoea, gastrointestinal distress, _____).

salivation, absorption, emesis, lacrimation, urination

10

What _____ is commonly used to treat patients who are the victims of organophosphate poisoning? Atropine sulfate.*
A large dose of atropine sulfate is used to _____ cholinergic poisoning from _____ and carbamates.

counteract, organophosphates, medication

11

A victim is unresponsive after a possible exposure to _____ _____ in a closed garage. Which of the following procedures should you do first?

- Wait for properly trained personnel to enter and evacuate the garage.*
- ____ the windows of the garage to ventilate the environment.
- _____ high-flow oxygen to the patient via positive-pressure ventilations.
- _____ the patient from the environment.

Safety first! Of the three _____ options, _____ _____ and protected rescuers can remove the patient safely.

extrication, Provide, carbon monoxide, properly trained, Open, Remove

12

Which finding is helpful __ _____ poisoning by spider venom from an acute abdominal condition?

- abdominal rigidity with no palpable tenderness*
- right lower-quadrant pain in the absence of fever
- diaphoresis accompanied by _____ ___ _____
- the presence of multiple ____ _____ on the stomach

This finding is helpful in ruling out acute abdomen as the cause.
_____ _____ generally always has pain associated with rigidity, whereas a _____ ____ may be painless initially due to the neurotoxicity of the _____. Spiders _____ bite more than once, ruling

out the last choice as a realistic clue.

> rarely, in distinguishing, spider bite, bite marks, chills and fever, Acute abdomen, venom

13
These are characteristic of a mild or moderate pit viper envenomation:
- _____ located around the wound site*
- _____ _____ like nausea or vomiting*
- localised _____ at the wound site*

Pit viper _____ is generally very painful. Little or no pain is characteristic of coral snake (_____) envenomation.

> neurotoxic, systemic effects, envenomation, bruising, oedema

14
The physiological cause of the anxiety and restlessness that make up the classic _____ _____ of shock is a _____ _____ of what phenomenon? The release of catecholamines.*
The release of catecholamines that results from the initial drop in blood pressure causes the feelings of _____ ___ _____.

> early signs, anxiety and restlessness, direct result

15
A patient who experienced a seizure, rather than a period of syncope, usually reports that the episode happened without any warning.*
_____, unlike syncope, do not usually have _____ _____ such as a period of light-headedness. Some seizures are _____ ___ a feeling or sensation of impending seizure called an aura.

> preceded by, Seizures, warning signs

16
During the initial phase of an acute stress reaction, what physiological response will occur? Increased pulse rate and papillary dilatation.*
Both good stress (_____) and bad stress (_____) will initially cause sympathetic stimulation such as _____ heart and respiratory rate, bronchodilation, _____ _____, and increased blood flow to the _____ _____.

> skeletal muscles, distress, increased, dilated pupils, eustress

17

Continual reexperiencing of a traumatic event is a characteristic of which of the following?
• an _____ disorder
• stress and _____
• cumulative stress reaction
• delayed stress reaction*

_____ _____ _____, or post-traumatic stress disorder, is characterized by reexperiencing of the traumatic event and diminished responsiveness to _____ ___, as well as physical and cognitive symptoms.

burnout, anxiety, Delayed stress reaction, everyday life

18

• What signs and symptoms are characteristic of a patient in compensated shock? Lethargy; confusion; pulse and blood, pressure normal to slightly elevated; skin, cool; and capillary refill, delayed.*

The signs and symptoms given – _____; _____; pulse and blood pressure, normal to slightly elevated; skin, cool; and _____ _____, delayed – are characteristic of early, or compensated, shock. The single characteristic signalling the change from compensated to uncompensated shock is

a drop in blood pressure that remains below normal despite _____ ___ _____.

You _____ _____ wait to see a decrease in BP to decide if shock is present or not since early __ ___ _____ _____; sympathetic stimulation during compensation may result in a slight elevation of the diastolic blood pressure.

intervention and treatment, lethargy, capillary refill, in the shock process, confusion, should never

19

What is the purpose of the body's _____ _____ to a stressor? To prepare for the most efficient reaction.*

All the components of the stress reaction – _____ ___ ACTH, relaxation of the young healthy adult, _____ _____, slowdown of _____, release of adrenaline – prepare the body to react to the _____ as efficiently as possible.

stressor, bronchial tree, physiological response, release of, digestion

20

Why are vital sign changes not a good early indicator of shock in a young, healthy adult? The

body attempts to compensate __
_____ normal vital signs.*
The body's physiological
mechanism _____ ___
the insult that causes shock.
Therefore, although changes in
_____ _____ are ominous late
signs in patients with poor tissue
perfusion, they are unlikely to
occur in a _____, _____ _____
who has just entered a state of
shock.

> young, healthy adult, by
> maintaining, compensate for,
> vital signs

Vocabulary 2
ACTH, **Adrenocorticotropic** /əˌdriː.nəʊˌkɔː.tɪ.kəʊˈtrɒf.ɪk/ **Hormone** /ˈhɔː.məʊn/ adrenokortikotropní hormon
actual /ˈæk.tʃu.əl/ skutečný, opravdový, současný
aldosterone /ˈɔːl.dəs.tər.əʊn/ aldosteron, mineralokortikoidní hormon vylučovaný nadledvinami
ataxia /əˈtæk.si.ə/ ataxie, ztráta kontroly volních pohybů
atropine /ˈæt.rə.pɪn/ **sulfate** /ˈsʌl.feɪt/ atropin-sulfát, lék
aura /ˈɔː.rə/ aura, předzvěst, bezprostřední známky blížícího se záchvatu
beta-2 /ˈbiː.tə.tuː/ **agonists** /ˈæg.ə.nɪsts/ beta-2 agonisté, uvolňují a otevírají dýchací cesty, které se během astmatického záchvatu zužují,

astma „uvolňovače" nebo bronchodilatátory
burnout /ˈbɜːnaʊt/ vyhoření, naprosté vyčerpání
carbamate /ˈkɑː.bəˌmeɪt/ sůl nebo ester kyseliny karbamové (karbamová kyselina – H_2N–COOH, kyselina, která se okamžitě rozpadá na oxid uhličitý a amoniak; její soli jsou karbamáty, otrava, stažení zorniček, svalový třes, salivace, ataxie, dyspnoe
cervical /ˈsɜː.vɪkəl/ **spine** /spaɪn/ krční páteř
cholinergic /kɒ.lɪn.ə.dʒɪk/ cholinergický
cluster /ˈklʌs.tər/ shluk, hlouček, skupinka, trs, hrozen
cognitive /ˈkɑg.nə.tɪv/ kognitivní, poznávací
coral /ˈkɒr.əl/ **snake** /sneɪk/ korálovec
counteract /ˌkaʊn.tərˈækt/ působit proti, potlačovat
crop /krɒp/ úroda, sklizeň
cumulative /ˈkjuː.mjʊ.lə.tɪv/ kumulativní, hromadící se
diarrhoea /ˌdaɪ.əˈriː.ə/ průjem
digestion /daɪˈdʒes.tʃən/ trávení, zažívání
dilatation /ˌdɪl.əˈteɪ.ʃən/ dilatace, rozšíření
disorder /dɪˌsɔː.dər/ porucha
efficiently /ɪˈfɪʃ.ənt.li/ efektivně, účinně
emesis /eˈmɪ.sɪs/ emeze, zvracení

envenomation /ɪn͵ven.ə'meɪ.ʃən/ vniknutí jedu do těla při kousnutí nebo štípnutí

eustress /juː.stres/ dobrý, pozitivní stres

evacuate /ɪ'væk.ju.eɪt/ evakuovat, vyklidit

event /ɪ'vent/ událost, případ, akce

examination /ɪg͵zæm.ɪ'neɪ.ʃən/ lékařská prohlídka, vyšetření

experienced /ɪk'spɪə.ri.ənst/ zkušený, zběhlý

general /'dʒen.ər.əl/ celkový, všeobecný

guideline /'gaɪd.laɪn/ směrnice, instrukce

history /'hɪs.tər.i/ anamnéza

illness /'ɪl.nəs/ nemoc

in order to /'ɔː.dər/ aby, kvůli

intake /'ɪn.teɪk/ příjem, přísun

lacrimation /͵læk.ri'meɪ.ʃən/ slzení

leading /'liː.dɪŋ/ vedoucí

lethargy /'leθ.ə.dʒi/ letargie, netečnost

medical /'med.ɪ.kəl/ léčebný, léčivý, lékařský

mnemonic /nɪ'mɒn.ɪk/ mnemotechnická pomůcka

moderate / 'mɒd.ər.ət/ mírný, nevelký, střední, umírněný, přiměřený

nature /'neɪ.tʃər/ povaha, podstata, charakter

neurotoxicity /͵njʊər.ə.tɒk'sɪs.ɪ.ti/ neurotoxicita, schopnost ničit nervovou tkáň

onset /'ɒn͵set/ nástup

OPQRST, Onset, Provocation, Quality, Radiation, Severity, Time cílená anamnéza, kdy bolest začala, co ji zhoršuje, jak je pociťována, zda se přemisťuje, jak je vážná, jak dlouho trvá

oral /'ɔː.rəl/ ústní, verbální

organophosphates /ɔː͵gæn.əʊ'fɒs.feɪts/ organofostáty, organické sloučeniny fosforu

palpable /'pæl.pə.bl̩/ hmatný, zřetelný

paramount /'pær.ə.maʊnt/ prvořadý, nejzásadnější

past /pɑːst/ minulý, dřívější

phenomenon /fə'nɒm.ɪ.nən/ pl

phenomena fenomén, jev, úkaz

physiological /͵fɪz.i'ɒl.ə.dʒi.kəl/ fyziologický

pit /pɪt/ **viper** /'vaɪ.pər/ chřestýšovec, chřestýšovitý had

portion /'pɔː.ʃən/ část, díl, rozdělit

positive /'pɒz.ə.tɪv/ pozitivní, kladný

pressure /'preʃ.ər/ tlak

previous /'priː.vi.əs/ předchozí, předešlý

provocation /͵prɒvə'keɪʃən/ vyprovokování

quadrant /'kwɒd.rənt/ kvadrant, čtvrtina kruhu

quality /kwɒlɪtɪ/ povaha, vlastnost

radiation /͵reɪ.di'eɪ.ʃən/ vyzařování

reexperience /͵riː.ɪk'spɪə.ri.əns/ znovu prožít, prodělat

refill /'riː.fɪl/ plnění, doplnění, doplnit, dolít, znovu se naplnit

responsiveness /rɪ'spɒn.sɪv.nəs/ schopnost reagovat, reakce

233

restlessness /'rest.ləs.nəs/ neklid, nepokoj

salivation /'sæl.ɪ.veɪ.ʃən/ salivace, slinění

SAMPLE, Signs and **Symptoms, Allergies, Medications, Past medical histor**y, **Last oral intake** mnemotechnická pomůcka (příznaky a symptomy, alergie, léky, minulá zdravotní anamnéza, poslední příjem ústy, události vedoucí k poranění či nemoci) pro klíčové otázky při posuzování stavu pacienta, užívá se spolu s hodnocením životních znaků, viz také OPQRST

severity / sɪ'ver.ɪ.ti/ vážnost, útrapy

signal /'sɪg.nəl/ signál, znamení, signalizovat, indikovat

skeletal /'skel.ɪ.təl/ skeletální, kosterní

slowdown /'sləʊ.daʊn/ zpomalení

sludge /slʌdʒ/ kal, usazenina

SLUDGE, Salivation, Lacrimation, Urination, Diarrhoea, Gastrointestinal distress, Emesis příznaky otravy, slinění, slzení, močení, průjem, zažívací potíže, zvracení

spray /spreɪ/ rozprašovač, postříkat

stressor /'strɛs.ə/ stresor, prostředek, stav či podnět, který způsobí stres

symptom /'sɪmp.təm/ symptom, příznak

tap /tæp/ poklepat, zaťukání

teary /'tɪə.r.i/ uslzený

time /taɪm/ čas

uncompensated /ˌʌnˈkɒmpənseɪtɪd/ nekompenzovaný

unlike /ʌnˈlaɪk/ na rozdíl od, odlišný od

vague /veɪg/ vágní, nejasný, neurčitý

venom /'venəm/ jed hadí ap.

warning /'wɔː.nɪŋ/ varování, upozornění

whereas /weərˈæz/ kdežto, zatímco

Unit 3

I

A patient presents with symptoms of _____, _____, hives, difficulty breathing, decreased blood pressure, and dizziness. What should you suspect? Anaphylaxis.*

_____, accompanied by difficulty breathing, strongly _____ anaphylaxis.

---

suggest, Hives, flushing, itching

2

While assessing a patient complaining of difficulty breathing, you note an _____ _____ _____, stridor, chest tightness, and tachycardia.

Based on these symptoms, you should suspect anaphylaxis.*

_____ indicates an upper-airway obstruction, in this case most likely from an allergic reaction. A patient with _____ would exhibit difficulty breathing with wheezing and rhonchi. A patient with _____ will exhibit wheezing respirations. A patient suffering from a CVA would have an altered mental status but would not have stridor.

Asthma, Stridor, altered mental status, emphysema

3

What is the first sign of _____ _____ in a patient _____ ____ anaphylaxis?

- wheezing
- coughing
- hoarseness*
- dyspnoea

The first sign of laryngeal oedema is usually a _____ _____.

---

hoarse voice, laryngeal oedema, suffering from

4

What are the two most common causes of _____ anaphylaxis? Penicillin and insect bites/stings.*

_____ antigens are likely to cause the most severe reactions; penicillin and insect stings are the two ____ _____ causes of severe anaphylaxis.

Injected, most common, severe

5

What is the _____ ____ for the management of acute anaphylaxis? Epinephrine.*

To manage _____ _____, epinephrine is the first medication used. Epinephrine is a potent antihistamine and immediately _____ the physiological effects of the reaction (vasodilation, bronchoconstriction, and _____ _____).

> airway swelling, primary drug,
> reverses, acute anaphylaxis

6

Epinephrine 1:1,000 may be
indicated in:
- asthma*
- epiglottitis
- pertussis
- emphysema

As a _____, epinephrine
1:1,000 is sometimes _____
in younger (ʿ 35 years old) _____
patients.

> indicated, asthma,
> bronchodilator

7

An important disadvantage
in using both nasal- and
oropharyngeal airway adjuncts is
that they are unable to protect the
lower airway from aspiration.*
Neither the nasopharyngeal nor
the oropharyngeal airway is long
enough to _____ the lower
airway from _____ _____.
Generally, the presence of
_____ __ _____ in the airway
does not affect their use since
suction is easily performed
through and around these
devices. The _____ come in a
wide variety of sizes and styles.
Use of the oropharyngeal airway
is limited to patients who do not
have a ___ _____.

> vomitus or blood, protect,
> gag reflex, devices, aspirated
> material

8

Your patient has suffered
_____ trauma to the neck
and is bleeding _____ from
several large vessels.
You should apply an occlusive
dressing, then apply pressure.*
Apply an _____ _____
(a gloved hand can be used in
the interim until the occlusive
dressing is applied), then
attempt to stop the bleeding with
_____, _____ _____, but do
not clamp neck vessels. Medical
control may also direct _____
with a gloved finger.

> profusely, tamponade, constant,
> direct pressure, occlusive
> dressing, penetrating

9

You are caring for a patient
whose finger was just cut off in an
accident.
What should you do with the
amputated finger? Place the
_____ finger in a plastic bag
and _____ the bag in cold
water.*
Do not allow the severed digit to
___ ___ because tissues will begin
to draw in the hypotonic fluid
and _____ __, which may make
reimplantation impossible. The

_____ _____ will help reduce
_____ _____ by the cells of the
severed digit and will help keep it
_____ longer.

> cold environment, get wet,
> severed, oxygen demand, swell
> up, immerse, alive

10

Assessment and care of a patient
who is a victim of sexual assault
should include the following:
place sterile dressings on any
wounds.*
Do not _____ a vaginal exam,
ask detailed questions about
the _____ in the field, or _____
the patient to change clothes
or bathe. You should not overly
_____ any wounds you encounter,
but instead wrap them up with
dry _____ _____. Place
any clothing or other evidence
removed from a patient in a clean
_____ ___ and take it with you to
the hospital.

> paper bag, assault, allow, sterile
> dressings, perform, clean

11

Your patient is hypothermic with
a body temperature of 93 °F
(33.9 °C). The patient is likely __
_____ which of the following
symptoms?
- severe shivering
- impaired judgement*

- respiratory depression
- bradycardia

This patient is experiencing early
to moderate _____ and
is likely to manifest _____
_____, _____ _____,
normal blood pressure, and
tachycardia. Severe _____
generally peaks around 95 °F
and continues to decrease in
intensity until ____ _____
reaches the high 80s; it then
stops altogether. Respiratory
depression and bradycardia occur
when the temperature _____ into
the mid 80s.

> shivering, impaired judgement,
> hypothermia, to exhibit,
> slurred speech, drops, body
> temperature

12

Shivering _____ in a hypothermic
patient when the body
temperature drops below 86 °F
(30 °C).*
_____ is the body's attempt
to _____ body temperature.
Shivering continues until the body
temperature reaches about 86
°F (30 °C). ____ __ shivering in
a hypothermic patient indicates
_____ _____.

> Lack of, regulate, severe
> hypothermia, Shivering, ceases

13

Which of the following patients shows signs and symptoms of heat exhaustion?

a) Male, age 34; severe _____ _____ in legs and abdomen; fatigue and dizziness

b) Female, age 45; rapid, shallow respirations; weak pulse; cold, clammy skin; dizziness*

c) Male, age 42; deep respirations; _____, _____ pulse; dry, hot skin; loss of _____

d) Female, age 70; shallow respirations; weak, rapid pulse; dilated pupils; _____

Patients c and d show signs and symptoms of heatstroke, and patient a shows signs of heat cramps.

> consciousness, rapid, strong, muscle cramps, seizures

14

Which of the following patient scenarios is the typical profile for a victim of classic ___ _____?

- a healthy young adult who has been _____ in hot, humid weather
- someone _____ profusely and drinking large amounts of water without salt

- an elderly person with chronic illness who __ _____ to a hot room*
- __ _____ who is exposed to overly high ambient temperatures indoors

Although any of these individuals could suffer from heatstroke, the _____ _____ represents the typical profile of a victim of classic heatstroke.

> is confined, sweating, elderly person, heatstroke, exercising, an infant

15

A patient begins to have a _____ _____ while running a marathon on a hot day. Which of the following procedures should you do first?

- Move the patient into the _____.
- _____ 5 mg diazepam intravenously.
- Establish an airway and ventilate the patient.*
- Place ____ _____ around the neck and under the arms.

While the other procedures are applicable to the treatment of a possible heatstroke victim, _____ the airway and _____ respirations should occur first.

> securing, ambulance, administer, cold packs, generalized seizure, ensuring

16

Which of the following patients is considered to be at ____ ____ for a heat-related emergency?
- 29-year-old _____
- 48-year-old police officer
- 17-year-old athlete
- 78-year-old diabetic*

The very young, the very old, those undernourished, and those with chronic illness are all predisposed to ____ _____ for a variety of reasons.

heat illness, high risk, amputee

17

You are called to the scene of a possible drowning at a local pool. Upon arrival, you discover that _____ have removed the patient from the pool and are performing _____ _____ since the patient is apnoeic with a pulse.

_____ should consist of defibrillation at 200 joules.*
The patient presents with pulseless ventricular tachycardia, a _____ _____. Immediate defibrillation is indicated to terminate this event.

Management, lifeguards, lethal rhythm, rescue ventilations

18

What is the most important treatment consideration for a patient who is suffering from _____ _____? Provide high-concentration oxygen with a nonrebreather mask.*
_____ _____ at 100% concentration and intubate if the patient is not breathing _____.

Provide oxygen, decompression sickness, spontaneously

19

What is the correct field treatment for a _____ body part? Transport the patient to the hospital.*
The correct treatment is _____ _____ in a water bath maintained between 100 °F (37.8 °C) and 106 °F (41 °C), although this treatment should not be attempted __ ___ _____ because of the danger of _____. Pain management is essential because the procedure is _____ _____.

in the field, gradual warming, extremely painful, refreezing, frostbitten

20

A patient presents with _____ _____ at a rate of 6 per minute. What should you do next?
_____ positive-pressure ventilation with a BVM.*

The respiratory rate is too slow and must __ _____ immediately with _____ assistance.

> ventilatory, Administer, be corrected, shallow breaths

Vocabulary 3
accident /ˈæksɪdənt/ nehoda, neštěstí
adjunct /ˈædʒ.ʌŋkt/ dodatek, doplněk, přidružený, pomocný
alive /əˈlaɪv/ živý, naživu
amputee /ˌæm.pjʊˈtiː/ osoba, která se podrobila amputaci
antigen /ˈæn.tɪ.dʒən/ antigen
applicable /əˈplɪk.ə.bl̩/ platný, použitelný
bathe /beɪð/ koupat, omýt, vymýt ránu
cease /siːs/ přestat, ustat, zastavit se
cerebrovascular / ˌser.ɪ.brəˈvæskjʊlə/ cerebrovaskulární, týkající se mozkových cév
cut st off /kʌt/ odříznout, přerušit, zastavit
CVA, **Cerebrovascular**/ ˌser.ɪ.brəˈvæskjʊlə/ **Accident** / ˈæksɪdənt/ mrtvice
digit /ˈdɪdʒ.ɪt/ prst na ruce i noze, číslice
dilated /daɪˈleɪtɪd/ rozšířený, dilatovaný
draw /drɔː/ pohybovat se, táhnout, natáhnout, načerpat

exercise /ˈek.sə.saɪz/ cvičit, cvičení, výkon
flush /flʌʃ/ propláchnout, pročistit
frostbitten /ˈfrɒstˌbɪt.ən/ omrzlý
gag /gæg/ navalovat se, téměř zvracet
gloved /glʌvd/ v rukavicích
heat /hiːt/ **cramp** /kræmp/ křeč z horka
heat /hiːt/ **exhaustion** /ɪgˈzɔː.s.tʃən/ vyčerpání z horka
heat /hiːt/ **stroke** /strəʊk/ úžeh, úpal
hives /haɪvz/ kopřivka
humid /ˈhjuː.mɪd/ vlhký
hypotonia /ˌhaɪpəʊˈtəʊ.niə/ hypotonie, snížené svalové napětí
immerse /ɪˈmɜːs/ ponořit se, potopit
impaired /ɪmˈpeəd/ oslabený, poškození
indoors /ˌɪnˈdɔːz/ uvnitř, v domě
insect /ˈɪn.sekt/ hmyz
intensity /ɪnˈten.sɪ.ti/ intenzita, síla, ostrost
interim /ˈɪn.tər.ɪm/ prozatímní, dočasný, interval, časový úsek
intravenously /ˌɪn.trəˈviː.nəs.li/ nitrožilně
lifeguard /ˈlaɪf.gɑːd/ plavčík na plážích ap.
manifest /ˈmæn.ɪ.fest/ projevit, projev
mental /ˈmen.təl/ duševní
mid /mɪd/ střední
occlusive /ɒˈkluː.sɪv/ **dressing** / ˈdres.ɪŋ/ okluzní obvaz, uzavřený obvaz
overly /ˈəʊ.vəl.i/ přespříliš, až moc

peak /piːk/ špička, vrchol maximum, nejvyšší stupeň
penetrate /ˈpen.ɪ.treɪt/ proniknout, vniknout, prorazit
penetrating /ˈpen.ɪ.treɪ.tɪŋ/ pronikavý
pertussis /pəˈtʌ.sɪs/ černý kašel
pool /puːl/ bazén
rapid /ˈræp.ɪd/ rapidní, rychlý, překotný
refreeze /ˌriː.ˈfriː.z/ znovu zmrznout
regulate /ˈregjʊˌleɪt/ regulovat, usměrňovat, řídit

sever /ˈsev.ər/ oddělit, přerušit, urvat, odseknout
slurred /ˈslɜːd/ nejasný
terminate /ˈtɜː.mɪ.neɪt/ ukončit, přerušit
tightness /ˈtaɪt.nəs/ tíseň, těsnost, napětí
undernourished /ˌʌn.dəˈnʌr.ɪʃt/ podvyživený, trpící podvýživou
weak /wiːk/ slabý, křehký, nedostatečný

Unit 4

I

Your patient is an adult female whom you suspect is unconscious as a result of an upper-airway obstruction. You use the head-tilt/chin-lift method __ ____ her airway and then attempt to give two _____, which are unsuccessful.

What is the next thing you should do? Reposition and attempt to ventilate again.*

During the initial _____ _____, the next step after two unsuccessful attempts at ventilation for an unconscious adult patient is to _____ the head and try again. Once you have confirmed _____, you do not need to repeat this step (repositioning) again.

Perform the blind finger sweep following the _____ _____ before attempting ventilation each time. _____ _____ for relieving airway obstruction are reserved for very obese and pregnant adults.

> Chest thrusts, obstruction, abdominal thrusts, resuscitation attempt, to open, reposition, ventilations

2

When _____ a patient, you should always begin suctioning after the catheter is placed in the airway.*

Attempts at suctioning should be limited to no more than 5-10 seconds (depending upon the level of _____). You should _____ the patient after each attempt, and you should not turn on the apparatus until the catheter is _____ _____.

In the case of a _____ _____ that has a hole in the system that allows you to control if suction is being applied or not by occluding the opening, you should only suction upon withdrawal. This system may remain turned on at all times as long as you _____ _____ when suction is actually being applied to the patient.

> placed properly, monitor closely, suction catheter, consciousness, suctioning, ventilate

3

You are called for a 54-year-old woman who is unconscious. Your assessment reveals the patient to be _____ ___ _____.

Initial management of this patient's airway should include the insertion of an _____ airway and ventilation with a bag-valve _____.*

device, oropharyngeal, apnoeic and pulseless

4

Your patient has a partial airway obstruction but adequate air exchange.

You should monitor the patient closely while he or she continues trying to clear the airway him- or herself.*

If a patient has a _____ airway obstruction but adequate ___ _____, allow her to continue her spontaneous efforts to clear the airway (_____), but monitor her carefully. Your _____ may actually worsen the obstruction by making it _____. If air exchange becomes inadequate, treat her as if the obstruction is total __ _____ the Heimlich, intubation, _____, or other efforts to relieve the

_____.

by performing, interference, coughing, partial, air exchange, suction, obstruction, complete

5

After inserting a blind insertion airway device, what step should you take before inflating the balloon to ensure that the tube is properly positioned? Look for chest rise and auscultate the lungs and abdomen.*

Regardless of which device you use, _____ of placement is generally advisable prior to _____ of any balloons on the device by looking for _____- ____ and fall and _____ ___ breath sounds in the chest and _____.

inflation, listening for, abdomen, chest rise, confirmation

6

What is the most definitive treatment of a patient with a flail chest injury? Intubation and positive-pressure ventilation.*

_____ _____ ventilation of the patient with a _____ _____ _____ reverses the mechanism that causes the _____ chest wall movement, restores _____ _____, and _____ _____ of chest wall movement.

reduces pain, Positive-pressure, paradoxical, tidal volume, flail chest injury

7

One breathing pattern is characterized by periods of apnoea followed by periods in which respirations first increase then decrease in both _____ ___ _____.

This _____ is called Cheyne-Stokes breathing.*

Cheyne-Stokes respirations are characterized by periods of

243

_____ lasting 10-60 seconds, followed by periods in which respirations gradually _____, then _____, in depth and rate.

decrease, apnoea, increase, pattern, depth and frequency

8
This statement regarding a _____ pneumothorax is true: it is usually limited to only 20% of the lung and is well tolerated by the patient.*
A spontaneous pneumothorax occurs when a ____ (cystic lesion on the lobe of the lung) ruptures, allowing air to enter the _____ _____ from within the lung. It usually occurs in otherwise healthy individuals age 20 to 40. They are usually well _____ and occupy less than 20% of the lung.

pleural space, tolerated, spontaneous, bleb

9
The paper bag effect occurs when the occupant of a car takes a deep breath just _____ _ _____, resulting in which of the following injuries?
• pneumothorax*
• pulmonary embolism
• shearing of the aorta
• lung laceration

The paper bag effect or the paper bag syndrome is thought to __ _____ for most pneumothoraces that result from car crashes. During this event the _____ _____ traps pressurized air in the _____. When compression occurs during the crash against the closed glottis, _____ _____ can occur to the hyperinflated _____ ___ _____, resulting in collapse.

chest, closed glottis, be responsible, alveoli and bronchioles, severe damage, before a collision

10
A patient is found lying supine on the floor with a ____ _____ to her right anterior chest just below the breast. The patient is having _____ _____, with cool, clammy skin signs. No JVD is noted. Breath sounds are absent over the right side.
This patient most likely is experiencing a haemothorax.*
The lack of jugular venous _____ in the supine position is very telling; it suggests a _____ ____ of volume from the circulatory system.

difficulty breathing, stab wound, large loss, distension

11

A patient was hit several times in the left chest with the large end of a pool cue. The patient is in severe respiratory distress with tachycardia and tachypnoea.
_____ can be felt over the left anterior fourth, fifth, sixth, and seventh rib areas. Lung _____ are clear and equal, but diminished.
What condition best describes the patient's presentation? Flail chest segment.*
_____ _____ is very possible in this case due to the _____ of injury. The lack of other signs or symptoms such as jugular venous distension or unequal or absent breath sounds minimizes the possibilities of a _____ __
_____.

> pneumothorax or tamponade, Flail segment, Crepitus, sounds, mechanism

12

This _____ in vital signs comprises Cushing's reflex, a sign of increasing _____ _____: respiratory rate increased, heart rate decreased, blood pressure increased.*
Cushing's reflex is also sometimes called Cushing's triad or Cushing's _____.

> response, intracranial pressure, change

13

The primary use of the Magill forceps in the field is to directly _____ a visible foreign-body obstruction.*
Magill forceps are used to remove an obstructing _____ _____ that is visible during laryngoscopy after _____ _____ have been unsuccessful.

> remove, foreign body, abdominal thrusts

14

- Progressively deeper, faster breathing _____ gradually with shallow, slower breathing is called Cheyne-Stokes.*

_____-_____ respirations are _____ ___ ____. Biot's breathing is an irregular pattern.

> alternating, regular and deep, Cheyne-Stokes

15

Which of the statements about the deflation of the PASG/MAST in the field setting is correct?

- Deflation should be accomplished rapidly in the field.

- Deflate the legs first and then the _____ compartment.
- _____ the garment if the patient begins to experience dyspnoea.
- Deflation should not be attempted in the field without medical direction.*

Because the PASG corrects a symptom and not the _____ _____, deflating should be _____ only in the hospital after the underlying _____ is corrected.

> attempted, underlying problem, hypovolaemia, abdominal, Deflate

16

The following conditions would result in an increase of a patient's PaO_2: airway obstruction, hypoventilation, and physical exertion.*
PaO_2 measures _____ _____ levels in the blood, which are influenced by _____ in CO_2 production or _____. Such levels would be increased by _____ _____ of muscles, by _____, or by an airway obstruction.

> carbon dioxide, hypoventilation, elimination, physical exertion, alterations

17

Which of the following factors would normally cause a _____ in a patient's respiratory rate?
- anxiety
- sleep*
- fever
- hypoxia

A patient will breathe more slowly when _____ than when _____; all the other factors listed increase _____ _____.

> awake, decrease, respiratory rate, asleep

18

The volume of air normally inhaled and exhaled during each respiration is called the tidal volume.*
Tidal volume is the amount of air that moves into and out of the lungs during the _____ _____; minute volume is the total amount of air exchanged in the lungs in one _____. Inspiratory _____ is the extra air that could be inspired in addition to the tidal volume. Total _____ _____ is the sum of the inspiratory reserve, tidal volume, expiratory reserve, and residual volume.

> lung capacity, respiratory cycle, reserve, minute

19

Which is the recommended
method when measuring
respiratory rate? Count
respirations while pretending to
take a radial pulse.*
Place your hand on the patient's
wrist as if you were measuring
his or her pulse and _____ ___
__ _____. This will prevent the
patient from consciously _____
the respiratory rate. Placing the
wrist and hand over the patient's
_____ ____ is called the pledge of
allegiance method.

chest wall, changing, count for 30 seconds

20

When using a peak flow meter
to measure peak expiratory
flow, the correct procedure is to
ask the patient to inhale deeply,
then exhale once as quickly as
possible, taking one reading.*
The correct procedure is to have
the patient _____ _____ and
_____ _____. Some meters ask
you to repeat the procedure and
_____ your findings, but you
would still have the patient inhale
deeply and quickly exhale with
each _____.

average, inhale deeply, exhale quickly, reading

Vocabulary 4

allegiance /əˈliː.dʒəns/ věrnost, loajalita
alternating /ˈɒl.tə.neɪ.tɪŋ/ střídavý, střídající se
asleep /əˈsliːp/ spící, usnout
average /ˈæv.ər.ɪdʒ/ průměr, činit v průměru
balloon /bəˈluːn/ balonek
bleb /bleb/ puchýřek
confirmed /kənˈfɜːmd/ potvrzený
consciously /ˈkɒn.ʃəs.li/ vědomě, úmyslně
count /kaʊnt/ počítat
cycle /ˈsaɪ.k|/ cyklus
deflation /dɪˈfleɪ.ʃən/ vyfouknutí
exertion /ɪgˈzɜː.ʃən/ úsilí, námaha
frequency /ˈfriː.kwən.si/ frekvence, četnost výskytu
garment /ˈgɑː.mənt/ oděv, šaty, svršky
haemothorax /ˈhiː.məˈθɔː.ræks/ hemotorax, nahromadění krve v dutině hrudní
hole /hoʊl/ díra, otvor, mezera
hypoventilation /ˌhaɪpəʊˌven.tɪˈleɪ.ʃən/ hypoventilace, omezené dýchání
increase /ɪnˈkriːs/ zvýšit, zvýšení
inflation /ɪnˈfleɪ.ʃən/ naplnění, nafouknutí
interference /ˌɪn.təˈfɪə.rəns/ interference, zasahování, rušení
JVD, Jugular /ˈdʒʌg.jə.lər/ **Venous** /ˈviː.nəs/ **Distension** /dɪˈsten.tʃən/ roztažení krční tepny
lasting /ˈlɑːstɪŋ/ trvalý, stálý
method /ˈmeθ.əd/ metoda, způsob

otherwise /'ʌð.ə.waɪz/ jinak, v jiném případě

peak /piːk/ **flow** /fləʊ/ vrcholový výdechový průtok

place /pleɪs/ místo, umístit, položit

pledge /pledʒ/ závazek, slib

pleural /'plʊə.rəl/ pleurální, pohrudniční

pool cue /kjuː/ tágo

pressurized /'preʃ.ər.aɪzd/ přetlakový, s regulovaným tlakem

pretend /prɪ'tend/ předstírat, tvrdit

progressively /prə'gres.ɪv.li/ progresivně, postupně

rate /reɪt/ frekvence

regular /'reg.jʊ.lər/ pravidelný, častý, obvyklý

relieve /rɪ'liːv/ utišit, zmírnit, pomoci

reserve /rɪ'zɜːv/ rezerva, vyhradit si, zamluvit

setting /'set.ɪŋ/ prostředí

shear /'ʃɪə.r/ nůžky, stříhat, utrhnout se

sweep /swiːp/ (swept, swept) shrnout, stáhnout, smést

take /teɪk/ **breath** /breθ/ vdechnout

tidal /'taɪ.dəl/ přílivový, týkající se respiračního vzduchu

total /'təʊ.təl/ celkem, úplný

unequal /ʌn'iː.kwəl/ nerovný, nedostatečný, neschopný zvládnout

visible /'vɪz.ɪ.bl̩/ viditelný, zřejmý

wrist /rɪst/ zápěstí

Unit 5

1

What is an assessment finding of pulsus paradoxus associated with? COPD*

_____ _____, or a drop in _____ _____ with each respiratory cycle, is associated with chronic obstructive pulmonary disease (____).

> COPD, Pulsus paradoxus, blood pressure

2

What is bronchiolitis caused by? The respiratory syncytial virus.*

The respiratory syncytial virus, which causes only _____ upper-respiratory infections in older persons, causes _____, a serious _____ _____ in infants and young children

> respiratory infection, mild, bronchiolitis

3

A disease that is associated with cigarette smoking and is related to, but distinct from, emphysema is chronic bronchitis.*

In addition to emphysema, _____ _____ is associated with cigarette smoking. Either condition can lead to CHF. A _____ _____ can be caused by cigarette smoking,

especially in young and thin males, but the disease process is unrelated to _____.

> emphysema, chronic bronchitis, simple pneumothorax

4

A dull sound heard during chest _____ may be associated with which condition? Pneumonia.*

A ____ _____ heard during chest percussion may be associated with pneumonia, _____, or_____ _____.

> haemothorax, dull sound, pulmonary oedema, percussion

5

What condition best suggests respiratory failure? Hyperextension of the neck.*

A patient in _____ _____ is compensating for the underlying condition, thereby preserving _____ to the brain. Once _____ _____ have collapsed, the loss of gas exchange at the brain will result in a change in _____ _____.

In a paediatric patient, hypertension of the neck can complicate ventilation. Hyperextending the neck of a small child may result in an unintentional _____ of

249

the airway, due to the softer
_____ _____ supporting the
trachea.

compensatory mechanisms, cartilage rings, respiratory distress, oxygenation, mental status, closure

6

These statements about airway obstruction caused by the tongue are correct:

- The tongue is the most common cause of _____ _____ in an unconscious patient.*
- Airway blockage does not depend on the _____ of the patient's head, neck, and jaw.*
- The _____ ___ _____ can contribute to airway blockage in an unconscious patient.*
- Blockage of the airway by the _____ can occur when the patient is in any position.*

airway obstruction, oesophagus and epiglottis, position, tongue

7

The hypoxic drive is regulated by low PaO$_2$.*
COPD patients can no longer ____ _____ normal regulatory mechanisms to control their _____. The hypoxic drive measures for low levels of oxygen in the _____ to increase respiratory rate.

rely upon, bloodstream, respirations

8

What is the condition that is present when the pleural space expands because air enters from an interior wound? A closed pneumothorax.*

_____ _____ occurs when air enters the pleural space from an _____ _____. An open pneumothorax occurs when the chest wall is open so that air can enter directly into the chest from ___ _____. A tension pneumothorax develops when a _____ _____ becomes large enough to cause pressure and structural changes within the chest.

Closed pneumothorax, the outside, simple pneumothorax, interior wound

9

What respiratory pattern is characteristic of Kussmaul's respiration? An _____ in both rate and depth.*
Kussmaul's respirations, which are associated with _____

_____, are characterized by increased rate and depth of _____.

> respirations, diabetic ketoacidosis, increase

10

What does the term *stridor* refer to? A ____-_____ sound upon inspiration from airway obstruction.*
Stridor is a sound made during _____ and is associated with croup and upper-airway _____. It is a harsh upper-airway sound that can be heard when the patient inhales and can usually be heard without a _____ and emanates from the area of the _____.

> throat, inspiration, obstruction, stethoscope, high-pitched

11

A whistling or musical sound heard on exhalation is referred to as what abnormal breath sound?
- snoring
- wheezing*
- stridor
- friction rub

_____, a whistling sound heard on _____, is generally associated with _____. Snoring and stridor are _____-_____ obstructions, and a friction rub sounds like rubbing.

> Wheezing, expiration, upper-airway, asthma

12

What condition is the pathophysiological result of near drowning in seawater? Pulmonary oedema.*
Because seawater is _____, fluid is drawn from the _____ into the _____, causing pulmonary oedema. Because of this, all near-drowning patients should be hospitalized and monitored for a short time.

> hypertonic, bloodstream, alveoli

13

Your patient is in respiratory distress. He is exhibiting jugular venous _____. Crackles are auscultated throughout his ____ _____. He is tachycardic, hypertensive, and tachypnoeic. What ___ __ _____ is indicated for this patient's presentation?
What are the correct _____ ___ _____ of the indicated medications? Oxygen, intravenous line at 30 cc/hr, nitroglycerin sL, and 40 mg furosemide IV.*
This patient appears to be experiencing _____ pulmonary oedema.

distension, lung fields, choices and routes, set of treatment, acute

14
Which of the following factors increases the amount of energy necessary for the patient to expend for respiration?
- loss of pulmonary surfactant*
- decrease in airway resistance
- increase in pulmonary compliance
- a decrease in body temperature

____ __ _____ _____, which can occur in pneumonia and other conditions, increases the tendency of the alveoli to _____ and, thus, increases the work _____ ___ respiration.

necessary for, Loss of pulmonary surfactant, collapse

15
Signs and symptoms of traumatic asphyxia include dyspnoea, bloodshot eyes, distended neck veins, and a cyanotic upper body.*
Traumatic asphyxia occurs when _____ ___ _____ pushes the chest wall inward, resulting in severe _____ and backflow of venous blood. Important signs and symptoms of

this include _____, bloodshot eyes, distended neck veins, and a _____ upper body.

dyspnoea, hypoventilation, cyanotic, serious rib injury

16
You note snoring sounds during your initial assessment of a semiconscious trauma patient. What is your next step? Perform the chin-lift/jaw-thrust manoeuvre.*
_____ indicates that the airway is partially obstructed by the patient's tongue. Clear the airway first by positioning with the ____-___/___-_____ manoeuvre or by inserting a nasopharyngeal airway. An oropharyngeal airway is ___ _____ due to the patient's LOC. Cervical stabilization takes place prior to beginning your ABC assessment, and head tilt/chin lift is not advisable due to the possibility of _-_____ _____.

C-spine, not indicated, Snoring, chin-lift/jaw-thrust, injury

17
When administering IV fluids to a trauma patient, it is critical to continuously monitor which _____ ____? Breath sounds.*
_____ _____ are particularly important to monitor during IV

fluid administration because of the danger of ____ _____, which will initially _____ __ pulmonary oedema.

> manifest as, fluid overload, vital sign, Breath sounds

18

A patient is found in a back bedroom lying supine on the bed with a hunting knife embedded in her anterior chest, midline below the right breast. The patient is in obvious _____ _____. She is cold, clammy, and diaphoretic with flat neck veins. You hear no breath sounds on the right side.
This patient is most likely suffering from haemothorax.*
____ ____ _____ while the patient is supine indicate a lower-than-normal pressure inside the vasculature, most likely due to _____ ____. This would indicate a haemothorax as the _____ _____ of the described signs and symptoms.

> blood loss, Flat neck veins, primary cause, respiratory distress

19

What is your first action for an adult patient who is conscious but who has a _____ _____ _____? Deliver rapid

_____ _____ until cleared or unconsciousness results.*
For the _____ patient, your first action would be abdominal thrusts.

> abdominal thrusts, conscious, complete airway obstruction

20

The most _____ cause of upper-airway obstruction is the relaxation of the tongue.*
The loss of lingual control during _____ occurs more commonly that the other _____.

> unconsciousness, conditions, common

Vocabulary 5
abbreviation /əˌbriːvɪˈeɪʃən/ zkratka slova
abnormal /æbˈnɔː.məl/ abnormální, neobvyklý
asphyxia /æsˈfɪksɪə/ asfyxie, zadušení
backflow /ˈbæk.fləʊ/ zpětný tok
blockage /ˈblɒk.ɪdʒ/ ucpání, neprůchodnost
bloodshot /ˈblʌd.ʃɒt/ krví podlitý (oči)
bronchiolitis /ˈbrɒŋ.ki.əˈlaɪ.tɪs/ bronchiolitida, zánět průdušinek
cartilage /ˈkɑː.təl.ɪdʒ/ **ring** /rɪŋ/ chrupavčitý prstenec
consciousness /ˈkɒn.ʃəs.nəs/ vědomí, povědomí

COPD, Chronic /ˈkrɒnɪk/
Obstructive /əbˈstrʌk.tɪv/
Pulmonary /ˈpʊl.mə.nə.ri/ **Disease**
/dɪˈziːz/ chronické obstruktivní
onemocnění plic
danger /ˈdeɪn.dʒər/ nebezpečí,
ohrožení
deliver /dɪˈlɪv.ər/ předat, doručit
diabetic /ˌdaɪəˈbet.ɪk/ **ketoacidosis**
/ˈkiːtəʊˌæs.ɪˈdəʊ.sɪs/ diabetická
ketoacidóza, acidóza způsobená
nadměrným množstvím ketolátek
v krvi
distinct /dɪˈstɪŋkt/ odlišný, zřetelný
emanate /ˈem.ə.neɪt/ vycházet,
proudit, vyzařovat
embedded /ɪmˈbed.ɪd/ pevně
usazený, zarytý
exhalation /ˌeks.h əˈleɪ.ʃən/
vydechnutí
expend /ɪkˈspend/ vydat, vynaložit,
spotřebovat
friction /ˈfrɪk.ʃən/ frikce, tření
furosemide /fjʊr.ɔsˈæm.aɪd/
furosemid, silné diuretikum
harsh /hɑːʃ/ drsný, výrazný
hyperextension /ˌhaɪ.pərˈɪkˈstenʃən/
nadměrné protažení
hypertonia /ˌhaɪ.pəˈtəʊ.niə/
hypertonie, zvýšené napětí
(svalové)
hypoxic /haɪˈpɒk.sɪk/ **drive** /draɪv/
stimulace dýchání nízkým stavem
PaO₂ (parciální tlak kyslíku v
tepenné arteriální krvi)
intravenous /ˌɪn.trəˈviː.nəs/ **line** /
laɪn/ nitrožilní linka
lingual /ˈlɪŋgwəl/ lingvální,
jazykový

LOC, Level /ˈlevəl/ **of consciousness**
/ˈkɒn.ʃəs.nɪs/ hladina vědomí
LOC, Loss /lɒs/ **of consciousness** /
ˈkɒn.ʃəs.nɪs/ ztráta vědomí
obstructive /əbˈstrʌk.tɪv/
obstrukční, bránící čemu,
obstruktivní, ucpávající
outside /ˌaʊtˈsaɪd/ vnejší strana,
venku
PaCO₂, partial /ˈpɑːʃəl/ **pressure** /
ˈpreʃ.ər/ **of carbon** /ˈkɑː.bən/
dioxide /daɪˈɒk.saɪd/ **in arterial** /
ɑːˈtɪərɪəl/ **blood** /blʌd/ parciální
tlak oxidu uhličitého v alveolu,
ovlivňuje jej alveolární ventilace
particularly /pəˈtɪk.jʊ.lə.li/ hlavně,
zejména, obzvlášť
primary /ˈpraɪ.mə.ri/ primární,
prvořadý
rely /rɪˈlaɪ/ **upon** /əˌpɒn/ spoléhat,
být odkázán na koho, co
semiconscious /ˌsem.iˈkɒn.ʃəs/
zpola při vědomí
stabilization /ˌsteɪ.bɪ.laɪˈzeɪ.ʃən/
stabilizace, ustálení
stream /striːm/ proud, pramínek,
téci
surfactant /sərfakˈtənt/
surfaktant, povrchově aktivní
látka, pokrývající vnitřek plicních
sklípků, nedostatečně vyvinut
u předčasně narozených dětí,
poškozován i v průběhu těžkých
plicních chorob dospělých
syncytial /sɪnˈsɪ.ʃɪ.əl/ **virus** /ˈvaɪrəs/
syncytiální virus, způsobuje
záněty dýchacích cest, množení
viru vede ke splývání sousedních
buněk a vzniku

syncytia

tendency /ˈten.dən.si/ tendence, sklon

traumatic /trɔːˈmæt.ɪk/ traumatický, úrazový

treatment /ˈtriːt.mənt/ léčení, ošetření

unintentional /ˌʌn.ɪnˈten.ʃən.əl/ neúmyslný, bezděčný

unrelated /ˌʌn.rɪˈleɪ.tɪd/ netýkající se, vzájemně nesouvisející

vasculature /ˈvæs.kjʊ.lə.tʃər/ vaskularita, cévnatost

Unit 6

I

These statements about airway obstruction caused by the tongue are correct:

- The tongue is the most common cause of _____ _____ in an unconscious patient.*
- Airway blockage does not depend on the _____ of the patient's head, neck, and jaw.*
- The _____ ___ _____ can contribute to airway blockage in an unconscious patient.*

Blockage of the airway by the _____ can occur when the patient is in any position.

> airway obstruction, oesophagus and epiglottis, position, tongue

2

An unconscious patient has snoring respirations. When should this condition be corrected?

_____ _____ the respiratory status.*

_____ respirations are indicative of an airway issue and should be _____ before further assessment __ _____.

> is completed, corrected, Before evaluating, Snoring

3

A patient is short of breath after impact with the _____ _____ in a motor vehicle crash. Breath sounds are diminished on the left. What condition is most likely the cause of the patient's _____? Simple pneumothorax.* The question does not provide any indication of a tension pneumothorax. A pulmonary _____ or cardiac tamponade should affect ____ _____.

> lung sounds, complaint, contusion, steering wheel

4

Before using nitrous oxide for a _____-_____ patient, you should exclude the possibility that the patient has:

- cervical spine injury
- flail chest
- pericardial tamponade
- pneumothorax*

Nitronox should not be used with patients with head injuries because it can increase _____ _____. It should not be used with patients who have _____ because the drug can move __ _____ to air spaces in the body.

> pneumothorax, by diffusion, chest-injury, intracranial pressure

5

Your trauma patient is _____ and apprehensive. She is increasingly _____, and breath sounds are rapidly diminishing over her left lung. She is exhibiting signs and symptoms of _____. You should suspect:
- haemothorax
- tension pneumothorax*
- cardiac _____
- flail chest

agitated, shock, tamponade, cyanotic

6

Distended neck veins, _____ unilateral breath sounds, and progressively _____ compliance are indications of tension pneumothorax.*
Excessive pressure inside the _____ _____ due to the tension pneumothorax will result in all of the described symptoms.

worsening, diminishing, thoracic cavity

7

The term *tracheal tugging* refers to which of the following?
- the use of _____ _____ during respirations
- retraction of intercostal muscles during inspiration
- cyanosis and _____ _____ with exhalation
- retraction of neck tissues during respiration*

Tracheal tugging refers to the _____ of neck tissues during respiratory _____.

effort, retraction, accessory muscles, nasal flaring

8

Your patient _____ cold, clammy skin; air hunger; distended neck veins; _____ displacement; and _____ breath sounds on one side.
You should suspect tension pneumothorax.*
The signs and symptoms of _____ _____, the presence of air in the _____ _____ and mediastinal shifting, are listed.

tension pneumothorax, pleural space, tracheal, absent, exhibits

9

You can reduce gastric distension during _____ _____ by providing ventilations deep enough to cause _____ _____ only.*
Quickly _____ a BVM may cause enough pressure to _____ ___ into the oesophagus.

squeezing, chest rise, artificial ventilations, force air

onset, chest pain, laboured, pulmonary embolism

10

Prehospital care of an ____ _____ includes occlusive dressing, high-flow oxygen, and rapid transport.*

The steps involved in the management of this injury are _____ _____, high-flow oxygen, and rapid transport. _____ is not necessary for each patient. Needle decompression is not necessary if tension pneumothorax develops. If dyspnoea _____, open the dressing __ _____ some of the pressure that is built up. An IV lifeline should be _____, but large-volume fluid resuscitation should be withheld.

established, Intubation, open pneumothorax, worsens, to relieve, occlusive dressing

11

The following are signs and symptoms of acute pulmonary embolism: rapid, laboured breathing and tachycardia.*

The most common signs of a _____ _____ (rapid, _____ breathing and tachycardia) are given; _____ is usually sudden, and there may be or may not be _____ ____.

12

Which of the following are signs and symptoms of air embolism?
  a) Pruritus, skin _____ and cyanosis, pitting oedema in the ankles
  b) Chest pain, sharp with sudden onset, dyspnoea with coughing*
  c) _____, auditory and vestibular disturbances, headache
  d) Fatigue, pain in chest and _____ _____, nausea, and vomiting

All other options list signs and symptoms of _____ _____, only choice b includes signs of ___ _____ (sharp chest pain with sudden onset, dyspnoea with coughing).

decompression sickness, pallor, lower abdomen, Dizziness, air embolism

13

After experiencing a sudden syncopal episode, a 41-year-old female is complaining of pleuritic chest pain and shortness of breath. Her vital signs are as follows: RR = 28, P = 126, and BP = 88/60. The pulse oximeter reads 89% on high-flow oxygen. Her breath sounds are clear.

Which of the following conditions best describes the patient's signs and symptoms?

- pulmonary embolism*
- pulmonary oedema
- chronic bronchitis
- acute asthma

The patient's presentation points to a _____ _____ as the likely cause. The other conditions are not normally associated with sudden _____, and adventitious lung sounds like _____ ___ _____ should be evident, unlike the patient's clear ones.

crackles or wheezes, pulmonary embolism, syncope

14

What is the most commonly used drug in the _____ setting for patients with asthma? Inhaled or nebulized albuterol.* Albuterol, a _____, is frequently given via _____ ___ _____ in the field.

inhaler or nebulizer, prehospital, bronchodilator

15

A patient presents with a sudden onset of _____ _____ ____ and respiratory distress. She has _____ lung sounds, a pulse rate of 110 and regular, BP of 112/76, and respirations of 28. Which of the following conditions best describes this patient presentations?

- Psychogenic hyperventilation
- Acute exacerbation of asthma
- Pulmonary embolism *
- Pulmonary oedema

The lack of findings is almost as important as the reported ones. For example, ___ _____ pedal oedema, crackles, or wheezes in the lung fields, or hypertension, reduces the _____ of pulmonary oedema. The lack of medical history or wheezes _____ asthma as a possible cause.

not having, possibility, sharp chest pain, minimizes, clear

16

What does the disease process of emphysema cause within the ____ _____? A loss of elasticity in the alveoli due to _____ _____.*

Patients with emphysema have a loss of _____ in the alveoli due to prolonged insult. Bleb formation results in decreased ability of the _____ to expand and contract and an overall decreased _____ ____ of the lungs. Ruptured blebs do not result in lung deflation.

| alveoli, surface area, prolonged insult, lung tissues, elasticity |

17

What is the primary treatment for a patient with chronic _____ who is NOT severely hypoxic? Administering low-flow oxygen via _____.*

Patients with emphysema or _____ _____ benefit from the _____ of low-flow oxygen and constant monitoring.

| cannula, chronic bronchitis, emphysema, administration |

18

What is the treatment for someone who is suffering an _____ of either emphysema or chronic bronchitis and is not too hypoxic? Establish an _____, position the patient seated or ____-_____, administer low-flow oxygen, establish an IV lifeline, and transport.*
___-____ _____ is appropriate for this patient if he or she is not too hypoxic. If a patient with emphysema or chronic bronchitis is _____, he or she needs more oxygen.

| semi-seated, Low-flow oxygen, exacerbation, hypoxic, airway |

19

Your patient, who has had a recent tracheotomy, tried to remove himself from the _____ and dislodged the trach cannula. Subcutaneous emphysema is now_____. What should you do next? _____ the tracheotomy tube and insert an _____ ____.*

If the trach tube has been dislodged, it may not be easy to reinsert, so rest it in its _____ _____. Placing an endotracheal tube into the stoma and _____ ___ ____ will help rapidly establish the patient's airway.

| original position, Remove, ventilator, endotracheal tube, inflating the cuff, evident |

20

Which technique should you use to open the airway of a trauma patient? The jaw thrust.*
The ___ _____ is used to open the airway of patients with suspected _____ _____ _____. Any trauma patient with questionable or unknown mechanism of injury should __ _____ to have a cervical spine injury until it is _____ ___.

| jaw thrust, be assumed, ruled out, cervical spine injury |

Vocabulary 6

agitated /ˈædʒ.ɪ.teɪ.tɪd/ rozrušený, nervózní

apprehensive /ˌæp.rɪˈhen.sɪv/ znepokojený

artificial /ˌɑː.tɪˈfɪʃ.əl/ **ventilation** /ˌven.tɪˈleɪ.ʃən/ umělé dýchání

ascites /æˈsaɪ.tɪːz/ ascites, abnormální hromadění tekutiny v břišní dutině

BVM, Bag Valve Mask, Ambu bag, manual resuscitator, self-inflating bag dýchací maska s ventilem

cannula /kæn.jʊl.ə/ kanyla, dutá jehla, trubička

displacement /dɪˈspleɪs.mənt/ vytlačení, odsunutí

evaluate /ɪˈvæl.ju.eɪt/ zhodnotit, ocenit, stanovit

exclude /ɪkˈskluːd/ vyloučit, vyřadit, zabránit vniknutí

inhaler /ɪnˈheɪ.lər/ inhalátor, inhalační přístroj

mediastinal /ˌmiː.di.əsˈtaɪ.nəl/ mediastinální, mezihrudní

nasal /ˈneɪ.zəl/ **flaring** /fleər.ɪŋ/ zvětšení nosních dírek při dýchání, klasický příznak zavažného astmatu

nebulizer /ˈneb.jə.laɪz.ər/ nebulizér, rozprašovač

Nitronox /ˌnaɪ.trə.nɒks/ nitronox

nitrous oxide /ˌnaɪ.trəsˈɒk.saɪd/ oxid dusný

overall /ˌəʊ.vəˈrɔːl/ celkový, celkově

pedal /ˈped.əl/ nožní, nohou se týkající

pitting /pɪt.ɪŋ/ **oedema** /ɪˈdiː.mə/ jamkovitý otok

pruritus /prʊəˈraɪ.təs/ svědění, projev alergie nebo způsobené emocionálním stresem

questionable /ˈkwes.tʃə.nə.bl̩/ pochybný, sporný

recent /ˈriː.sənt/ nedávný, poslední

reinsert /ˌriː.ɪnˈsɜːt/ znovu vložit, vsunout

rest /rest/ spočívat, záviset, ležet

semi /ˌsem.i/ -**seated** /ˈsiː.tɪd/ zpola posazený, v polosedě

squeeze /skwiːz/ zmáčknout, stisknutí

stoma /ˈstəʊ.mə/ ústa, malý otvor, pór, uměle vytvořený otvor mezi dutinami

thoracic /θɔːˈræs.ɪk/ **cavity** /ˈkæv.ɪ.ti/ dutina hrudní

tracheostomy /ˌtræk.iˈɒst.ə.mi/ tracheostomie, chirurg. vytvoření otvoru do průdušnice k umožnění dýchání

tug /tʌg/ trhnutí, cuknutí

unilateral /ˌjuː.nɪˈlæt.ər.əl/ unilaterální, jednostranný

vestibular /vesˈtɪb.jə.lər/ vestibulární, předsíňový

Unit 7

1

An endotracheal tube that has been advanced ___ ___ is prone to enter the right main bronchus.* Because of the _____ appearance of the distal trachea, it is most common for an ET tube that has been inserted too far to enter the ____ ____ _____, resulting in atelectasis and _____ of the left lung.

anatomical, insufficiency, right main bronchus, too far

2

To ensure the proper placement of the endotracheal tube, you should confirm the placement of the tube by two different methods.*

To ensure proper placement, always confirm __ ___ _____ _____. After watching the tube pass through the ____ _____, assess the chest for breath sounds in numerous locations and ____ _____, then check the proximal end of the tube for breath condensation. You may also use one of the several commercial _____ _____ that monitor end-tidal CO2 or provide an audible whistling sound to confirm ___ _____.

confirmation devices, air movement, by two different methods, chest expansion, vocal cords

3

You are _____ the tracheal tube when you begin to hear the sound of the patient's breathing. Your next action would be to wait for the patient to inhale and insert the tube farther.*

As the tip of the nasotracheal tube reaches the glottic opening, you should hear the _____ _____ of the patient. Inserting of the tube past the vocal cords is timed to the _____ _____ in order to minimize _____ against the tube itself.

resistance, inhalation phase, respiratory effort, inserting

4

After placing an endotracheal tube, you note that breath sounds are much stronger on the right side of the chest than on the left. What does this suggest? The ET has been inserted into the right main stem bronchus.*

If breath sounds are _____ on one side than on the other or absent __ ___ ____, this suggests that the tube has been inserted ___ ___ and is resting in one bronchus.

stronger, on one side, too far

5

After you orally intubate a patient, your partner _____ the patient with a bag-valve device. You _____ the lung sound to confirm the placement. __ _____ are heard over the _____; breath sounds are present on the right side of chest and are decreased over the left. What should you do next? Withdraw the tube slightly after deflating the cuff, reinflate the cuff, and reevaluate lung sounds.* The original breath sounds indicated that the tube was placed in the trachea, but perhaps ___ ____. Adjusting the depth of the tube so that the _____ ___ is sitting just above the carina will likely resolve this situation.

No sounds, epigastrium, distal end, ventilates, too deep, auscultate

6

Which of the following is a sign of oesophageal intubation?
- a) air leak heard over the trachea
- b) breath sounds absent on the left
- c) bilateral chest wall expansion
- d) abdominal movement with ventilation*

Right-side-only breath sounds are a sign of right _____ _____, ruling out choice b. Air leak over the trachea may be the sign of an _____ _____ ____, ruling out choice a. Bilateral chest wall expansion is a _____ _____, ruling out choice c. These findings point to the need to have a good baseline assessment of ____ _____ and respiratory status prior to performing any _____.

interventions, improperly inflated cuff, normal finding, lung sounds, mainstem intubation

7

You use end-tidal carbon dioxide _____ as a tool to determine if endotracheal intubation has been _____ obtained.
The absence of _____ _____ in exhaled air after six ventilations indicates that the endotracheal tube has been placed in the oesophagus.*
No carbon dioxide after six ventilations indicates either that the tube is in the _____ or that the patient has been ____ long enough that no carbon dioxide is being produced.

oesophagus, dead, carbon dioxide, detector, correctly

8

While ventilating a patient with a bag-valve mask, you note decreasing compliance.
How should you react to this finding? Assess the cause of this finding and try to correct it.*
_____ refers to how easily air flows ____ ___ ___ ___ the lungs. If compliance is _____, look for the cause by first reassessing (with look, auscultate, and feel) the _____ and ___ _____ and then looking for signs that the patient is developing a tension pneumothorax; once you find the cause, try to correct it.

decreasing, head position, Compliance, into and out of, airway

9

Ventilating a patient at 30 breaths per minute with a ____-____ ____ and high-flow oxygen may result in alkalizing the _____.*
_____ may result in respiratory _____, a harmful condition to the patient.

alkalosis, bag-valve mask, bloodstream, Hyperventilation

10

To adequately ventilate a patient with a partial laryngectomy through a stoma, you should _____ the nose and _____ the mouth.*

A patient with a partial _____ has an ability to exhale through the mouth and nose. Therefore, you will have to close them in order to _____ air into the lungs while providing artificial ventilations.

direct, laryngectomy, pinch, close

I I

Minute respiratory _____ is best described as the _____ __ ___ moved in and out of the _____ in 1 minute.*

lungs, volume, amount of air

12

Stroke volume can be increased by all of the following:
- Increasing _____ _____
- Increasing _____ _____
- Decreasing afterload*

Preload can be increased by increasing venous return, by increasing the contractile force of the heart, or by decreasing _____.

venous return,* afterload, contractile force*

13

What is the _____ treatment for patients with suspected ____ _____

thrombosis? Immobilization and elevation of the extremity.*
Prehospital treatment is limited to _____ ___ _____ of the extremity and transportation.

> elevation and immobilization, prehospital, deep venous

14
A patient with nonperfusing _____ _____ would receive the same treatment as a patient with ventricular fibrillation.* Treatment for both conditions consists of _____ defibrillation; _____ treatment includes ___ and drugs.
_____ therapy depends upon whether a normal rhythm is initiated.

> CPR, immediate, continued, Additional, ventricular tachycardia

15
You are managing a patient with _____ _____ and multifocal PVCs. Suddenly, your patient slumps _____ and goes into ventricular fibrillation.
You _____ that your patient is pulseless.
Your next action would be to defibrillate at 200 joules.*
Immediate defibrillation has been proven to be effective in terminating _____

_____. Even stopping for CPR in a witnessed event such as this may be more _____ than _____.

> ventricular fibrillation, confirm, symptomatic bradycardia, harmful, unconscious, beneficial

16
How does the Valsalva manoeuvre improve a ___-_____ heartbeat? It stimulates the vagus nerve to slow the ____ _____.*
The Valsalva manoeuvre (bearing down against a closed glottis) stimulates the _____ _____, which innervates the heart.

> heart rate, vagus nerve, too-rapid

17
What rhythm might indicate a ____ ___ cardioversion?
Ventricular tachycardia at a rate of 120.*
If the tracheal tube has been dislodged, it may not be easy to reinsert, so rest it in its _____ _____. Placing an endotracheal tube into the _____ and _____ ___ ____ will help rapidly establish a patient's _____.

> inflating the cuff, airway, original position, stoma, need for

18
What is often the first sign of the _____ of the development of a potentially lethal dysrhythmia in an MI patient? Changing pulse rate.*
A change in the _____ _____ may be the first sign that a _____ is developing; this is why recording baseline _____ _____ is particularly important.

dysrhythmia, vital signs, pulse rate, onset

19
What is the purpose of performing the Sellick manoeuvre?
- to _____ the upper-airway structures during BVM
- to prevent the tongue from _____ the airway
- to protect a patient with possible spinal injury
- to prevent vomiting during attempts at intubation*

_____ _____ is used to prevent patients from _____ during intubation.

visualize, vomiting, Sellick manoeuvre, blocking

20
Traumatic aortic rupture usually occurs as a result of _____ of the aorta at the:
- pulmonary artery

- ligamentum teres
- _____ nuchae
- ligamentum arteriosum*

Ligamentum arteriosum is the most common area for an _____ _____ secondary to trauma.

aortic rupture, transection, ligamentum

Vocabulary 7
adjust /əˈdʒʌst/ přizpůsobit se, upravit, nastavit
alkalize /ˈælkəˌlaɪz/ alkalizovat
arteriosum /ɑːˌtiə.riˈɒs.əm/ ligamentum arteriosum, lat. vazivový pruh, na který se po svém uzavření mění ductus arteriosus, Botallova dučej
atelectasis /ˌætəˈlek.tə.sɪs/ atelektáza, neúplné roztažení části plic, spojené se ztrátou jejich vzdušnosti
carina /kəˈraɪn.ə/ člunek, výběžek
condensation /ˌkɒn.denˈseɪ.ʃən/ orosení, opocení, kondenzace páry
continue /kənˈtɪn.juː/ pokračovat, zůstat
contractile /kənˈtræk.taɪl/ kontraktilní, stažitelný
CPR, Cardiopulmonary /ˌkɑː.di.əʊˈpʊl.mə.nə.ri/ **Resuscitation** /rɪˌsʌs.ɪˈteɪ.ʃən/ kardiopulmonární resuscitace
end-tidal /ˈtaɪ.dəl/ přílivový, týkající se respiračního vzduchu, hodnota CO_2 na konci výdechu (ETCO$_2$)

farther /'fɑː.ðər/ dále
hear /hɪər/ (heard, heard) slyšet
heartbeat /'hɑːt.biːt/ tlukot srdce
improperly /ɪm'prɒp.ər.li/
nesprávně, nevhodně
initiate /ɪ'nɪʃ.i.eɪt/ zahájit, započít
innervate /'ɪn.ə.veɪt/ inervovat,
povzbudit (nerv nebo orgán k
činnosti)
laryngectomy /ˌlær.ɪn'dʒek.təm.i/
laryngektomie, odstranění hrtanu
leak /liːk/ unikání, otvor,
prosakovat
ligament /'lɪg.ə.mənt/ vaz mezi
kostmi, kloubu ap.
main /meɪn/ hlavní, nejdůležitější
mainstem /meɪn.stəm/ **bronchus** /
'brɒŋ.kəs/ hlavní průduška
MI, Myocardial /maɪ.əˌkɑː.di.əl/
Infarction /ɪn'fɑːk.ʃən/ infarkt
myokardu
multifocal /mʌl.ti'fəʊ.kəl/
víceohniskový
nonperfusing /ˌnɒn.pər.fjuːz.ɪŋ/
neprosakující, nepronikající
nucha /njuːkə/ šíje, vaz
oesophageal /iːˌsɒfə'dʒiːəl/
ezofageální, týkající se jícnu
orally /'ɔː.rə.li/ ústně
original /ə'rɪdʒ.ɪ.nəl/ originální,
prvotní, původní
pass /pɑːs/ projít, minout
position /pə'zɪʃ.ən/ pozice, poloha,
umístit
proven /'pruːvən/ prokázaný,
ověřený
PVCs, Premature /'preməˌtjʊə/
Ventricular /ven'trɪk.jə.lər/

Contractions /kən'trækʃəns/
předčasné stahy srdečních komor
reach /riːtʃ/ dorazit, dosáhnout,
dostat se
recording /rɪ'kɔː.dɪŋ/ záznam,
nahrávka
resolve /rɪ'zɒlv/ vyřešit, vstřebat se
slump /slʌmp/ prudce poklesnout,
propadnout se, krize
stroke /strəʊk/ **volume** /'vɒl.juːm/
tepový objem, objem krve, který
srdce vypudí při jednom srdečním
stahu tepu, systole
teres /tiː.riːz/ pl **teretes** sval nebo
vazivo cylindrického tvaru
through /θruː/ přes, skrz, napříč,
po celém
tip /tɪp/ naklonit se, sklonit se
visualize /'vɪʒ.u.əl.aɪz/ zviditelnit,
vizualizovat
watch /wɒtʃ/ sledovat, pozorovat,
dávat pozor

Unit 8

I

What is the clinical significance of a first-degree AV block?

- It signals the onset of rapid cardiovascular

  _____.

- It indicates that the ____ ____ may drop if action is not taken.
- It can lead to syncope and angina if not corrected quickly.
- It may foreshadow the development of a ____ _____ dysrhythmia.*

First-degree AV block in itself calls for _____ only; however, it may indicate the development of a more advanced heart block.

> heart rate, observation, decompensation, more advanced

2

In the _____ of baseline neurological status, these should be included: _____ to sensory stimulation, _____ reaction, and _____ function.*

> response, pupillary, documentation, motor

3

These are signs/symptoms of an _____ cerebrovascular accident: _____ of the speech, facial _____, drooling, weak _____ _____ on the affected side.

> slurring, motor response, droop, acute

4

Which term best describes the following definition? Disease of arterial vessels marked by _____, _____, and loss of elasticity in the arterial walls. Arteriosclerosis.*

_____ is the most common form of arteriosclerosis, usually involving medium-sized and large arteries.
Arterionecrosis is the destruction (_____) of the arteriole.
Angina is chest _____ associated with a deficiency of oxygen supply to the heart muscle.

> thickening, hardening, necrosis, discomfort, Atherosclerosis

5

The point of maximal impulse (PMI) can usually be felt on the:
1. left _____ chest
2. in the _____ line
3. at the fifth intercostal space

This is an excellent place to auscultate heart sounds and _____ _____.

> apical pulse, anterior, midclavicular

6

Central neurogenic hyperventilation is commonly associated with CNS trauma.*

_____ _____ hyperventilation is characterized by rapid, deep, noisy breathing and is associated with lesions of the central _____ _____. Cheyne-Stokes is the pattern commonly seen with _____ _____.

> Central neurogenic, diabetic emergencies, nervous system

7

The _____ of Type II diabetes mellitus includes polydipsia, polyuria, and polyphagia.*
Polydipsia (excessive _____), polyuria (excessive _____), and polyphagia (excessive _____) are just a few symptoms of _____ diabetes mellitus.

> hunger, urination, untreated, thirst, pathophysiology

8

Diabetic patients may _____ hypoglycaemia if they take too much _____ or if they exercise too much with limited food intake.* Hypoglycaemia develops in patients with diabetes when they take too much insulin or get too much _____ for the _____ __ ____ they eat.

> amount of food, exercise, insulin, develop

9

You are called to treat a patient who is unconscious and responsive to painful stimuli only. Which of the following treatment modalities is appropriate for this patient?
- _____ _____ test *
- dextrose (if indicated)
- thiamine
- monitor, _____, IV
- rapid transport

This choice gives the most appropriate treatment protocol for this patient. Because he is _____, he may be treated under _____ _____. Treatment in this case is _____ __ ruling out the most treatable cause for diabetec-coma.

> aimed at, unconscious, oxygen, implied consent, blood glucose*

10

A risk factor for the formation of atherosclerosis is diabetes mellitus.*

_____ _____ for atherosclerosis include diabetes, _____ ___, obesity, ____ __ _____, hypertension, and smoking.

lack of exercise, Risk factors, advanced age

11

A patient with hypoglycaemia may present with which of the following signs or symptoms?

- bizarre behaviour*
- blurred vision
- gradual onset
- bradycardia

Changes in behaviour are the ____ _____ signs of hypoglycaemia. Other signs and symptoms include _____, tachycardia, and _____.

diaphoresis, headache, most common

12

You have _____ the airway and _____ the cervical spine for your patient with an altered mental status.
What is your next priority of care? ____ _____ for glucose assessment and _____ __ __.*

The first priority for patients with _____ _____ _____ of unknown cause is a blood glucose determination to ____ ___ hypoglycaemia as a potential cause.

rule out, Draw blood, altered mental status, secured, immobilized, establish an IV

13

General management for a patient with altered mental status should include the following procedure: _____ blood glucose levels.*
Patients who _____ ____ altered mental status should __ _____ high-flow oxygen, IV access, and blood glucose levels _____. D50 should be administered when hypoglycaemia __ _____.

present with, be provided, is suspected, Determine, measured

14

What are the _____ _____ for the development of hyperosmolar hyperglycaemic nonketotic coma (HHNK)?

- old age, type II diabetes, coexisting cardiac or renal disease, and increased insulin requirements*

- _____ age, type I diabetes, coexisting cardiac or respiratory disease, and decreased insulin requirements
- _____, type II diabetes, viral infections, chronic alcoholism, and poor carbohydrate metabolism
- coexisting kidney disease, type I diabetes, narcotics use, and _____ with insulin regimen

The most significant predisposing factors are old age, type II diabetes, coexisting cardiac or renal disease, and increased insulin requirements.

young, predisposing factors, noncompliance, obesity

15

This statement about hypoglycaemia is correct: hypoglycaemia may occur in _____ patients, especially in chronic alcoholics.*
Hypoglycaemia may occur in nondiabetic patients, especially in _____ _____ who have poor diet and the inability to properly _____ carbohydrates. Except in cases of alcoholism and prolonged lack of ____ _____, nondiabetics seldom have problems with hypoglycaemia. Signs and symptoms of hypoglycaemia have

a _____ _____. In the early stages of hypoglycaemia, the patient may complain of extreme _____ ___ _____.

rapid onset, hunger and thirst, metabolize, food intake, nondiabetic, chronic alcoholics

16

For which of the following conditions would you be likely to receive an order to administer intravenous thiamine?

- in status _____
- in _____ shock
- hyperventilation
- profound intoxication*

Intravenous thiamine is used to reverse the effects of acute thiamine deficiency, which may lead to seizures and encephalopathy in _____.

alcoholics, metabolic, epilepticus

17

A patient in a very _____ _____ of hypoglycaemia may complain of hunger.*
The earliest _____ of hypoglycaemia are hunger, anxiety, and _____.

restlessness, manifestations, early stage

18

In a patient with_____
_____, assessment of the
abdomen should be performed
in the following order: inspect,
auscultate, palpate, percuss.
_____ is the obvious first
step since you are going to
look before you do anything.
_____ may not provide
much useful information, but
if you are going to auscultate,
it must be performed before
palpation. _____ is the
third step. You can gain a lot of
information through palpation.
_____ (if performed) is the
last assessment step.

> Auscultation, Percussion,
> Palpation, Inspection, abdominal
> pain

19

You respond to a 20-year-old
female complaining of dizziness
and weakness. She is slow to
_____ to your questions but
admits to taking several diet pills
a day in an effort to quickly ____
_____. Vitals are blood pressure
98/54, pulse 184, respirations 32,
the skin ____ ___ _____.
Immediate treatment should
include IV, oxygen, Adenocard 6
mg rapid IV push.

> lose weight, pale and moist,
> respond

20

Focused examination of the
abdomen of a patient who is
complaining of abdominal pain
should consist of gentle palpation
of the entire abdomen.*
Use only gentle palpation __
___ _____. Properly performed
auscultation for _____ _____
takes several minutes and is
of little value to your overall
treatment _____. Correctly
performed _____ requires a
relatively quiet environment and
an experienced hand to be of
any diagnostic value. Continued
assessment for rebound
tenderness will aggravate the
patient's _____ and is
unnecessary once you have
determined the patient has
abdominal distress.

> discomfort, in the field, regimen,
> percussion, bowel sounds

Vocabulary 8
Adenocard, adenosine /ə.den'ə.sin/
lék, s tlumivým účinkem na srdce,
vazodilátor, proti arytmii
advanced /əd'vɑːnst/ provedený
předem, před
aggravate /'æg.rə.veɪt/ ztížit,
zhoršit
aim /eɪm/ **at** /ət/ zaměřit se, snažit
se, mít v úmyslu, chtít
apical /'eɪ.pɪ.kəl/ apikální, ležící v
okolí hrotu

arrhythmia /əˈrɪð.mi.ə/ arytmie, nepravidelný rytmus
carbohydrate /ˌkɑː.bəʊˈhaɪ.dreɪt/ uhlovodan
coexist /ˌkoʊ·ɪgˈzɪst/ koexistovat, žít vedle sebe
consent /kənˈsent/ souhlas, svolení
decompensation /diːˌkɒm.penˈseɪ.ʃən/ dekompenzace, selhání kompenzačních mechanismů, udržujících určitou chorobu v přijatelných mezích, vzniká postupem nemoci, následkem přidružení jiné choroby nebo nedodržením léčby
depressant /dɪˈpres.ənt/ látka s tlumivým účinkem
determination /dɪˌtɜː.mɪˈneɪ.ʃən/ určení, stanovení
dextrose /ˈdek.strəʊs/ dextróza, D-glukóza
encephalopathy /enˌsef.əˈlɒp.ə.θi/ encefalopatie, mozkové onemocnění různého původu
female /ˈfiː.meɪl/ žena
foreshadow /fɔːˈʃæd.əʊ/ naznačovat, předznamenat
formation /fɔːˈmeɪ.ʃən/ formování, vytvoření, útvar
gentle /ˈdʒen.tl̩/ jemný
HHNK, Hyperosmolar Hyperglycaemic Nonketotic Coma hyperosmolární diabetické kóma bez ketoacidózy, vysoká hladina krevního cukru, která způsobuje výraznou hyperosmolaritu se ztrátami tekutin a minerálních látek močí při výrazné polyurii,

projevuje se zejm. nervovými a oběhovými příznaky až kómatem
hyperglycaemic /ˌhaɪ.pə.glaɪˈsiː.mɪk/ s nadměrným množstvím glukózy v krvi
hyperosmolar /ˌhaɪ.pə.ɒz.mɒ.lər/ **coma** /ˈkəʊmə/ hyperosmolární kóma, akutní komplikace cukrovky
hypertension /ˌhaɪ.pəˈten.ʃən/ hypertenze, vysoký krevní tlak
hypoglycaemia /ˌhaɪ.pəʊ.glaɪˈsiː.mi.ə/ hypoglykémie, snížená koncentrace glukózy v krvi
implied /ɪmˈplaɪd/ implicitní, nepřímo vyjádřený
insulin /ˈɪn.sjʊ.lɪn/ inzulín
intercostals /ˌɪn.təˈkɒs.təlz/ mezižeberní svaly
interior /ɪnˈtɪə.ri.ər/ interiér, vnitřek, vnitřní
intoxication /ɪnˌtɒk.sɪˈkeɪ.ʃən/ intoxikace, otrava, opilost
loose /luːs/ **weight** /weɪt/ ubrat na váze
maximal /ˈmæk.sɪ.məl/ maximální
medium /ˈmiː.di.əm/ středné velký, průměrný, medium, přenašeč, střed, prostřední
metabolize /mɪˈtæbəˌlaɪz/ metabolizovat, přeměňovat, trávit
modality /məʊˈdæl.ə.ti/ modalita, možný způsob
noncompliance /ˌnɒn.kəmˈplaɪəns/ nedodržování, nesoulad
nonketotic /ˌnɒn.ke.tɒt.ɪk/ neketotický
obesity /əʊˈbiː.sɪ.ti/ obezita

observation /ˌɒb.zəˈveɪ.ʃən/
pozorování, postřehy
pathophysiology /ˌpæθ.ə.ˌfɪz.
iˈɒl.ə.dʒi/ patofyziologie, nauka
o chorobných pochodech a
změnách funkcí organizmu
během nemoci
polydipsia /ˌpɒl.ɪˈdɪp.sɪ.ə/
polydipsie, chorobná žíznivost
polyphagia /ˌpɒl.ɪˈfeɪ.dʒə/
polyfagie, zvýšená chuť k jídlu,
pojídání velkého množství jídla
present /ˈprez.ənt/ projevovat
rebound/ˌriːˈbaʊnd/ **tenderness** /
ˈten.dər.nəs/ zvýšená bolestivost
při náhlém uvolnění tlaku
regimen /ˈredʒ.ɪ.mən/ režim,
životospráva
requirement /rɪˈkwaɪə.mənt/
požadavek, podmínka

significance /sɪgˈnɪf.ɪ.kəns/
význam, důležitost, hodnota
thiamine /ˈθaɪ.ə.miːn/ thiamin,
vitamin B 1
untreated /ʌnˈtriː.tɪd/ neléčený,
neošetřený
vasodilator /ˌveɪ.zə.daɪˈleɪ.tər/
vazodilátor, vyvolávající rozšíření
cévy

Unit 9

I

Which is the best way to examine a patient with abdominal pain? Begin palpation of all four quadrants, ending with the painful area.*

_____all quadrants of the abdomen, ending where the patient says it _____. Because of the need for a quiet environment and several minutes to _____ this successfully, you should not perform abdominal _____ or _____ in the field.

Palpate, perform, auscultation, hurts, percussion

2

Which organs are contained in the right upper quadrant of the abdomen? Liver, gallbladder, head of the _____, part of the _____, and part of the _____.*

duodenum, colon, pancreas

3

A patient who complains of pain in the left upper abdominal quadrant may be suffering from which of the following?
- pancreatitis*
- appendicitis
- hepatitis
- diverticulitis

Pain in the left upper quadrant is most often due to _____, _____, or diseases of the ____ _____.

Appendicitis often results in right lower-quadrant pain, but the actual location of the area of the appendix that is _____ may result in left lower-quadrant or even flank pain. _____ results in dull right upper-quadrant pain that is independent of the presence of food in the GI tract. Diverticulitis presents much like appendicitis, but it is generally localized to the left lower abdomen.

inflamed, pancreatitis, gastritis, left kidney, Hepatitis

4

What do orthostatic vital sign changes suggest for a patient with acute abdominal pain?
- the patient has

  _____
- the patient is hypovolaemic*
- the patient has

  _____
- the patient is a diabetic

A positive tilt test in a patient with acute abdominal pain suggests that the patient is _____ and may have impending shock.

hypovolaemic, appendicitis, peritonitis

5
A patient with left shoulder pain may have a ruptured spleen.* Bleeding within the abdominal cavity can _____ the abdominal surface of the _____, causing _____ _____ to the shoulder.

irritate, referred pain, diaphragm

6
A patient with an acute abdomen who shows no signs of _____ and has stable vital signs should be positioned in whatever position is _____ _____ for the patient.* Medical patients who are _____ should be in a position of comfort.

stable, haemorrhage, most comfortable

7
An unrestrained driver of a small car struck a tree at high speed. He has a distended abdomen that is tender when palpated. Vital signs are as follows: pulse, 120 beats per minute; respirations, 20 per minute; and blood pressure, 116/90 mmHg.
What would most likely be the cause of the _____ _____? Organ damage.* _____ _____ from the mechanism of injury may _____ __ inflammation and bleeding,

resulting in the _____ vital signs.

Organ damage, result in, abdominal tenderness, compensatory

8
If your patient has an open abdominal wound with a loop of bowel obtruding, you should treat this with a wet, sterile dressing and an occlusive dressing.* The most appropriate dressing for an evisceration is the application of a ___, _____ _____ (which keeps the organs moist) and an _____ dressing (which provides a barrier against further contamination and ___ _____).

wet, sterile dressing, occlusive, heat loss

9
A patient has been stabbed in the back. Which of the following signs would most likely make you suspect that the patient has a _____ _____?
• abdominal tenderness
• haematuria*
• thirst
• ecchymosis to the flank
Frank blood in the _____ is a strong sign of injury to the kidney. _____ _____ is unlikely, since the kidneys are located in the retroperitoneal

space. _____ may provide indirect information about organ involvement but is not as specific as haematuria.

> kidney injury, Bruising, urine, Abdominal tenderness

10

The signs of uraemia resulting from chronic renal failure include which of the following?

- pale skin, diaphoresis, and oedematous extremities
- pasty, yellow skin and wasting of the extremities*
- anxiety, delirium, nausea, and hallucinations
- anorexia, watery diarrhoea, nausea, and vomiting

Signs of _____ _____ are pasty, yellow skin and thin extremities; urea frost is a late sign. These signs result from jaundice, poor nutrition, and _____ ____ in the tissues. In _____ _____, the potassium level can be _____ _____. Pericardial tamponade and uremic encephalopathy may also be present. Coupled with _____ _____, non-cardiac pulmonary oedema, severe dyspnoea, ascites, neck vein distension, and rales in the bases may also be seen.

> uraemia, extreme cases, kidney failure, dangerously elevated, protein loss

11

Patients with _____ inflammatory disease often complain of which of the following?

- diffuse lower-abdominal pain*
- severe vaginal _____
- tearing pain in the _____
- _____ upon urination

The most common presentation of PID is _____, moderate to severe lower-abdominal pain, which makes _____ difficult.

> pelvic, uterus, itching, ambulation, bleeding, diffuse

12

You respond for a 44-year-old male diabetic who is complaining of a general feeling of weakness. During your questioning, you learn that he has been constantly _____ ___ _____. His breath has a _____ _____, and his level of consciousness appears to be diminishing.

What _____ _____ is this patient most likely suffering from? Diabetic ketoacidosis.*

What vital signs would you expect from this patient? Warm, dry skin; tachycardia; _____* _____.

This patient's symptoms are most likely due to low levels of _____.
This statement is the most accurate: he has not taken his _____ ____ of insulin or is ill.*
During transport, this patient slips into unconsciousness, and his breathing becomes very deep and rapid.
What is this pattern called? Kussmaul's respirations.*
Kussmaul's respirations are very ____ ___ _____ and represent the body's attempt to _____ ___ the metabolic acidosis produced by the ketones and organic acids in the blood.
What does the appropriate treatment for this patient include? A _____ _____ test, IV normal saline, and a fluid bolus.*

---

deep and rapid, compensate for, blood, glucose, diabetic emergency, insulin*, thirsty and hungry, correct dose, fruity odour, increased respirations

---

14
Signs of _____ include:
- ____, rapid pulse*
- cold, clammy skin*
- headache*
- _____
- coma*

---

hypoglycaemia, irritability,* weak*

15
Which rhythm is likely to foreshadow the development of other, more serious _____? Accelerated junctional rhythm.*
Because the _____ _____ is usually ischaemia, _____ junctional rhythm can _____ into more serious dysrhythmias.

---

deteriorate, accelerated, underlying cause, dysrhythmias

13
What is the primary treatment of metabolic acidosis? Ventilating the patient adequately with oxygen.*
Treatment of _____ _____ consists mainly of adequate _____. Identification of the cause of acidosis is not as critical as identifying that it is present and beginning _____ _____ to prevent its worsening.

16
What is a possible cause of pulseless electrical activity? Hypovolaemia.*

_____ _____ _____ may occur secondary to a variety of _____ and carries a grave prognosis.
_____ _____ are: pulmonary embolus, tension pneumothorax,

acidosis, cardiac tamponade, hypovolaemia, hypoxia, hypothermia, hyperkalaemia, AMI, and drug overdose. Hypokalaemia may cause dysrhythmias but does not usually cause PEA. Tachycardia is not considered a cause of PEA simply because the definition of PEA is a pulseless patient with a rhythm that you would normally expect to find a pulse with. In other words, tachycardia _____ a pulse is PEA.

> conditions, without, Common causes, Pulseless electrical activity

17

Paroxysmal _____ _____ (PND) is commonly a sign of left-side heart failure.*
Left-side heart failure with pulmonary oedema is often _____ ____ PND. PND manifests as difficulty _____ when the patient ____ ____. As the condition worsens, many patients will report the need to sleep _____ __ in a recliner.

> lies flat, sitting up, associated with, nocturnal dyspnoea, breathing

18

Which set of _____ _____ is suggestive of left ventricular heart failure with pulmonary oedema?
BP elevated, pulse fast and _____, respirations rapid and _____.*

> vital signs, laboured, irregular

19

What feature distinguishes dissecting aortic aneurysm from acute myocardial infarction?
- The pain of dissecting aortic aneurysm is severe from the outset.*
- The pain of dissecting aortic aneurysm usually migrates to the right arm.
- Patients with dissecting aortic aneurysm have equal peripheral pulses.
- Patients with dissecting aortic aneurysm show signs of periacdial tamponade.

Patients with _____ _____ _____ describe their pain as _____ severe from the outset, whereas the pain of AMI tends to build _____.

> extremely, dissecting aortic aneurysm, slowly

20

These statements about the pain that accompanies a myocardial infarction are correct:
- Patients often describe the pain as 'crushing'.*

- The pain is present only during exertion or stress.*
- Pain due to AMI radiates like anginal pain.*

The pain of MI is not generally relieved by sublingual nitroglycerin, and intravenous morphine or nitroglycerin is usually necessary. It may have all of the ____ _____ of angina, making a diagnosis by ____ _____ relatively difficult. The pain caused by myocardial infarction is usually relieved only by the use of _____.

---

morphine, same characteristic, EMS providers

Vocabulary 9

accelerate /ə k'sel.ə.reɪt/ zrychlit, přidat rychlost, vzrůst

acute /əˈkjuːt/ akutní

ambulation /ˈæm.bjʊ.lən.ʃən/ chůze

AMI, Acute /əˈkjuːt/ **Myocardial** /ˌmaɪ.ə'kɑː.di.əl/ **Infarction** /ɪnˈfɑː.ʃən/ akutní infarkt myokardu

barrier /ˈbær.i.ər/ překážka, zábrana

breathing /ˈbriː.ðɪŋ/ dýchání, dýchací

build /bɪld/ (built, built) posílit, upevnit, vybudovat

colon /ˈkoʊ.lən/ trakčník

constantly /ˈkɒn.stənt.li/ neustále, nepřetržitě

contamination /kənˌtæm.ɪˈneɪ.ʃən/ kontaminace, zamoření

corrective /kəˈrek.tɪv/ korekční, nápravný

crushing /ˈkrʌʃ.ɪŋ/ drtivý

dangerously /ˈdeɪn.dʒər.əs.li/ nebezpečně

delirium tremens /dɪˌlɪr.i.əmˈtrem.ənz/ kvalitativní porucha vědomí při chronickém alkoholismu

dissecting /daɪˈsekt.ɪŋ/ **aortic** /eɪˈɔː.tɪk/ **aneurysm** /ˈæn.jʊə.rɪ.zəm/ disekující aneurysma aorty

duodenum /ˌdjuː.əˈdiː.nəm/ dvanácterník

dyspnoea /dɪs.pniː.ə/ dyspnoe, dušnost, porucha dýchání

ecchymosis /ˌeki'məʊ.sɪs/ ekchymóza, tečkovité krvácení na sliznicích

evisceration /ɪˌvɪs.əˈreɪ.ʃən/ eviscerace, vynětí orgánů z těla

fruity /ˈfruː.tɪ/ ovocný

gastritis /gæsˈtraɪ.tɪs/ gastritida, zánět žaludku

grave /greɪv/ závažný, smrt, hrob

haematuria /ˌhiː.mə.t'jʊə.ri.ə/ hematurie, krev v moči

hallucination /həˌluːˈsɪˈneɪ.ʃən/ halucinace, přelud

hurt /hɜːt/ (hurt, hurt) zranit, poranit

identification /aɪˌden.tɪ.fɪˈkeɪ.ʃən/ identifikace, určení, rozpoznání

infarction /ɪnˈfɑː.k.ʃən/ infarkt

involvement /ɪnˈvɒlv.mənt/ účast, zapojení se, vztah

irritate /ˈɪr.ɪ.teɪt/ dráždit kůži, ránu

itching /ˈɪtʃ.ɪŋ/ svědění, svědící

jaundice /ˈdʒɔː.n.dɪs/ žloutenka

late /leɪt/ pozdní, pokročilý, ke konci

loop /luːp/ smyčka, obtočit

migrate /maɪˈɡreɪt/ migrovat, stěhovat se

morphine /ˈmɔː.fiːn/ morfium, morfin

nitroglycerin /ˌnaɪ.trəʊˈɡlɪs.ər.iːn/ nitroglycerin, lék pro zklidnění srdečních arytmií a snižování krevního tlaku

nocturnal /nɒkˈtɜː.nəl/ noční

normal /ˈnɔː.məl/ normální, obvyklý

obtrude /əbˈtruːd/ narušovat, rušit

odour /ˈəʊdə/ odér, pach

orthostatic /ˌɔː.θəˈstæt.ɪk/ ortostatický, ve vzpřímené poloze

outset /ˈaʊt.set/ začátek, počátek

pasty /ˈpæs.ti/ bledý, bílý

PEA, Pulseless /pʌls.ləs/ **Electrical** /ɪˈlek.trɪ.kəl/ **Activity** /ækˈtɪv.ɪ.ti/ bezpulzní elektrická aktivita

PID, Pelvic /ˈpel.vɪk/ **Inflammatory** /ɪnˈflæm.ə.tər.i/ **Disease** /dɪˈziːz/ zánětlivé onemocnění pánve

PND, Paroxysmal /ˌpær.ɒk.ˈsɪz.məl/ **Nocturnal** /nɒkˈtɜː.nəl/ **Dyspnea** /dɪs.pniː.ə/ záchvatovitá (paroxysmální) noční dušnost

protein /ˈprəʊ.tiːn/ protein, bílkovina

provider /prəˈvaɪ.dər/ poskytovatel, dodavatel

pulseless /pʌls.ləs/ bez pulzu

recliner /rɪˈklaɪ.nər/ polohovací, sklápěcí křeslo

retroperitoneal /ˌret.rəʊˌper.ɪ.təʊ.ˈniː.əl/ ležící za pobřišnicí

slip /slɪp/ sklouznout, protáhnout, vsunout

stable /ˈsteɪ.bl̩/ stabilní, stabilizovaný, stálý

suggestive /səˈdʒes.tɪv/ připomínající, nasvědčující

unrestrained /ˌʌn.rɪˈstreɪnd/ nespoutaný, nevázaný

uraemia /jʊəˈriː.mɪ.ə/ uremie, chronické selhání činnosti ledvin

urea /jʊəˈriː..ə/ **frost** /frɒst/ klinický nález při chronickém renálním selhání, koncentrace močoviny je výrazně zvýšená v potu a způsobuje srážení krystalizované močoviny v pokožce

uremic /jʊəˈriː.mɪk/ uremický, týkající se uremie

ventilate /ˈven.tɪ.leɪt/ ventilovat, větrat

Unit 10

1

Which of the following conditions would result in an increase in a patient's $PaCO_2$?

- airway obstruction*
- hypoventilation*
- physical exertion*

$PaCO_2$ measures carbon dioxide levels in the _____, which are influenced by alterations in CO_2 production or _____. Such levels would be increased by physical _____ of muscles, by hypoventilation, or by an airway _____.

elimination, obstruction, blood, exertion

2

The pharyngotracheal lumen airway should be removed if the patient regains consciousness.* If the patient is unconscious and vomits, the PTL will help prevent _____. Instead, if a gag reflex returns, the PTL will have to _____ before the patient _____.

vomits, aspiration, be removed

3

Which of the following patient presentations would best be managed by a nasal intubation?

- The patient is unconscious and apnoeic with a pulse.
- The patient is unconscious, apnoeic, and pulseless.
- The patient is unconscious, is breathing slowly, and has a gag reflex.*
- The patient is semiconscious, is breathing slowly, and has a pulse.

There must be some _____ respiratory effort for the _____ _____ to have a good chance of successful _____. The presentation in the last choice can probably be managed by basic airway manoeuvres.

placement, spontaneous, blind insertion

4

The digital intubation method is used for patients who have suspected spinal injury.* Because the _____ _____ does not require hyperextending the patient's _____, it is used for patients with suspected _____ __ _____ injury.

spinal or cervical, digital method, neck

5

You are called to the home of a 26-year-old male who is having difficulty breathing. Your assessment reveals a pulse rate of 100 with a strong and regular radial pulse, a blood pressure of 132/78, and a respiratory rate of 36, laboured with audible wheezes.

The patient's skin is pale, moist, and at a normal temperature. He is having difficulty exhaling and says that he has experienced this before. He rates this event as a 9 on a 1-10 severity scale. He states that this event was unprovoked and that he has been having dyspnoea for 20-30 minutes.

This patient is most likely suffering from which condition? Asthma.*

This patient shows the clinical symptoms of _____. Due to the repeat nature of this episode, it is _____ that this is pulmonary oedema, upper-airway obstruction, or simple pneumothorax. If he were suffering from _____ _____, you would also expect haemoptysis.

A spontaneous (or _____) pneumothorax would also present with a sudden _____ but would most likely not also have wheezing or a history of _____.

Treating this patient with nebulized steroids would provide no immediate relief of the bronchospasm.*

_____ _____ would provide no immediate relief of this patient's bronchospasm as they will not prevent or lessen attacks in progress. Steroid therapy is useful as a long-term _____ treatment.

This patient's respiratory distress is due to constriction of the smaller airways.*

_____ of the smaller airways is causing air to be trapped in the alveoli.

This patient's disease is regarded as a chronic inflammatory disease.*

Asthma is regarded as chronic _____ _____. Chronic obstructive pulmonary diseases commonly include emphysema and chronic bronchitis.

This patient's respiratory distress may have been caused by one of several triggers. These _____ include allergens, irritants, and which of the following?

- viral infections
- hot weather
- exercise*
- bee stings

_____, exercise, and irritants are common triggers of asthma attacks. Cold weather, _____, and anxiety are lesser triggers.

pulmonary oedema, triggers, simple, Constriction, inflammatory disease, stress, asthma, onset, Nebulized steroids, recurrence, suppressive, unlikely, Allergens

6

Your patient is a 51-year-old male with a history of COPD. He states that he has called EMS because he can hardly breathe. On _____ assessment you _____ that the patient is in obvious respiratory _____ but not too hypoxic.

You should _____ low-flow oxygen at a rate of 2-6 l/min. via _____ cannula.*

determine, administer, distress, nasal, initial

7

You patient is a 29-year-old female complaining of the sudden onset of severe shortness of breath and chest pain. She indicates that she __ _____ from surgery to her left femur after an automobile crash. What is this patient most likely suffering from? Pulmonary embolism.*

You would expect to find bradycardia.*

You would expect to see this patient in tachycardia rather than in bradycardia due to the increasing dyspnoea and hypoxia

resulting from the _____ _____.

This patient's physiological problems are most likely due to what cardiac problem? The right side of the heart pumping against increased resistance.*

The pulmonary embolism has caused the right side of the heart to have to pump harder against a _____ caused by the _____ _____. This result is the severe shortness of breath and hypoxia.

Proper management for this patient includes transport in shock position.*

- This patient should be transported in the position in which it is easiest for her to breathe (i.e. the _____ _____).

What condition is a common cause of this patient's problem? Placement of a central line.*

pulmonary embolism, is recovering, partial blockage, pumping, shock position, resistance

8

You are called by the police department to a neighbourhood where you encounter a male patient approximately 20-30 years old. The police officer states that neighbours called because the patient was freaking out. _____ say they saw him smoking something just before he started acting in a _____ _____.

During your assessment, you notice that the patient is _____ and anxious. His pupils are _____, and he is hypertensive and tachycardic.

Dilated pupils, hyperactivity, tachycardia, and hypertension are classic signs of _____ ___. (Narcotic use would result in lethargy, stupor, and respiratory depression.)

The appropriate treatment for this patient consists of oxygen, IV, ECG, monitoring and transport.* Transport is the only other treatment required for this patient. Be prepared to provide _____ _____ if needed.

Naloxone is used with narcotic ingestion to restore respirations and is not indicated in this patient. Activated charcoal and ipecac are indicated for _____ __ _____ via the oral route. This patient was reported to have inhaled (smoked) something that appears to be a _____.

When treating this patient, you should be prepared for which of the following complications?

- Tachycardia and _____ _____
- ___ _____ and hypoglycaemia
- Dysrhythmias and seizures*
- Bradycardia and tachypnoea

Dysrhythmias and seizures are both serious possible _____ of stimulation effects from cocaine use.

Witnesses, hyperactive, CNS depression, complications, stimulant, septic shock, dilated, respiratory support, cocaine use, bizarre manner, poisoning or overdose

9

Which of the following requires intermediate-level _____ through the use of a solution of bleach and water?

- routine _____ _____ measures in your station and bunkroom
- any items that have come into contact with _____ _____
- any _____ that were used in any invasive procedures
- all items that have come into contact with intact skin*

Intermediate-level disinfection is used for all instruments and supplies that have come into contact with _____ ____.

> mucous membranes, intact skin, house cleaning, disinfection, instruments

10
Why must your assessment be especially diligent in an intoxicated patient?
- Alcohol can decrease pain tolerance in the patient.
- Alcohol can mask signs and symptoms of injury.*
- Alcohol can increase the patient's willingness to _____.
- Alcohol can _____ an injury's effect on the patient's level of consciousness.

As a mild anaesthetic, ethanol can reduce the patient's _____ of pain. It will be important to carefully and completely _____ the patient for any _____ _____.

> unnoticed injuries, examine, perception, cooperate, decrease

11
Early symptoms of overdose of tricyclic _____ include which of the following?
- tachycardia and a wide QRS complex*

- _____, vomiting, and severe diarrhoea
- psychosis and bizarre behavioural changes
- altered mental status and _____ _____

_____ with wide QRS complex is an important early sign of _____. High doses of sodium bicarbonate IV drip will help control dysrhythmias.

> toxicity, antidepressants, Tachycardia, slurred speech, nausea

12
What do the symptoms of acetaminophen _____ include?
- _____, vomiting, malaise, diaphoresis, and right upper-quadrant pain*
- nausea, _____, confusion, lethargy, seizures, and dysrhythmias
- altered _____ _____, hypotension, slurred speech, and bradycardia
- nausea, dilated _____, rambling speech, lethargy, headache, and dizziness

> mental status, overdose, vomiting, nausea, pupils

13
_____ administration of sodium bicarbonate may be

ordered for a patient who has overdosed on which of the following drugs?
- acetaminophen
- benzodiazepines
- narcotics
- antidepressants*

_____ _____ is sometimes ordered in the field for ingestions of tricyclic _____ with cardiac symptoms (wide complex tachycardias).

> Prehospital, Sodium bicarbonate, antidepressants

14

An adult patient has overdosed on an unknown medication in a _____ _____. She is _____, oriented, and refusing treatment and transport.

What is your most appropriate next action? Consult with _____ _____ to transport the patient.*

This patient may not have the right to _____ _____ and transport due to the actions she has taken. Consulting with medical direction on how to ____ _____ this patient may be helpful.

> best approach, medical direction, suicide attempt, refuse treatment, alert

15

What are the classic symptoms of _____ overdose? Respiratory depression and constricted pupils.*

_____ _____ and _____ (pin-point) pupils are classic symptoms of narcotic overdose.

> constricted, Respiratory depression, narcotic

16

Chest pain associated with stable angina may be caused by a built up of lactic acid and CO_2.*

_____ _____ is caused by a temporary low-flow state in the _____ _____ that does not lead to ____ _____ __ _____ (infarction). During hypoperfusion, lactic acid and excessive carbon dioxide are not _____ ____, causing irritation and pain.

> Stable angina, coronary, carried away, arteries, cell injury or death

17

The pain of _____ _____ is brought on by:
- exercise or stress*
- imminent AMI
- difficulty breathing
- _____ of nitroglycerin

_____ of stable angina are brought on by exercise or by

stress and are usually easily managed.

Oxygen, increasing, prevent, anxiety

Attacks, overuse, stable angina

18
A patient's signs and symptoms include orthopnoea, spasmodic coughing, agitation, cyanosis, rales, jugular vein distension, and elevated blood pressure, pulse, and respirations. What _____ should you suspect?
- left-side heart failure*
- right-side heart failure
- _____ infarction
- _____ shock

Listed are _____ signs and symptoms of left heart failure with _____ oedema.

cardiogenic, classic, pulmonary, condition, myocardial

19
A primary reason for administering oxygen to a patient with AMI is to:
- help limit the infarct size*
- _____ pulmonary oedema
- reduce _____ and fear
- treat ventricular dysrhythmias

_____ can help limit the size of the infarct by _____ oxygen delivery to the heart muscle.

20
You have just started an IV lifeline, but the fluid is not flowing properly.
What is the first thing you should do to troubleshoot this situation?
Make sure the constricting band has been removed.*
Proper flow cannot be achieved if the constriction band (_____) is not removed.
Care of the patient with _____ _____ is similar to care for the patient with _____ _____. Patients with cardiac contusion can present with the symptoms of myocardial infarction, including ____-_____ dysrhythmias.
Care is similar to care of any cardiac patient.

myocardial infarction, tourniquet, life-threatening, cardiac contusion

Vocabulary 10
acetaminophen /əˌsiː.təˈmɪn.ə.fen/ paracetamol
anaesthetic /ˌæn.əsˈθet.ɪk/ anestetický, anestetikum
antidepressant /ˌæn.ti.dɪˈpres.ənt/ antidepresivum, lék
asthma /ˈæs.mə/ astma
attack /əˈtæk/ útok, napadení, záchvat

band /bænd/ páska, pásek

bee /biː/ včela

benzodiazepines /benˈzɒ.dɪ.azˈe.piːnz/ benzodiazepiny

bleach /bliːtʃ/ odbarvit, bělicí prostředek

bunkroom /bʌŋk.rʊm/ lůžko, nocovat

carry /ˈkær.i/ nést, vézt

charcoal /ˈtʃɑːr.koʊl/ živočišné uhlí

cocaine /kəʊˈkeɪn/ kokain

cooperate /kəʊˈɒp.ər.eɪt/ kooperovat, spolupracovat

diligent /ˈdɪl.ɪ.dʒənt/ svědomitý, pečlivý

disinfection /ˌdɪs.ɪnˈfek.ʃən/ dezinfekce

drip /drɪp/ kapat, kapka, kapačka

ethanol /ˈeθ.ə.nɒl/ etanol, etylalkohol

freak /friːk/ bizarní, neobvyklý, ztratit hlavu, šílet

haemoptysis /hiːˈmɒ.ptɪ.sɪs/ hemoptýza, vykašlávání krve

instead /ɪnˈsted/ místo toho, raději

instrument /ˈɪn.strə.mənt/ nástroj, přístroj

intermediate /ˌɪn.təˈmiː.di.ət/ prostřední, středně pokročilý

invasive /ɪnˈveɪ.sɪv/ invazivní, šířící se, narušující

ipecac /ˈɪp.ɪ.kæk/ ipecac, lék způsobující zvracení, používaný např. při otravě

irritant /ˈɪr.ɪ.tənt/ iritující, obtíž, dráždidlo

item /ˈaɪ.təm/ položka, věc, předmět, bod, záležitost

life-threatening /ˈlaɪfˌθret.ən.ɪŋ/ životu nebezpečný, život ohrožující

lumen /ˈluː.mən/ pl **lumina** lumen, průchod, průsvit

malaise /mælˈeɪz/ malátnost, nevolnost

manner /ˈmæn.ər/ chování, styl, zvyk

Naloxone /nəˈlɒksəʊn/ naloxon, antidotum narkotik

narcotic /nɑːˈkɒt.ɪk/ narkotikum, omamná látka

ordered /ˈɔː.dəd/ nařízený, předepsaný

overuse /ˌəʊ.vəˈjuːz/ nadužívat, nadměrné používání

perception /pəˈsep.ʃən/ vnímání, vjem, pohled

progress /ˈprəʊ.gres/ postup, vývoj, probíhat

rambling /ˈræm.blɪŋ/ nesouvislý, zmatený

rate /reɪt/ ohodnotit, řadit

recover /rɪˈkʌv.ər/ zotavit se, uzdravit se

recurrence /rɪˈkʌr.əns/ recidiva, opakování, opětovný výskyt

refuse /rɪˈfjuːz/ odmítnout, nepřijmout

relief /rɪˈliːf/ úleva, pomoc

restore /rɪˈstɔːr/ obnovit, znovu zavést, vrátit

scale /skeɪl/ škála, rozsah

septic /ˈsep.tɪk/ septický, zanícený, zhnisaný

spasmodic /spæzˈmɒd.ɪk/ spazmický, křečovitý

station /'steɪ.ʃən/ být umístěný,
pozice, stanoviště
stimulant /'stɪm.jʊ.lənt/ stimulant,
povzbuzující prostředek
stupor /'stju:.pər/ mrákoty,
otupělost, bezvědomí
suppressive /sə'pres.ɪv/ potlačující,
zatajující
surgery /'sɜ:.dʒər.i/ operace,
chirurgický zákrok
tourniquet /'tʊə.nɪ.keɪ/ škrtidlo,
tlakový obvaz
troubleshoot /'trʌb.ḷ.ʃu:t/ řešit
problémy, odstraňovat závady

unnoticed /ʌn'nəʊ.tɪst/
nepozorovaný, nepovšimnutý
unprovoked /ˌʌn.prə'vəʊkt/
nevyprovokovaný, ničím
nevyvolaný
willingness /'wɪl.ɪŋ.nəs/ ochota

Unit 11

1

What factor would _____ a patient from receiving thrombolytic therapy after an AMI? He or she has had recent ulcer or gastrointestinal bleeding.* Any condition that would present a significant _____ _____ excludes a patient from receiving _____ therapy.

> thrombolytic, bleeding hazard, exclude

2

In which of the following situation should a paramedic perform an _____ _____ first?
- during cardiac arrest at a swimming pool*
- when the patient is in a toxic environment
- when the scene is not yet secured by law enforcement
- during a rescue from a fully involved structure fire

Before assessing _____, _____, ___ _____, it is necessary to remove the patient (and yourself) to a place of relative _____.

> safety, airway, breathing, and circulation, initial assessment

3

What are the signs of _____ _____ in a patient who is receiving IV fluids? Dyspnoea, rales, and rhonchi.* _____, rales, and rhonchi are classic signs of fluid overload, which is usually first _____ __ pulmonary oedema.

> manifested as, Dyspnoea, circulatory overload

4

When caring for a patient with a pulmonary contusion, it is essential not to overload the patient with IV fluids.* _____ _____ involves bruising of the lung tissue. It is essential not to _____ a patient suffering from pulmonary contusion with fluids as this can quickly lead to pulmonary _____. The patient should be given high-flow oxygen and intubated if necessary. Immobilization on a _____ may be necessary depending on the mechanism of injury. If so, the head of the board may be elevated slightly to improve _____ _____.

> Pulmonary contusion, respiratory effect, overload, backboard, oedema

5

A single-lead ECG tracing is useful for obtaining information about the heart.

What can be determined from a single-lead ECG tracing? Timing of electrical impulse travel.*

A single-lead ECG, used for_____ _____, can be used to determine the _____ ____, _____, and the length of time it takes for the _____ to travel through the heart.

> heart rate, impulse, routine monitoring, regularity

6

What does the treatment for a patient whose ECG shows premature _____ _____ include? Observation only as long as the patient remains asymptomatic.*

If the patient is _____, this arrhythmia requires _____ only.

> observation, asymptomatic, atrial contractions

7

Why are _____ _____ and _____ ____ considered major goals for prehospital care of MI patients? Both anxiety and pain increase heart rate and myocardial oxygen demand.*

Anxiety and pain can increase the heart rate and, therefore, the _____ _____ of the myocardium.

> oxygen demand, relieving pain, easing anxiety

8

Some treatments for suspected __ _____ mask the elevated cardiac enzyme levels that are used to diagnose MI in the hospital setting.

To prevent this, you should NOT administer any drugs via the IM route.*

_____ injections can injure muscle tissues, causing the release of _____ that may mask the cardiac enzymes that are locked to confirm a _____ of MI.

> Intramuscular, diagnosis, enzymes, MI patients

9

Patients who ____ _____ and have altered mental status are best transported left-lateral recumbent.*

There is significant opportunity for the loss of _____ _____ for this patient. A lateral recumbent position will allow _____ _____ of the airway in the case of vomiting, as well as ____ _____ for suctioning.

easy access, airway control,
passive draining, have
overdosed

10

Blood flows from the pulmonary
veins into which structure?

- left atrium of the heart.*
- right atrium of the heart
- capillaries of the lungs
- right ventricle of the heart

Oxygenated blood flows from
the lungs, ___ the pulmonary
veins, into the ____ _____. From
there, it passes through the mitral
(_____) valve into the left
_____. It passes through the
aortic _____, then enters into the
_____.

via, ventricle, left atrium, valve,
bicuspid, aorta

11

Blood enters the right atrium of
the heart through which of the
following structures?

- tricuspid valve
- right ventricle
- left pulmonary arteries
- superior and inferior vena
  cava*

Blood enters the right atrium
through the superior and inferior
____ ____ and is pumped through
the _____ _____ into the right
ventricle. From there, it passes
through the pulmonic valve into

the _____ _____ and into
the lungs.

Simultaneous palpation of the
apical impulse and the _____
_____ allows you to assess the
relationship between the ventricular
contractions and the pulse.

Determining the relationship
between the _____ _____
and the carotid pulse may give
you the first indication of a
_____ _____, such as a
dysrhythmia. To assess central
and _____ circulation, you
should assess _____ (central)
and _____ (peripheral) pulses.

Remember that the
cardiovascular system requires
three factors to work effectively:
an intact and functioning pump,
an adequate circulating blood
volume, and a container (vascular
vessels) of the appropriate size to
_____ the blood effectively.

An apical pulse indicates that
the pump is functioning, and a
carotid pulse shows you that
the circulating blood volume is
reaching target tissues.

peripheral, apical impulse,
circulate, tricuspid valve, carotid,
cardiac irregularity, carotid
pulse, pulmonary arteries, vena
cava, radial

12

What do the signs and symptoms of hypertensive crisis include?

- _____ oedema, tachycardia, tachypnoea, and venous _____
- paralysis, seizures, headache, and _____ level of consciousness
- severe _____ distress, apprehension, cyanosis, and diaphoresis
- restlessness, confusion, blurred vision, nausea, and vomiting*

---

congestion, respiratory, pitting, altered

13

These statements are true regarding _____:

- It may cause a reflex hypothermia.*
- _____ may result which can lead to a rise in core temperature.*
- 101.84 °F (38.8 °C) should be used as a target temperature to prevent overcooling.*

Using ice or cold water may cause a _____ _____ and cause the patient to shiver which will raise the body temperature again. Hypothermia can result from an increase in ___ ____, a decrease in ___ _____, or a combination of these two factors.

---

heat loss, reflex hypothermia, heat production, overcooling, Shivering

---

14

In case of _____, do not ____ if there is any possibility of refreezing.*
A golden rule for the treatment of _____ _____ is to never thaw it if there is any possibility of _____.

---

refreezing, frostbite, frozen flesh, thaw

15

A 17-year-old male complains of a steadily worsening headache several days after being struck in the head during football practice. What injury best describes this patient's presentation? Subdural haematoma.*
A subdural bleed occurs when a _____ ____ bleeds into the area below the ____ _____. It may take some time before _____ from the bleeding is high enough __ _____ clinical signs and symptoms.

---

dura mater, pressure, to cause, small vein

16

_____ _____ allows you to continuously record pulse rate and oxygen saturation.*

Once it is attached to the patient's _____, the pulse oximeter will continuously record the _____ ____ and oxygen saturation level.

| pulse rate, finger, Pulse oximetry |

17
What would a pulse oximetry reading of 88% indicate for your patient with acute respiratory distress?
- normal oxygenation
- mild hypoxia
- moderate _____
- severe hypoxia*

A pulse oximetry _____ around 90% for a patient in a normal _____ indicates that severe hypoxia is present. _____ pulse oximetry readings are from 93% to 100%, with 93-95 considered the lower end of normal.

| atmosphere, reading, Normal, hypoxia |

18
Pulsus paradoxus means an abnormal decrease in the systolic pressure during inspiration compared with expiration.*
Pulsus paradoxus is an _____ _____ in systolic blood pressure that drops more than 10 to 15 mmHg during inspiration _____ ____ expiration.
Normally, the systolic pressure decreases 5 to 10 mmHg during

inspiration. However, in patients with asthma, COPD, pericardial tamponade, pulmonary embolism, or tension pneumothorax, the _____ _____ may decrease 10 to 20 mmHg or more during _____.

| systolic pressure, inspiration, compared with, abnormal decrease |

19
Bradycardia refers to a heart rate that is less than how many beats per minute? 60.
What _____ is considered normal in an athletic adult? Bradycardia.*
Sinus _____, or a heartbeat slower than 60 bpm, is often _____ _____, particularly in an _____ adult.

| athletic, considered normal, dysrhythmia, bradycardia |

20
The wheezing associated with left-side ____ _____ results from fluid in the lungs.*
The wheezing, due to _____ of smooth muscle in the lung, is a reaction to _____ in the lung spaces.
Which of the following are signs and symptoms of right-side heart failure? Tachycardia, _____

_____, and _____ ____ distension.

```
fluid, heart failure, jugular vein,
bronchoconstriction, peripheral
oedema
```

Vocabulary 11

aorta /eɪˈɔː.tə/ aorta, srdečnice

asymptomatic /əˌsɪmp.təˈmæt.ɪk/ asymptomatický, bezpříznakový

atmosphere /ˈæt.mə.sfɪər/ atmosféra, ovzduší, prostředí

atrial /ˈeɪ.tri.əl/ síňový, týkající se předsíně

bicuspid valve /baɪˈkʌs.pɪdˌvælv/ dvojcípá chlopeň

board /bɔːd/ deska

circulate /ˈsɜː.kjʊ.leɪt/ cirkulovat, obíhat, šířit se

continuously /kənˈtɪn.ju.əs.li/ nepřetržitě, neustále

core /kɔːr/ střed, jádro

drain /dreɪn/ odvést, odtéct, vysušit

dura mater /ˌdjuə.rəˈmeɪ.tə/ dura mater, tvrdá plena

easing /ˈiːz.ɪŋ/ zmírnění, uvolnění

frostbite /ˈfrɒst.baɪt/ omrzlina

golden /ˈgəʊl.dən/ **rule** /ruːl/ zlaté pravidlo

hypertensive /ˌhaɪ.pəˈten.sɪv/ hypertenzní, se zvýšeným krevním tlakem

impulse /ˈɪm.pʌls/ impuls, podnět

irregularity /ɪˌreg.jəˈlær.ə.ti/ nepravidelnost, nesouměrnost

law /lɔː/ **enforcement** /ɪnˈfɔːs.mənt/ prosazování práva, prosazování zákona

lead /liːd/ svod (EKG)

mitral valve /ˈmaɪ.trəlˌvælv/ mitrální, dvojcípá chlopeň

overcooling /ˌəʊ.vəˈkuː.lɪŋ/ nadměrné zchlazení

paralysis /pəˈræl.ə.sɪs/ paralýza, ochrnutí

production /prəˈdʌk.ʃən/ produkce, tvoření, tvorba

pulse /pʌls/ pulz, rytmus, tepat

pump /pʌmp/ pumpovat, čerpat

regularity /ˌreg.jʊˈlær.ə.ti/ pravidelnost, pravidelný jev

relationship /rɪˈleɪ.ʃən.ʃɪp/ vztah, příbuznost

routine /ruːˈtiːn/ rutina, běžná praxe

saturation /ˌsæt.jʊˈreɪ.ʃən/ saturace, nasycení

severe /sɪˈvɪə/ závažný

simultaneous /ˌsɪm.əlˈteɪ.ni.əs/ souběžný, současně probíhající

smooth /smuːð/ hladký, klidný

steadily /ˈsted.ɪ.li/ stále, plynule

structure /ˈstrʌk.tʃər/ struktura, stavba

superior /suːˈpɪə.ri.ər/ horní, vyšší

target /ˈtɑː.gɪt/ cíl, úkol

thrombolytic /ˌθrɒm.bɒˈlit.ɪk/ **therapy** /ˈθer.ə.pi/ trombolytická léčba, rozpuštění trombu

timing /ˈtaɪ.mɪŋ/ načasování

tracing /ˈtreɪ.sɪŋ/ sledování, zjišťování

travel /ˈtræv.əl/ cestovat, putovat, pohybovat se

tricuspid valve /traɪˈkʌs.pɪdˌvælv/ trikuspidální (trojcípá) chlopeň

ulcer /ˈʌl.sər/ vřed

vena cava /ˌviː.nəˈkeɪ.və/ dutá žíla

Unit 12

1

Why is _____ sulphate used in the management of AMI patients? To relieve pain and reduce myocardial _____ _____.*
Morphine relieves pain, decreases venous return, and reduces the oxygen demand of the _____.

> oxygen demand, morphine, myocardium

2

If it is not treated, left ventricular failure results in:
- ischemic heart disease
- pulmonary oedema*
- chronic hypertension
- cor pulmonale

Because the left ventricle fails to function as an effective forward _____, left ventricular failure results in pulmonary oedema as blood _____ __ _____ the pulmonary circulation. Left-side failure is common _____ an _____ myocardial infarction and can also lead to cardiogenic _____.

> acute, shock, following, pump, backs up into

3

What is the most common cause of cardiogenic shock? Left ventricular failure.*

Cardiogenic shock _____ most often from ____ _____ _____ following acute MI. Management of left-side heart failure _____ high-flow oxygen, IV of crystalloid solution, ECG monitoring, and the administration of morphine sulphate and nitroglycerin.*

> includes, left ventricular failure, results

4

Which of the following indicates that an ___ _____ is developing cardiogenic shock?
- increasing pain
- narrowing pulse pressure
- falling blood pressure*
- sinus bradycardia

_____ _____ _____, especially a systolic pressure lower than 80 mmHg together with decreasing level of consciousness, is a sign of _____ _____ in an AMI patient. Reflex _____ may develop as the patient's body attempts to compensate for the shock.

> AMI patient, Falling blood pressure, cardiogenic shock, tachycardia

5

A patient is complaining of chest pressure and shortness of breath.

He has jugular venous distension and pedal oedema. His lung sounds are clear and equal. What condition most likely causes these findings? _____-____ heart failure.*
Reduced _____ _____ of the right ventricle causes _____ ____ to back up into the _____ vascular system, causing _____ as evidenced by the pedal oedema and JVD. Lung fields that are past the cardiac _____ remain free from fluid.

systemic, congestion, pumping capacity, Right-side, insufficiency, blood flow

6
What is the most common complication of an acute _____ _____? The onset of a dysrhythmia.*
The most common complication of MI is _____, and some dysrhythmias are or become ____ _____. Cardiogenic shock may develop _____ an AMI, especially when the site of infarction is the ____ _____. _____ is a complication of arterosclerosis and coronary artery vasoconstriction or vasospasm.

left ventricle, life-threatening, myocardial infarction, following, dysrhythmia, Angina

7
What is the _____ ____ of management for a patient with left ventricle failure and pulmonary oedema? Decrease venous return.*
The primary goal for patients with left ventricular failure and pulmonary oedema is to reduce _____ _____ to the heart, or preload, and thus reduce pressure on the _____ _____.
What set of vital signs is suggestive of left ventricular ____ _____ with pulmonary oedema? BP elevated, pulse ____ ___ _____, and respirations _____ ___ _____.*

fast and irregular, pulmonary circulation, heart failure, rapid and laboured, venous return, primary goal

8
You arrive at a golf course to find a 45-year-old male unconscious and _____ __ ____ but only with movement. The patient was _____ in the head by a golf ball travelling at ____ _____. His eyes are closed; _____ _____ reveals his left pupil is 2 mm, and the right is 8 mm and not reactive to light. This patient moves upper extremities to localized pain and moves lower extremities spontaneously. He is breathing

full, deep respirations at a rate of 24 per minute.

You would expect the vital signs of this patient generally to follow the following grouping: RR increased, HR decreased, and BP increased.*

This set of vitals, known as Cushing's _____ (respiratory rate increased, heart rate decreased, blood pressure increased) is common in closed-head injuries. Treatment of this patient would include placing the patient in the sniffing position to facilitate airflow.* Placing the victim in the _____ _____ manipulates the head and neck, facilitating airflow.

A patient with a closed-head injury should be closely _____ ___ all of the following: hypovolaemic shock, respiratory alkalosis, and hypoxic seizures.*

monitored for, triad, pupil examination, responsive to pain, sniffing position, high velocity, struck

9

Which group of vital sign changes is associated with Cushing's reflex? Increased _____ pressure, decreased _____ ___, decreased _____ ____, and increased temperature.*

blood, pulse rate, respiratory rate

10

For which of the following procedures is a gown most necessary?

- emergency childbirth*
- drawing blood
- suctioning the airway
- cleaning instruments

Wearing a ____ is considered part of your BSI precautions with _____ _____. It may be recommended in some circumstances when _____ instruments or _____ _____ but is not generally needed.

drawing blood, cleaning, emergency childbirth, gown

11

All of the following statements about the use of disposable gloves and infection control are true:

- Gloves should be worn for _____ _____ contact.*
- Gloves should be _____ for each new patient contact.*
- Gloves cannot protect health-care workers from _____ _____.*

Gloves cannot protect you from food- or airborne-infectious agents. _____ should not eat or drink inside the ambulance.

changed, needle sticks, Personnel, every patient

12
- How should you maintain respiratory isolation when transporting a patient _____ __ having tuberculosis? Have both patient and personnel wear the appropriate masks.*

Both the patient and all _____ who come in contact with him or her should wear the appropriate masks in order to maintain _____ _____. For your own legal protection and for the optimal patient care, you should never transport a patient unattended in your unit.

> suspected of, personnel, respiratory isolation

13
For which procedure is it necessary to wear gloves, gown, mask, and protective eyewear? _____ with an emergency childbirth.*
Childbirth can be extremely messy and involve blood, _____ _____, urine, and _____, so maximum _____ should be taken to include gloves, gowns, mask, and ___ _____. For routine IV starts and IM drug administration, gloves alone should be appropriate BSI.

> amniotic fluid, faeces, eye protection, precautions, Assisting

14
The use of alcohol-based wash is encouraged in the ____ _____ when hot water and soap are not readily available. To be most effective, you should also _____ gross matter from your hands since alcohol cannot penetrate protein.*
Alcohol can never take the place of thorough hand washing, but when ____ _____ is not possible, it can offer some protection. To be ____ _____, you should first remove debris, as alcohol cannot penetrate large protein molecules. Saturate your hands and use _____ to remove particulate matter. Let your hands ___ ___ immediately, but do not wipe them dry, as this _____ the effectiveness of the alcohol.

> friction, diminishes, hand washing, field setting, most effective, air-dry, remove

15
For what procedure is it necessary to wear a mask and protective eyewear? Endotracheal intubation.*
Commonly accepted infection-control guidelines call

for all personnel to wear _____
and _____ _____ for any
procedure that carries the risk of
_____ __ blood, _____, or
other fluids.

---

vomitus, splashing of, masks,
protective eyewear

16

When you are _____ ___ more
than one _____ _____ at a
time, you should change your
gloves for each new patient.*
Changing gloves for ____
new patient contact prevents

_____-_____.

---

each, caring for,
cross-contamination, trauma
patient

17

Which form of hepatitis poses
the lowest risk to paramedics?
Hepatitis A.*
Hepatitis A is _____ (or
food-borne) and poses the least
risk for _____-____ _____.
Hepatitis B virus (HBV) is the
_____ occupational blood-borne
pathogen risk for paramedics.
Hepatitis C occurs most
frequently in __ ____ _____,
and paramedics are at risk of
contracting this disease from
accidental needle sticks.
Hepatitis D occurs only in
individuals who currently have

or had HBV infection and who
therefore also pose a ____ ____ to
EMS providers.

IV drug abusers, enteric, high
risk, health-care providers, major

18

Which type of hepatitis is spread
via the faecal or oral route?
Hepatitis A.*
Hepatitis A is spread by the
_____-____ _____ and is most
commonly acquired from eating
_____ ____. Hepatitis
B, C, and D are all _____-_____
diseases.

---

blood-borne, contaminated food,
faecal-oral route

19

Which infection is transmitted
through contact with blood or
body secretions? Hepatitis B.*
_____ _ is a blood-borne
disease that is transmitted
through contact with blood or____

_____.
What is the most common
job-related source of HIV
infections among health-care
workers? An accidental needle
stick.*

_____ _____ _____ are
the most common source of
work-related ___ and hepatitis B
infections in health-care workers.

Accidental needle sticks,
Hepatitis B, HIV, body secretions

20
What does the initial symptom of
infection with HIV primarily consist
of? Mild fatigue and ____.*
Although symptoms of full-blown
AIDS include Kaposi's sarcoma
and opportunistic infections,
____ ____ of infection with
the AIDS virus often consist only
of ____ ____ and fever.

initial symptoms, mild fatigue,
fever

Vocabulary 12
accidental /ˌæk.sɪˈden.təl/
náhodný, nepředvídaný,
neúmyslný
acquire /əˈkwaɪər/ získat, nabýt
ambulance /ˈæm.bjʊ.ləns/ sanitka,
záchranka
blood-borne /bɔːn/ nesený krví
blow /bləʊ/ (blew, blown) foukat,
vyfouknout, vanout, vyletět
BSI, British /ˈbrɪt.ɪʃ/ Standards
/ˈstæn.dədz/ Institution /
ˌɪnstɪˈtjuːʃən/ Britský úřad pro
standardizaci
capacity /kəˈpæs.ə.ti/ objem,
schopnost, výkonnost
childbirth /ˈtʃaɪld.bɜːθ/ porod,
narození dítěte
common /ˈkɒmən/ společný
consist /kənˈsɪst/ skládat se, být
složen z čeho

contract /kənˈtrækt/ stáhnout,
zúžit se
cor /kɔːr/ pulmonale /ˈpʊl.mə.nə.l/
lat. plicní srdce, chorobné
zvětšení pravé srdeční komory
effectiveness /ɪˈfek.tɪv.nəs/
účinnost, efektivnost
eyewear /ˈaɪweər/ oční optika
faeces /ˈfiː.siːz/ fekálie, výkaly
food /fuːd/ -borne /bɔːn/ přenášený
potravou
full-blown /ˌfʊlˈbləʊn/ zralý,
plnohodnotný, rozvinutý
gross /grəʊs/ hrubý, drsný
ischemic /ɪsˈkiː.mɪk/ ischemický,
nedokrvený
Kaposi's /kæˈpəʊ.sɪz/ sarcoma /
sɑːˈkəʊ.mə/ Kaposiho sarkom,
kožní onemocnění nádorového
charakteru, u nemocných s
AIDS, červenofialové kožní uzly,
postiženy bývají i vnitřní orgány
matter /ˈmæt.ər/ hmota
messy /ˈmes.i/ nepořádný,
neuspořádaný, špinavý
needle /ˈniː.dl/ stick /stɪk/ píchnutí
jehlou
occupational /ˌɒk.juˈpeɪ.ʃən.
əl/ pracovní, zaměstnanecký,
profesní
opportunistic /ˌɒp.ə.tjuːˈnɪs.tɪk/
oportunistický
particulate /pəˈtɪ.kju.lət/ z
drobných částic
primarily /praɪˈmer.ɪ.li/ především,
hlavně
sarcoma /sɑːˈkəʊ.mə/ sarkom,
zhoubný nádor pojivové tkáně

saturate /ˈsæt.jʊ.reɪt/ saturovat, nasytit, nasáknout
splash /splæʃ/ postříkat, šplíchnutí
sulphate /ˈsʌl.feɪt/ sulfát, síran
triad /ˈtraɪ.æd/ triáda, trojice
wear /weər/ vzít si na sebe, nosit oblečení
wipe /waɪp/ otřít, utřít, ubrousek
wiper /ˈwaɪp.ər/ utěrka
worker /ˈwɜː.kər/ pracovník, zaměstnanec

Unit 13

1

When performing _____-_____
rescues, the use of a personal
_____ _____ is required
when the rescuer works in any
and all water.*
No matter the _____ _____
of the rescuer, personal safety is
absolute.

competency level, flotation
device, water-related

2

_____ may be best defined as a
general feeling of uneasiness.*
Anxiety is a general feeling of
uneasiness or _____ that
results from _____ _____.

apprehension, Anxiety,
continued stress

3

Hyperventilation syndrome most
often occurs in a patient who is:
- anxious and upset*
- asthmatic
- in shock from _____
- a heavy smoker
_____ syndrome,
which is characterized by rapid
breathing, is most often caused
by _____, though it is also
associated with many organic
diseases.

anxiety, Hyperventilation, trauma

4

When interviewing patients who
are distraught or potentially
violent, you should do all of the
following:
- Remove the patient from
  the crisis situation as
  quickly as possible.*
- _____ the patient to
  explain the situation in his
  or her own words.*
- Avoid _____ ____ or
  shouting at the person
  who is distraught.*
The purpose of the interview is to
____ the patient and to _____
as much information as possible,
not to tell the patient what you
think. There is a time to reorient
patients to reality, but first, you
must work to calm them down
and ____ _____ _____.

gain their trust, calm, obtain,
arguing with, Encourage

5

Your partner and you are
evaluating a patient experiencing
a behavioural emergency. Your
patient is visibly _____ and is
pacing back and forth. He is
verbally confrontational, and his
hands are in fists. At times, he
displays _____ _____,
both physical and verbal.
What action is most appropriate
for this situation? Observe the
scene for danger.*

Given the circumstances, not enough personnel are available __ _____ this patient if he becomes violent. _____ a hands-on assessment may not be possible given the state of the patient's _____. Constantly being aware of your surroundings will provide the greatest _____ __ _____.

level of safety, aggressive actions, upset, behaviour, to restrain, Conducting

6

This is an example of _____ and labelling the patient's feelings: 'You seem angry. Do you want to tell me about it?'*
This is one way to acknowledge what a patient is feeling and to _____ him or her to _____ those feelings without passing _____ or getting too personal.

encourage, judgement, express, acknowledging

7

Your patient is a 46-year-old male with a ____ _____ of mental illness. He appears depressed and _____. Suddenly, he begins to sob uncontrollably. What should you do? Maintain _ ____, _____, and non-judgemental attitude.*

a quiet, listening, long history, withdrawn

8

Your friend experiences severe _____ when crossing bridges. She _____ to cross any bridges and alters her travel routes accordingly. This is an example of which of the following conditions?
- psychosis
- neurosis
- delirium
- phobia*

An intense fear of something is called a phobia. A _____ can be disabling, and its _____ is often unknown.

cause, phobia, anxiety, refuses

9

Depression is an example of a(n):
- psychiatric _____
- psychosis
- mood disorder*
- _____ disease

Depression is a ____ _____; depressed patients feel _____ and helpless and manifest many physical symptoms as well.

hopeless, illness, mood disorder, organic

305

10

What term best describes a patient who talks non-stop and is restless and _____?
- manic*
- depressed
- demented
- schizophrenic

A patient who is displaying manic symptoms is _____ or extremely active and _____ constantly. The patient may be extremely _____ or violent. If the patient has bipolar disorder, he or she may swing between periods of _____ and depression.

talks, overactive, suspicious, restless, mania

11

A patient with bipolar disorder usually suffers from which of the following?
- frequent _____
- delusional behaviour
- wide mood swings*
- _____ thoughts

A patient with _____ _____ (manic-depressive disorder) suffers from wide mood swings from _____ to debilitating depression.

euphoria, bipolar disorder, hallucinations, psychotic

12

You are interviewing a 43-year-old woman with a long history of schizophrenia. She appears to try to cooperate, but there are long periods of _____ in your conversation while she listens to her 'voices'. How should you respond during her silence?
- _____ your last question.
- Restate her last _____.
- Remain quietly attentive.*
- Tell her an interesting _____.

During silences, remain relaxed and attentive and wait to hear what the patient has to say. This will _____ the patient to talk.

story, Repeat, response, encourage, silence

13

What is the difference between bulimia and anorexia nervosa?
- They are basically the same disorder.
- Bulimia is an intense fear of _____, whereas anorexia is the insatiable _____ for food.
- Anorexia is less severe and rarely life-threatening.
- Bulimia is more often associated with binge eating.*

Bulimia and anorexia nervosa are both common _____ _____. They both have similar features

such as misperceptions of ____
_____. Bulimia is characterized
by _____ _____ followed by
self-induced vomiting.

eating disorders, binge eating, body image, obesity, craving

14

Which statement about suicide is correct?

- People who talk about suicide rarely attempt it by deadly means.
- Suicidal patients are _____ ___ and require institutionalization.
- The _____ ____ is lowest during holiday seasons or birthdays.
- There is a high correlation between suicide attempts and alcohol consumption.*

_____ is a CNS depressant. People who do not frequently drink often do so before killing themselves; furthermore, alcoholics are _____ __ commit suicide. Suicidal patient may or may not openly discuss suicide, but you should ____ _____ any discussion of it by your patient. Most _____ _____ are depressed, not mentally ill. Holidays and important personal times such as anniversaries, birthdays, or death days are high times for suicide.

suicide rate, take seriously, prone to, suicidal patients, mentally ill, Alcohol

15

There are many factors to consider when assessing a patient for suicide risk. Which of the following accurately accounts for one _____ ____ factor?

- Young women _____ _____ more often than young men do.
- Generally, men _____ suicide more often than women do.
- Caucasian males over 85 years of age have the highest suicide rate.*

Women attempt suicide more often, but men are ____ _____ at it. Also, men choose more _____ ____.
About 60% of the people who successfully commit suicide have a history of _____ attempts.

more successful, deadly means, commit suicide, suicide risk, attempt, previous

16

Hyperextension of the neck, followed by hyperflexion, is common in rear-end impacts.*
A strong force _____ the car from behind causes the head to ____ _____. If the head restraint is not properly placed,

it can actually act as a fulcrum, causing the neck to _____. Then the head snaps forward, with the chin pointing toward the chest. This _____ __ a severe _____ of the neck.

hyperextend, results in, hyperflexion, move backward, striking

17

On reaching the scene of a single-motor vehicle accident, you note that the driver is pinned behind the _____ _____. You also note the presence of two sets of spiderweb patterns on the _____.

What does this alert you to? Look for a second _____ in this accident.*

The spiderweb pattern is made when a victim's head ____ the windshield. Two spiderweb patterns _____ that there is a second victim somewhere on the scene.

victim, windshield, hits, indicate, steering wheel

18

Your unit is dispatched to a single automobile crash. The patient's car hit a large tree ____-__. The patient, a young adult woman, is found conscious and alert but _____ in the car. The ___ ___ deployed, and she denies any head or neck pain, although she does _____ of hip and leg pain. After a difficult 20-minute _____, the patient is finally released from the car. Suddenly, your patient's vital signs begin to _____.

This patient is most likely transitioning from compensated shock to decompensated shock.* This patient's body is showing signs that it can no longer _____ for the damage done by the traumatic event. In addition, _____ metabolic products may have been trapped in the injured tissues and now are circulating back toward the heart. These toxins may result in cardiac dysrhythmias or cardiac arrest.

extrication, head-on, air bag, collapse, trapped, complain, toxic, compensate

19

Your patient is a middle-aged female who has been in a car accident. Because the initial assessment showed no immediate ____ _____, you are now treating her most serious injuries, which include a _____ broken femur and kneecap.

After _____ the injured leg and rechecking the pulse, motor responses, and sensation,

you should repeat the initial assessment.*
Quickly repeat the initial assessment after every
_____ _____. You and your partner have had your attention on her lower extremity for a few minutes and now you should refocus and repeat an ___ _____.
Cervical immobilization with a collar should be completed _____ ___ the treatment of the leg. Proximal pulse check is part of the reassessment that occurs immediately after stabilizing and _____ the leg.

---

life threats, prior to, stabilizing, significant intervention, suspected, splinting, ABC assessment

---

20
Cardiogenic shock can result in all of the following: _____, respiratory failure, an elevated heart rate.*
_____ _____ is the most severe form of pump _____ that often results in dysrhythmias, hypotension, respiratory failure, and possibly organ failure. The heart rate is initially elevated as the body attempts to _____ for the shock.

---

compensate, Cardiogenic shock, failure, dysrhythmias

Vocabulary 13
acknowledge /əkˈnɒl.ɪdʒ/ přiznat, uznat, brát na vědomí
angry /ˈæŋ.gri/ rozzlobený
anniversary /ˌæn.ɪˈvɜː.sər.i/ oslava výročí, jubileum
anorexia nervosa /æn.əˌrek.si.ə.nəˈvəʊ.sə/ mentální anorexie
argue /ˈɑː.gju:/ hádat se, přít se, argumentovat
attentive /əˈten.tɪv/ pozorný, věnující pozornost
attitude /ˈæt.ɪ.tjuːd/ postoj, stanovisko, přístup
aware /əˈweər/ bdělý, vnímající, uvědomovat si
back /bæk/ **and forth** /fɔːθ/ pohyb sem a tam
backward /ˈbæk.wəd/ zpět, zpětný, dozadu
binge eating /bɪndʒˌiː.tɪŋ/ záchvatovité přejídání
bipolar disorder /baɪˈpəʊ.lə.dɪˌsɔː.dər/ bipolární afektivní porucha, psychická porucha, která se projevuje nadměrnými změnami nálad, vitality a psychických funkcí
bulimia /bʊˌlɪm.i.ə/ bulimie, porucha příjmu potravy
calm (sb) /kɑːm/ **down** /daʊn/ uklidnit, utišit, upokojit
Caucasian /kɔːˈkeɪ.ʒən/ běloch
collar /ˈkɒl.ər/ límec
commit /kəˈmɪt/ spáchat, dopustit se
competency /ˈkɒmpɪtənsɪ/ schopnost, odborná způsobilost

confrontational /ˌkɒn.frʌnˈteɪ.ʃən.əl/ konfrontační

consumption /kənˈsʌmp.ʃən/ spotřeba, konzumace

correlation /ˌkɒr.əˈleɪ.ʃən/ korelace, vzájemná souvislost

craving /ˈkreɪ.vɪŋ/ bažení, chuť na co

crossing /ˈkrɒs.ɪŋ/ přejezd, přechod, křížení

deadly /ˈded.li/ smrtící, smrtelný

debilitating /dɪˈbɪl.ɪ.teɪt.ɪŋ/ oslabující, vysilující

decompensated /diːˈkɒmpenˌseɪt.əd/ dekompenzovaný

delusional /dɪˈluː.ʒən.əl/ klamný

demented /dɪˈmen.tɪd/ dementní, vyšinutý

deploy /dɪˈplɔɪ/ nasadit, rozmístit

disable /dɪˈseɪbl/ zmrzačit, vyřadit z činnosti

distraught /dɪˈstrɔːt/ silně rozrušený

euphoria /juːˈfɔː.ri.ə/ euforie, radostná nálada

feeling /ˈfiː.lɪŋ/ pocit, citlivost

fist /fɪst/ pěst, praštit pěstí

fulcrum /ˈfʊl.krəm/ opora, podpora

furthermore /ˌfɜː.ðəˈmɔːr/ navíc, kromě toho

hands-on /ˌhænd.ˈzɒn/ praktický, osobní, přímý

helpless /ˈhelplɪs/ bezmocný, bezradný

hit /hɪt/ zasáhnout, trefit, narazit, udeřit, uhodit

hopeless /ˈhəʊp.ləs/ zoufalý, beznadějný

image /ˈɪm.ɪdʒ/ představa, obraz, dojem

insatiable /ɪnˈseɪ.ʃə.bl̩/ nenasytný

institutionalization /ˌɪnt.stɪˌtjuː.ʃən.əl.aɪˈzeɪ.ʃən/ hospitalizace, umístění do léčebného ústavu

kneecap /ˈniː.kæp/ kolenní čéška

label /ˌleɪ.bəl/ nálepka, označit, opatřit štítkem

manic /ˈmæn.ɪk/ maniakální, šílený

means /miːnz/ možnosti, prostředky

mentally /ˈmen.təl.i/ psychicky

misperception /ˌmɪs.pəˈsep.ʃən/ klamné vnímání

mood /muːd/ nálada

mood /muːd/ **swing** /swɪŋ/ výkyv nálady (prudký)

neurosis /njʊəˈrəʊ.sɪs/ neuróza

no matter /ˈmætə/ nehledě na co

overactive /ˈəʊ.vərˈæk.tɪv/ nadměrně aktivní, čilý

pace /peɪs/ tempo, rychlost, krok, chůze

phobia /ˈfəʊ.bi.ə/ fobie, chorobný strach

psychiatric /ˌsaɪ.kiˈæt.rɪk/ psychiatrický, psychický

psychosis /saɪˈkəʊ.sɪs/ psychóza, porucha myšlení a jednání s následným rozpadem osobnosti

psychotic /saɪˈkɒt.ɪk/ psychotik, psychotička

rate /reɪt/ frekvence

rear-end /ˈrɪə.rend/ zadní část auta, nabourat zezadu

recheck /riːˈtʃek/ znovu zkontrolovat

relaxed /rɪˈlækst/ uvolněný

reorient /riːˈɔː.ri.ənt/ přeorientovat se

restate /ˌriːˈsteɪt/ jinak formulovat, přeformulovat

restrain /rɪˈstreɪn/ zadržet, potlačovat

schizophrenic /ˌskɪt.səˈfren.ɪk/ schizofrenický, schizofrenik

self-induced /ˌself.ɪnˈdjuːst/ způsobený sám sebou

seriously /ˈsɪə.ri.əs.li/ vážně, těžce

silence /ˈsaɪ.ləns/ ticho, mlčení

snap /snæp/ zapadnout, prasknout

sob /sɒb/ vzlykat, vzlyk

spiderweb /ˈspaɪ.də.web/ pavoučí síť

striking /ˈstraɪ.kɪŋ/ nápadný, výrazný

suicidal /ˌsuːˈɪˈsaɪdəl/ se sklony k sebevraždě, sebevražedný

surroundings /səˈraʊn.dɪŋz/ prostředí, okolní podmínky

swing /swɪŋ/ prudká změna, obrat, kývat

thought /θɔːt/ myšlenka, myšlenkový

toward /təˈwɔːd/ směrem k, ve vztahu k

toxin /ˈtɒk.sɪn/ toxin, jedovatá látka

trust /trʌst/ důvěra, věřit

uncontrollably /ˌʌn.kənˈtrəʊ.lə.bli/ neovladatelně

uneasiness /ʌnˈiː.zi.nəs/ neklid, znepokojení, nepříjemný pocit

upset /ʌpˈset/ podráždění, rozrušený, znepokojený, narušit

visibly /ˈvɪz.ɪ.bli/ viditelně, očividně

windshield /ˈwɪnd.ʃiːld/ čelní sklo

withdrawn /wɪðˈdrɔːn/ uzavřený, odtažitý

Unit 14

1

Why are patients who present
with pulmonary oedema
usually assumed to have had a
_____ _____? An AMI
is frequently a _____ _____ of
left ventricle failure.*
Myocardial infarction is a common
cause of left ventricular failure,
which is closely associated with

_____ _____.

> pulmonary oedema, common
> cause, myocardial infarction

2

A patient suspected of showing
early signs of shock should
usually be placed _____ with his
or her feet _____.
When is this position
_____? When a head
injury is suspected.*
The shock position is used only if
____ _____ is not suspected.

> contraindicated, elevated, head
> injury, supine

3

What is a differential sign or
symptom of _____ _____
associated with trauma? Warm,
dry skin distal to the _____ ____.*
This condition reflects a
specific sign that points directly
to the _____ _____ of
hypoperfusion.

> underlying cause, spinal shock,
> injury site

4

You are called to a rooftop for
a 17-year-old female who was
sunbathing. She is alert and
oriented and states she was using
lotion without any SPF protection
to speed up her tan. She was
in the sun from 9 a.m. to 2 p.m.
She is in _____ ____ and
requests that you help her off the
rooftop. She has blisters _____
the entire front of her body. You
should _____ this patient to
have:
- first-degree burns
- minor burns
- critical burns*

This should be classified as a
_____ ____ with over 50%
body surface area containing
_____-_____ ____.

> critical burn, consider,
> second-degree burns, significant
> pain, covering

5

This statement is true regarding
_____ burns: both _____
___ _____ cause burns by
_____ cell membranes and
damaging tissues on contact.*

> chemical, disrupting, acids and
> alkalis

6

The first step in managing a burn patient is to stop the burning process.*

The first step __ _____ a burn is to stop the _____ _____, or the burn will continue to _____ more tissue. Then attention should be turned toward ensuring and maintaining an _____ _____.

destroy, in managing, adequate airway, burning process

7

A burn wound that blisters is an example of a second-degree burn.*

_____ _____ is characteristic of _____-_____ burns.

second-degree, Blister formation

8

An adult who has burns over both sides of one arm and both sides of one leg would be _____ to have total burns over what percentage of body surface area? 27%.*

Using the ____ __ _____, this patient has burns over 27% of her body _____ ____ (both sides of one arm = 9%, ____ _____ of one leg = 18%).

both sides, surface area, rule of nines, estimated

9

Your patient has a chemical burn to her face and eyes. How should you treat this? Brush the chemical away and then flush the area with _____ _____ of clean cold water.*

The correct treatment for most chemical burns is to _____ the area with ____ _____ immediately and to continue this treatment even during the transport.

cool water, copious amounts, flush

10

A child has _____-_____ burns over the front of her trunk and the entire front of her right leg. According to the rule of nines, what _____ of her body surface area is affected? 25%.*

According to the rule of nines as applied to _____ _____, the front or back of the trunk each represents 18% of the body surface, and the front of one leg represents 7% with the entire leg _____ ___ 14%.

counting for, paediatric injuries, percentage, third-degree

11

How should you treat a patient who has sustained dry lime burns to the hand and arm? Brush the lime away and then flood the skin with cool water.*

Brush away as much of the _____ as possible, then flood the _____ _____ with water. _____ chemicals are generally not recommended because the use of one chemical to neutralize another usually _____ __ the release of heat and the _____ of a third chemical.

formation, Neutralizing, burned area, results in, lime

12

An adult patient has burns _____ her _____ and upper back.

Using the rule of nines, this patient's burns cover 18% of her body surface area.*

The head and _____ _____ are each equal to 9% of body surface area.

covering, upper back, head

13

How would you _____ a burn that is pearly white and almost _____? Third-degree burn.*

This is often the appearance of a _____-_____ burn, which is painless because of the _____ of nerve cells.

third-degree, classify, destruction, painless

14

In a patient with a _____ _____ to the airway, it is _____ to watch for signs and symptoms of the development of:
- laryngeal oedema*
- shock
- respiratory arrest
- bronchiolitis

A burn to the highly vascularized tissue of the airway can lead to _____ _____ and a _____ airway.

blocked, laryngeal oedema, critical, thermal burn

15

An adult with burns over the front of both arms and the chest is burned over what percentage of her body area (BSA)? 18%.*

Using the rule of nines, the _____ of each arm _____ 4.5% BSA, and the _____ _____ equals 9%; the _____ _____ covers 18% of the BSA.

total burn, anterior chest, equals, front

16

How will the skin over a second-degree burn appear?

- bright red
- mottled red*
- pearly white
- charred black

The skin over a second-degree burn will most frequently appear _____ ___ and contain _____. A first-degree burn will appear _____ ___, and a third-degree burn will be _____ __ _____.

> charred or white, bright red, blisters, mottled red

17

Which patient is most likely to need burn centre care versus _____ _____ care?

- female, age 34, second-degree burn over 10% of BSA (body surface area)
- male, age 46, third-degree burn over a small area of the back
- female, age 52, second-degree burns to face and right hand*
- male, age 27, second-degree burn over entire left arm excluding hand

Severe partial-_____ or full-thickness burns to the face, hands, feet, and perineum often _____ burn centre care, even if they are ___ _____.

> not extensive, warrant, thickness, trauma centre

18

Prehospital care for a patient who has moderate to severe burns includes dry sterile dressings and two IV lines with large-bore catheters held at a TKO rate.* Cover the burns with dry _____ _____ and be ready to institute aggressive _____ _____ as ordered. ___ _____ offer comfort but _____ the body temperature in a severely burned patient. ___-____ dressings are being used with some success, but the standard of care is still dry sterile dressing.

> Gel-type, lower, fluid therapy, sterile dressings, Wet dressings

19

What _____ _____ involves a fracture of both the _____ and _____ bone? Le Fort II.*

> maxillary, facial injury, nasal

20

The next two questions are based on the following scenario:
You are called to the scene of a 22-year-old man who was playing in a softball tournament. He was

hit in the eye with a hard-hit line-drive softball. According to his teammates, he was knocked to the ground and had a brief ____ __ _____ that lasted approximately 7 seconds.

While assessing the injured eye, you notice a collection of blood in front of the patient's pupil and iris. What is your differential diagnosis? Hyphaema.*

_____ is a collection of blood in the _____ _____ of the eye due to trauma. This type of injury is a potential threat to the patient's _____ and requires _____ by an ophthalmologist.

How would you transport this patient to the hospital? Immobilized on a _____ with the head of backboard elevated.* A C-spine injury should be suspected with any injury to the head. Treatment of this patient would include ___ ____ _____. The preferred position of transport of a hyphaema is with the head elevated; therefore, you should _____ the head of the backboard.

```
backboard, anterior chamber,
full body immobilization, elevate,
Hyphaema, evaluation, vision,
loss of consciousness
```

Vocabulary 14
bright /braɪt/ jasný, světlý, zářivý
brush /brʌʃ/ vyčistit kartáčkem, otřít
BSA, Body /ˈbɒd.i/ **Surface** /ˈsɜː.fɪs/ **Area** /ˈeərɪə/ oblast povrchu těla
charred /tʃɑːd/ ohořelý, spálený
classify /ˈklæs.ɪ.faɪ/ klasifikovat, třídit
count /kaʊnt/ **for** hrát roli, znamenat
covering /ˈkʌv.ər.ɪŋ/ pokrývající
degree /dɪˈgriː/ stupeň, míra, postupně
drive /draɪv/ odpal
ensure /ɪnˈʃɔːr/ zajistit, postarat se
excluding /ɪkˈskluː.dɪŋ/ vyjma, kromě
extensive /ɪkˈsten.sɪv/ rozsáhlý, značný
flood /flʌd/ záplava, povodeň
gel /dʒel/ gel
hard /hɑːd/ silně, tvrdě
held /held/ držený, ovládaný
institute /ˈɪn.stɪ.tjuːt/ zahájit, započít
iris /ˈaɪrɪs/ oční duhovka
large-bore /lɑːdʒ/, /bɔː/ jehla s velkým průměrem
last /lɑːst/ trvat
LeFort II fracture / ˈfræk.tʃə/ poranění střední obličejové etáže (nosní kůstky, nazomaxilární komplex), hlavní linie zlomeniny se setkávají v bodu nad nosními kostmi a tvoří trojúhelníkový úsek, oddělený od lebky
lime /laɪm/ vápno
line /laɪn/ čára, linie

lotion /ˈləʊ.ʃən/ pleťové mléko, pleťová voda

maxillary /mækˈsɪl.ər.i/ čelist, čelistní

ophthalmologist /ˌɒf.θælˈmɒl.ə.dʒɪst/ oftalmolog, oční lékař

painless /ˈpeɪn.ləs/ bezbolestný

pearly /ˈpɜː.li/ perlový, růžový

percentage /pəˈsen.tɪdʒ/ procento, procentní podíl

rooftop /ˈruːf.tɒp/ střecha, vršek střechy

rule/ ruːl/ **of nines** /naɪnz/ pravidlo devíti, pravidlo pro přibližné posouzení rozsahu popálenin, povrch těla je rozdělen na zóny představující 9 % tělesného povrchu (BSA)

speed up /ˈspiːd.ʌp/ zrychlit, zvýšit rychlost

tan /tæn/ opálit se, opálení

therapy /ˈθer.ə.pi/ terapie, léčba

TKO, **To Keep** (**venous** /ˈviː.nəs/ **infusion** / ɪnˈfjuː.ʒən/ **line** /laɪn/) **Open** udržovat otevřený vstup pro žilní infuzi

trunk /trʌŋk/ trup

317

Unit 15

1

You are called to a scene
of a motor vehicle collision
(MVC). During your initial
assessment, you find an
_____32-year-old male
with multiple _____ to his
face and head. He has _____
respirations and a weak, _____
peripheral pulse.
Your first action would be to open
the airway with a jaw thrust and
immobilize the _____ _____.*
Always remember ABCs.

> thready, cervical spine,
> contusions, snoring,
> unresponsive

2

Intracranial haemorrhage
can cause vital sign changes
characterized by an _____
systolic blood pressure and
_____ pulse pressure,
bradycardia, and _____
respiratory rate.
These changes are collectively
_____ Cushing's reflex.*
Change in vital signs that are
associated with increased
_____ _____ is termed
Cushing's reflex.

> widening, intracranial pressure,
> termed, increasing, irregular

3

A patient suspected of showing
early signs of shock should
usually be placed _____ with his
or her feet _____.
When is this position
_____? When a head
injury is suspected.*
The shock position is used only if
____ _____ is not suspected.

> contraindicated, elevated, head
> injury, supine

4

Your patient is a victim of an
assault and is experiencing
malocclusion and numbness
to the chin. There is also a
suspected nasal fracture and
significant facial bleeding and
bruising.
What treatment is appropriate for
this patient? _____ the cervical
spine, control the airway but avoid
the use of a nasopharyngeal
airway, control bleeding, and
transport.*
Patients with _____ _____
also have suspected _____
_____ and should be immobilized
appropriately.
Avoid the use of any _____
_____ manipulations in a patient
with facial fractures as the device
could be introduced directly into
the brain __ _____ through
the area of the fracture.

Cardiac (___) monitoring, pulse oximetry, and other _____ _____ are always appropriate when you have a _____ injured patient.

> monitoring devices, nasopharyngeal airway, by perforating, spinal trauma, Secure, ECG, facial fractures, seriously

5

The presence of marked purplish-red racoon eyes on a patient in prehospital environment should lead you to suspect significant previous head injury.* Periorbital ecchymosis, or _____ ___, presents as bruises _____ _____ the eyes. It often indicates basal or other _____ _____, but when seen in the prehospital environment, it suggests significant _____ _____ because this condition takes time to develop after injury.
The earliest finding you would note with a newly developing skull injury is _____ _____ of the soft tissues around each eye that may make it difficult even to open the eyes to check the _____.

> extreme swelling, skull fracture, previous injury, racoon eyes, circling around, pupils

6

The collective change in vital signs associated with the ____ _____ of increasing _____ pressure consists of slowing pulse rate, deep or erratic respirations, and _____ blood pressure.*

> intracranial, increasing, late stages

7

Your patient is a car-crash victim who was unconscious prior to your arrival but is now awake. As you examine the patient, you notice that he is becoming _____.
What should you suspect? Epidural haematoma formation.* The symptoms are indicative of a mass-forming _____ in the head, such as an epidural or subdural _____. When a patient has a simple concussion, his or her mental status will continue to _____ with time.

> improve, lesion, haematoma, disoriented

8

The _____ _____ of a patient experiencing the later stages of increased intracranial pressure will be characterized by increased blood pressure, _____ pulse, and _____ ____.*

respiratory rate, decreased, vital signs

9
Your patient suffers a head trauma that results in a _____ loss of consciousness followed by a complete _____ __ _____. What is the term for this condition? Cerebral concussion.*
A concussion is a _____ loss of consciousness in response to

____ _____.

head trauma, brief, transient, return of function

10
An injury to the brain _____ the site of a blunt force impact is called contrecoup.*
During significant force to the head, the brain can _____ ___ _____ the opposite side of the skull away from the _____ _____. This mechanism can cause a contrecoup injury.

opposite, original force, shift and strike

11
A _____ _____ is a brain injury that is on the opposite side of the head from the impact site.*
A contrecoup injury is an injury to the brain opposite the _____ ____; it results from the brain's

_____ movement against the skull wall following the initial impact. The ____ _____ is noted at the site of the actual impact.

coup injury, impact site, contrecoup contusion, rebounding

12
What is the management for a patient with a head injury and an unusual respiratory pattern? Rapid transport because of possible brain stem injury.*
_____ respiratory patterns indicate the possibility of _____ ____ injury and call for rapid transport of the patient. Hyperventilation should be used only when you strongly suspect herniation is _____. It is not indicated for the _____ _____ of increasing ICP. You should ventilate the patient at a normal rate with 100% oxygen.

brain stem, Unusual, routine treatment, occurring

13
Battle's sign and periorbital ecchymosis are classic signs of a basilar skull fracture.*
Battle's sign is the _____-___-____ discoloration just behind the ears. _____ _____, also known as raccoon eyes, is the black-and-blue discoloration

around the eyes. Both are classic signs of a _____ _____ _____.

> basilar skull fracture, Periorbital ecchymosis, black-and-blue

14

What is a positive Battle's sign an indication of? Basilar skull fracture.*

_____ _____ is noted as discoloration of the _____ _____ behind the ear. It is an indication that blood has collected there following a _____ _____ _____. Periorbital ecchymosis (racoon's eyes) is noted with _____ ___ _____ trauma and fractures. _____ _____ may have no external manifestations or signs.

> Subarachnoid bleeding, basal skull fracture, facial and orbital, mastoid area, Battle's sign

15

The signs and symptoms of _____ _____ include which of the following?
- disorientation and confusion, decreased pulse and blood pressure, and cyanosis
- transient loss of consciousness, headache, _____, nausea, and _____*

- _____ of cerebrospinal fluid, headache, and bleeding from the nose or ears
- headache, Battle's sign, confusion, lethargy, and rapid loss of _____

> consciousness, vomiting, drowsiness, cerebral haemorrhage, leakage

16

What is the greatest concern when a person experiences blunt force trauma to the head?
- It can interrupt the integrity of the blood brain barrier.
- It can cause a significant increase in intracranial pressure.*
- It can cause significant ringing in the ears.
- It can lacerate the scalp, causing bleeding.

Increased ICP after a _____ _____ trauma to the head is potentially _____ and will need close monitoring and management both _____ and within the _____ department.

> emergency, lethal, prehospital, blunt force

17
A patient who complains of a
_____ ___ _____ complete
loss of vision in one eye is
most likely suffering from retinal
detachment.*
The _____ captures the image
that is projected by the ____ of
the eye. It can spontaneously
_____ from the inner surface
of the eye, causing sudden and
painless loss of vision.

> lens, separate, retina, sudden
> and painless

18
Your patient, a car accident
victim, _____ __ seeing a
"dark curtain" in front of one eye.
What should you suspect? Retinal
detachment.*
A patient with a detached _____
will often complain of _____ a
dark curtain in front of part of the
field of vision.

> seeing, retina, complains of

19
An unconscious patient who has
one _____ _____ that is reactive
to light is showing early signs of
increased intracranial pressure.*
A unilaterally dilated pupil may
be an _____ ____ of increased
intracranial pressure. As _____
increases in the brain, it puts
pressure on the _____ _____

that is located near the area of
swelling.

> swelling, early sign, optic nerve,
> dilated pupil

20
Lifting improperly may most likely
result in an injury to the lumbar
part of the back.*
The _____ _____ will be most
impacted from an _____
_____ ____; the _____
_____ is also at risk for injury,
although such injuries are less
likely.

> cervical spine, unevenly
> distributed load, lumbar spine

Vocabulary 15
basal /beɪsəl/ bazální, spodní
Battle's /ˈbætəl/ **sign** /saɪn/
Battleův příznak, modravé
zabarvení kůže nad výběžkem
spánkové kosti, naznačuje
frakturu lební baze
brief /briːf/ krátký, stručný
capture /ˈkæp.tʃər/ zajmout, získat
cerebrospinal /ˌser.ɪ.brəˈspaɪ.nəl/
cerebrospinální, mozkomíšní
circle /ˈsɜː.kl̩/ kruh, vrátit se zpět
collectively /kəˈlek.tɪv.li/ společně,
celkově, dohromady
curtain /ˈkɜː.tən/ opona
department /dɪˈpɑːt.mənt/
oddělení, úsek, obor
detached /dɪˈtætʃt/ oddělený,
samostatně stojící

discoloration /dɪˌskʌl.əˈreɪ.ʃən/ zabarvení, změna barvy

distribute /dɪˈstrɪb.juːt/ rozdávat, distribuovat

environment /ɪnˈvaɪ.rən.mənt/ prostředí pro činnost, životní prostředí

examine /ɪgˈzæm.ɪn/ prohlédnout, vyšetřit

external /ɪkˈstɜː.nəl/ externí, vnější, zevní

ICP, Intracranial /ɪn.trəˈkreɪ.ni.əl/ **Pressure** /ˈpreʃ.ər/ nitrolebeční tlak

integrity /ɪnˈteg.rə.ti/ integrita, celistvost

interrupt /ˌɪn.təˈrʌpt/ přerušit, narušovat, překážet

introduce /ˌɪn.trəˈdjuːs/ zavést, přijít, představit

jaw /dʒɔː/ **thrust** /θrʌst/ předsunutí čelisti

lacerate /ˈlæs.ər.eɪt/ potrhat, rozervat

leakage /ˈliː.kɪdʒ/ únik, ucházení

lens /lenz/ čočka, kontaktní čočka

lumbar /ˈlʌm.bər/ lumbální, bederní

malocclusion /mæl.əˈkluː.ʒən/ špatný skus

manipulation /məˌnɪp.juˈleɪ.ʃən/ manipulace, ovládání, zacházení

mastoid /ˈmæs.tɔɪd/ mastoidní, bradavkový

MVC, Motor /ˈməʊtə/ **Vehicle** /ˈviː.ɪ.kl/ **Collision** /kəˈlɪʒ.ən/ srážka motorového vozidla

numbness /ˈnʌm.nəs/ necitlivost, znecitlivění, ochromení, pocit necitlivosti

opposite /ˈɒp.ə.zɪt/ proti, protilehlý, protějšek

perforate /ˈpɜː.fər.eɪt/ propíchnout, proděravět

periorbital /ˌper.ɪ.ˈɔːbɪtəl/ periorbitální

projected /prəˈdʒek.tɪd/ promítaný

purplish /ˈpɜː.pl.ɪʃ/ nafialovělý

reactive /riˈæk.tɪv/ reaktivní (chemicky)

respiratory /rɪˈspɪr.ə.tər.i/ **pattern** /ˈpæt.ən/ dechový vzorec

ringing /ˈrɪŋ.ɪŋ/ zvonění

showing /ˈʃəʊ.ɪŋ/ výsledek, vykázaná hodnota

subarachnoid /ˌsʌb.əˈræk.nɔɪd/ subarachnoideální, ležící pod pavučnicovou blánou

term /tɜːm/ termín, název

transient /ˈtræn.zi.ənt/ přechodný, nestálý

unevenly /ʌnˈiː.vən.li/ nestejně, nerovnoměrně

unilaterally /juːˈnɪˈlæt.ər.əl.i/ unilaterálně, jednostranně

widen /ˈwaɪ.dən/ rozšířit (se)

Unit 16

1

A patient has fallen off a 20-foot (6.1 m) ladder, striking his back on a railing. He is experiencing pain at the injury site and a loss of bladder control.
Which part of the _____ ____ is most likely affected by this mechanism? Sacral.*
Nerves that assist in _____ _____ exit from the _____ _____, located above the _____.

sacral spine, bladder control, spinal cord, coccyx

2

Your patient is a 65-year-old male who is complaining of pain in his abdomen, back, and flanks. His blood pressure is 90/60. On examination, you note that the _____ _____ are markedly the weaker than the radial pulses. What should you do next? Treat for hypovolaemia and transport rapidly.*
The patient is showing signs and symptoms of abdominal _____ _____. Do not palpate the abdomen _____; treat decreased tissue perfusion and transport.

unnecessarily, aortic aneurism, femoral pulses

3

Moving the outstretched forearm so that the anterior surface is facing downward is called pronation.*
Pronation is rotating the forearm so that the _____ _____ is facing down.
Supination is the _____ movement.
Rotation is the type of movement required to _____ the extremity.
_____ occurs when the arm is moved out from the midline of the body.

Extension, reposition, anterior surface, opposite

4

The posterior tibial pulse can __ _____ near the medial ankle bone.*
The posterior tibial pulse is assessed just _____ ___ _____ to where the _____ bone protrudes medially. The pulse located on the top of the foot is the _____ _____. The popliteal pulse is located _____ the knee.

dorsalis pedis, behind, below and posterior, be palpated, ankle

5

Where would you expect to see a wound that is described as _____ to the knee? Calf.*

Distal refers to a location that is _____ from the trunk of the body than the _____ _____.

| reference point, further, distal |

6

Which type of wound would most likely require a tourniquet?

- _____ of the hand at the forearm
- bilateral open _____ of the femurs
- below-the-knee amputation by a machine
- tearing injury of the upper arm*

Because a tearing wound can tear multiple large _____ _____, bleeding may be particularly difficult to control, and a _____ may be necessary. Clean amputations often do not require a tourniquet.

| tourniquet, blood vessels, amputation, fractures |

7

Your patient has a suspected hand injury.

How can you best immobilize the hand in the position of function?

Place a roll of _____ _____ into the palm and _____ the hand to a splint.*

The _____ _____, or position of function, for the hand __ _____ by using a gauze roller bandage (or similar material) placed inside the ____ with the _____ curled around it. The hand, _____, ___ _____ should then be splinted with a board, wire ladder, or _____-____ splint.

| palm, neutral position, vacuum-type, gauze bandage, wrist, and forearm, secure, fingers, is achieved |

8

A greenstick fracture is one that is partial.*

A _____ _____ is a partial fracture that is on only one side of the ____ ____. These fractures are noted most frequently __ _____ but may also be seen in adults.

| long bone, in children, greenstick fracture |

9

An injury to the _____ surrounding a joint that is marked by pain, swelling, and bruising is called a sprain.*

A sprain is a partial tearing of a ligament caused by a sudden twisting or _____ of a joint beyond its normal range of motion. It results in _____ and discoloration caused by bleeding into the _____.

A strain is an injury to the muscle or _____ and usually does not result in discoloration.

A dislocation occurs when the normal _____ of two bones is disrupted.

Arthritis is _____ of joints characterized by pain and swelling but does not result in discoloration.

articulation, inflammation, stretching, ligaments, tissue, swelling, tendon

10

When _____ a limb with a suspected fracture, one caregiver applies the splint while another holds the limb and monitors distal pulse, motor, and sensation.*

_____ of a suspected fracture is best accomplished with two _____. After positioning the limb properly, one EMS provider _____ the splint, while the other holds the ____ in position and _____ the distal pulse, motor, and _____ _____.

limb, rescuers, splinting, Immobilization, sensory responses, applies, monitors

11

What is the proper _____ for aligning a fractured long bone? Stabilize the proximal portion and then bring the distal portion into alignment.*

Use gentle _____ to bring the distal part of the limb ____ _____ with the proximal part.

into alignment, procedure, traction

12

When would you _____ ___ _____ limb injuries on the scene? Only if the patient does not need rapid transport.*

If the patient's condition is such that _____ _____ is necessary, you would care for limb injuries while __ _____ rather than completing a detailed physical exam and bandaging and splinting on the scene.

en route, rapid transport, bandage and splint

13

What should you always do if your _____ of a limb suggests that it is fractured? Treat it as if a fracture exists and immobilize it to prevent further injury.*

You cannot ____ a patient by immobilizing a limb properly, but you may possibly _____ further injury __ _____ __ immobilize a fracture. Always assess the _____ _____ before and after_____.

by failing to, harm, distal pulse, cause, splinting, examination

14

A wrestler feels his shoulders pop when his opponent _____ his arm during a hold. There is immediate pain and loss of _____ __ _____ in the shoulder. What is the patient's likely injury?
- Subluxation*
- Muscle _____
- ____ ligament
- Torn rotator cuff

A _____ of the shoulder is a partial dislocation of the _____ due to injuries sustained by the _____ ____ during a severe twisting force to the joint.

subluxation, strain, rotator cuff, twists, range of motion, Torn, joint

15

A driver who follows a 'down and under' pathway of injury after a collision is most likely to have what type of injury?
- fractured ribs
- ruptured diaphragm
- fractured femur*
- lacerated liver or spleen

The '____ ___ _____' pathway results in injury to the _____ ___ ____ rather than to the

abdominal and thoracic organs. These injuries are caused as the patient's knees strike the lower part of the _____ and energy forces travel along the _____ to the pelvis and maybe even into the _____ _____.

femur, dashboard, pelvis and legs, down and under, lower spine

16

Which of the following patients is most critical in terms of age and mechanism of injury?
- An 86-year-old female with a fractured clavicle
- A 28-year-old male with a fractured femur
- A 43-year-old female with a fractured rib
- A 56-year-old male with a pelvic fracture*

Each fracture has a potential _____ ____ of one or more units per fracture site. Because of its ring shape, the _____ frequently has two or more fractures present. In addition, nerve and blood vessel _____ and injury to _____ organs can complicate the severity of this injury.

Patients with pelvic fractures are always considered ____-_____ patients and should be rapidly _____ and transported.

If a patient has bilateral _____

327

_____, he or she is also a high-priority patient.

> high-priority, genitourinary, femur fractures, blood loss, damage, stabilized, pelvis

17
Which patient is most likely to require _____ transport?
- 25-year-old male, _____ wrist
- 45-year-old male, fractured pelvis*
- 38-year-old female, fractured _____
- 52-year-old female, fractured _____

Because of the possibility of severe _____ _____, patients with fractures of the pelvis are most likely to need immediate transport.

> fractured, blood loss, immediate, tibia, humerus

18
The patient has a closed fracture of the left ankle, and the pelvis is stable. There is no penetrating trauma noted in the chest or abdomen, and the patient denies pregnancy. Which of the following chambers of the PASG should be inflated?
- Both legs and the abdominal compartment

- The right leg and the abdominal compartments
- The left leg and the abdominal compartments
- None. PASG is not indicated in this patient.*

PASG is no longer indicated for the _____ _____ of shock patients. If this patient has an unstable _____ _____ in addition to the presence of shock, PASG could be used as an ___ _____ to assist in stabilizing the fractured pelvis.
Because the pelvis is intact, it would be better to rapidly transport her (after full-body and _____ _____ immobilization) to a well-padded long _____ _____.

Shock can be managed with oxygen, positioning (elevate lower end of long board), rapid transport, and careful _____ _____.
Some services use pulmonary oedema and penetrating _____ _____ as the only contraindications to the use of PASG. If that is the case in your service area, then PASG could be used for this patient, but in that case, all compartments should be _____.
You would never inflate only the leg and then the abdominal section. Most likely, the _____ would not help stabilize the ankle

fracture and additional _____
would be required.

---

pelvic fracture, splinting, air splint, cervical spine, garment, inflated, spine board, fluid administration, routine, management, chest trauma

19

Knee, femur, and hip dislocation and fracture caused by the _____ hitting the firewall and absorbing initial impact are common in _____ _____ with a 'down and under' pathway.*
'__ __ ____' refers to injuries sustained in the head, neck, and chest region. In the 'down and under' pathway, the body _____ forward and downward. This can be limited by the correct use of

___ _____.

---

slides, frontal collisions, seat belts, Up and over, Knees

20

What should you do to care for a patient with a suspected pelvic fracture? Apply the PASG/MAST, titrate two IVs to effect, and monitor for _____ __ _____.*
This is the current field treatment regimen for _____ _____.
The PASG/MAST is used as an ___-_____ to contain the fractured pelvis and _____ further injury.

---

prevent, air-splint, pelvic fractures, signs of shock

Vocabulary 16
align /əˈlaɪn/ sblížit se, spojit se, připojit se
alignment /əˈlaɪn.mənt/ podpora, postavení, pozice, poloha
amputation /ˌæm.pjʊˈteɪ.ʃən/ amputace
arteria /ɑːˈtiə.riə/ **dorsalis** /dɔr.sə.lɪs/ **pedis** /ped.ɪs/ lat. hřbetní tepna nohy, je pokračováním a. tibialis anterior
arthritis /ɑːˈθraɪ.tɪs/ artritida, zánět kloubů
articulation /ɑːˌtɪk.jʊˈleɪ.ʃən/ kloub, skloubení
bandage /ˈbæn.dɪdʒ/ obvaz, obinadlo, bandáž, obvázat
caregiver /ˈkeəˌɡɪv.ər/ pečovatel, opatrovatel
coccyx /ˈkɒk.sɪks/ kostrč, kostrční kost
curl /kɜːl/ natočit, stočit
dislocation /ˌdɪs.ləˈkeɪ.ʃən/ dislokace, vykloubení, narušení
face /feɪs/ **down** /daʊn/ směřovat dolů
firewall /ˈfaɪə.wɔːl/ protipožární přepážka, požární zeď
forearm /ˈfɔː.rɑːm/ předloktí
genitourinary /ˌdʒen.ɪ.təʊˈjʊə.rɪ.nər.i/ močopohlavní
greenstick /griːn.stɪk/ **fracture** /ˈfræktʃə/ nalomená kost
ligament /ˈlɪɡ.ə.mənt/ vaz mezi kostmi, kloubu ap.
limb /lɪm/ končetina

markedly /ˈmɑː.kɪd.li/ zřetelně

medial /ˈmiː.di.əl/ středový

opponent /əˈpəʊ.nənt/ oponent, soupeř, protihráč

outstretched /ˌaʊtˈstretʃt/ roztažený, natažený, napřažený

palm /pɑːm/ dlaň

pathway /ˈpɑːθ.weɪ/ cesta, dráha pohybu

pelvis /ˈpel.vɪs/ pánev

pop /pɒp/ prasknout

popliteal /ˌpɒp.lɪˈtiː.əl/ podkolenní, zákolenní

pronation /prəʊˈneɪ.ʃən/ pronace, stočení ruky s vnitřní polohou palce, stočení končetiny dovnitř podle podélné osy

railing /ˈreɪ.lɪŋ/ zábradlí, ohrada

roller /ˈrəʊ.lər/ **bandage** /ˈbæn.dɪdʒ/ obinadlo

rotate /rəʊˈteɪt/ točit se, obíhat, střídat se

rotator /rəʊˈteɪt.ər/ **cuff** /kʌf/ rotátorová manžeta, pouzdro ramenního svalu je zesíleno kloubními vazy a šlachami kolemjdoucích svalů (m. subscapularis, m. supraspinatus, m. infraspinatus, m. teres minor)

rotator /rəʊˈteɪt.ər/ rotátor, sval, který provádí rotaci

sacral /ˈseɪ.krəl/ sakrální, křížový

strain /streɪn/ nápor, zátěž, namáhat, přetěžovat

subluxation /ˌsʌb.lʌkˈseɪ.ʃən/ subluxace, neúplné vykloubení, posuntí

supination /ˈsuː.pɪn.əɪ.ʃən/ supinace, lat. supinus, obrácený vzhůru, rotace předloktí, kterou se u končetiny visící podél těla otočí dlaň dopředu, tzn. malíkem k tělu

tendon tendines /ˈten.dən/ šlacha

titrate /ˈtaɪ.treɪt/ titrovat, (titrace, metoda určení přesné dávky léku pomocí zkusmého dávkování od nižší k vyšší dávce s pečlivým sledování efektu)

twist /ˌtwɪst/ zkroutit, stočit, vyvrtnout si

wire /waɪər/ **ladder** /ˈlæd.ər/ typ dlahy

wrestler /ˈres.lər/ zápasník

Unit 17

1

Knee injuries and ___
_____ that occur during a
motor vehicle crash are often the
result of what pathway of _____
_____? Down and under.*
During a frontal crash, the 'down
and under' pathway causes
the _____ __ _____ the lower
dashboard violently, causing the
described _____ _____.

> knees to strike, injury pattern,
> energy transfer, hip dislocations

2

You suspect that a trauma patient
has a pelvic injury. She is cool
and diaphoretic, with a heart rate
of 134 and blood pressure of
100/72.
What _____ is most
appropriate in the management
of her condition? Application of
PASG.*
The use of the MAST/PASG
as a splint in the stabilization
of suspected pelvic fractures is
_____ for this patient.
Since the systolic blood pressure
is greater than 90-100 mmHg,
any IV fluid should __ _____
__ a slow, of 'keep open', rate.
This may _____ any additional
bleeding from the dilution of
_____ _____.

> clotting factors, reduce,
> indicated, be restricted to,
> procedure

3

A conscious adult who falls _
_____ of 20 feet (6.1 m) is
most likely to ____ __ his or her:
- head
- hands
- back
- feet*

Conscious adults who fall more
that three times their height tend
to land on their feet; this tends
to cause bilateral _____
fractures, hip _____, and
_____ _____ of the
spinal column.

> compression fractures,
> dislocations, a distance land on,
> calcaneous

4

A 25-year-old female complains
of _____ lower-abdominal pain,
vaginal _____, and low-grade
fever.
What condition best describes
the patient's presentation? Pelvic
_____ disease.*
PID causes lower-abdominal
_____ that is difficult to localize
and often has an associated fever.
Pain associated with an ectopic
pregnancy is more _____, as is
the pain associated with solid organ
involvement.

inflammatory, localized, discharge, discomfort, diffuse

5

A 28-year-old woman is complaining of a sudden onset of _____ abdominal pain that _____ to her shoulder. Her BP = 88/60, P = 110, and R = 20. Her skin is cool, pale, and _____. She states that her last normal menstrual period was six to eight weeks ago.

What condition best describes the patient presentation? Ectopic pregnancy.*

A sudden rupture of an ectopic pregnancy would result in a loss of blood that would place the patient in _____ shock.

compensatory, radiates, severe, clammy

6

Your patient is a 28-year-old female who reports that she is nine weeks pregnant. She is complaining of severe abdominal pain, shoulder pain, and vaginal _____. Vital signs are within normal limits, and a physical exam reveals _____ in the lower left quadrant.

What should you suspect is occurring? Ectopic pregnancy.*

Most ectopic pregnancies implant within the _____ ____ and have attained a large enough size

around nine weeks to _____ the tube, resulting in intense pain and bleeding.

The bleeding may or may not be present from the vagina. Most cases of spontaneous _____ are undetected by the mother, who doesn't even know she is pregnant, and present as an abnormal menstrual cycle.

abortion, bleeding, rupture, fallopian tube, tenderness

7

Your patient is a 32-year-old woman who reports that she is nine weeks pregnant. She is complaining of _____ abdominal pain, slight vaginal bleeding, and _____ pain. Abdominal examination reveals _____ tenderness in the lower right quadrant. The patient is somewhat _____ and tachycardic.

You should suspect developing _____ from what condition? Ectopic pregnancy.*

Signs and symptoms of ectopic pregnancy include lower-abdominal pain that is often referred to the shoulder, abdominal tenderness, and rapidly developing shock.

significant, shock, agitated, shoulder, severe

8

Your patient is a 33-year-old woman who is nine months pregnant. She _____ of severe abdominal pain and _____ tenderness. She _____ that there is no vaginal bleeding at this time.

What should you suspect?

Abruptio placentae (premature _____ of the placenta).*

> reports, separation, abdominal, complains

9

Answer the next three questions on the basis of the following information.

You respond to a 25-year-old female who is complaining of vaginal bleeding and abdominal pain.

The patient states that she is thirty-three weeks pregnant and that this is her first pregnancy. She says that when the pain started, it felt like something was tearing. She _____ vaginal bleeding during the pregnancy prior to this event. Upon _____, you notice what appears to be approximately 500 cc of dark, almost black, blood.

What _____ is this patient most likely suffering from?

Abruptio placentae*

The tearing feeling and the ____-_____ blood are classic signs and symptoms of abruptio placentae.

Placenta praevia often has bleeding that is contained within the uterus due to the placenta blocking the os (opening or mouth) of the _____.

This condition is _____ to both the mother and the baby.* Both lives are at stake. Oxygen is passed from the mother to the baby via the placenta. A separation greatly decreases the blood _____ to the infant, and the uncontrolled bleeding is dangerous to the mother.

In addition to high-flow oxygen and continuous _____ of the mother's vital signs and the baby's foetal heart tones, you should treat this patient with one or two large-bore IVs of normal saline or Ringer's lactate.*

Administering one or two large-bore IVs of normal saline or Ringer's lactate is _____ when combined with rapid transport.

You should titrate the BP to 100-110 so as not to _____ the circulation, causing pulmonary oedema and further compromising the oxygen supply to the infant.

> condition, denies, overload, dangerous, assessment, uterus, dark-coloured, supply, monitoring, appropriate

10
What is the usual clinical
_____ of placenta
praevia? _____ bright red
bleeding.*
Placenta praevia usually presents
as painless bright red bleeding
that occurs in the _____ trimester
of pregnancy. The blood may be
_____ within the uterus.

Painless, contained, third,
presentation

11
Your patient is a 32-year-old
woman who reports that she is
fourteen weeks pregnant. She
complains of abdominal _____
and vaginal bleeding.
How should you proceed? Treat
for signs and symptoms of
_____, provide _____
support, and transport.*
The patient is most likely suffering
a _____. Treat her for signs
and symptoms of shock due to
_____ ____, provide emotional
support, retain any clumps of
tissue she passes, and transport.

miscarriage, emotional,
cramping, blood loss,
hypovolaemia

12
Which are the only two
_____ in which a prehospital
provider should place a gloved

hand into the vagina? _____
cord and _____ presentation*
In both of these cases, relieving
pressure off the trapped umbilical
cord (prolapsed) or the face and
airway passages (trapped breech)
may be the ____ _____ measure
provided by the paramedic.

Prolapsed, breech, life-saving,
situations

13
Signs and symptoms of
a pregnant patient with
preeclampsia include elevated
BP, visual disturbance, headache,
and oedema.*
Common signs and symptoms of
_____ include headache,
_____, confusion, _____
_____, nausea, vomiting,
proteinuria, hypertension, and
_____.

dizziness, blurred vision,
oedema, preeclampsia

14
The normal _____ period is
forty weeks.*
___ ____ delivery usually occurs
within the fortieth week of
pregnancy. These are normal
_____ changes that
occur in vital signs during
pregnancy: a woman's blood
pressure usually _____ during the

first two trimesters, and her pulse rate _____.

> gestation, Full-term, physiological, rises, falls

15

You are recording vital signs for a 34-year-old woman who is eight months pregnant. Her blood pressure is 100/70, pulse rate is 80, and respirations are 17 per minute and normal. Upon _____ of her chest, you hear a mild systolic flow _____. How should you treat this patient? The murmur is not a _____ of concern; document these findings on the patient-care report.* A mild systolic murmur in a pregnant patient whose vital signs are normal is not a cause of

_____.

> murmur, finding, concern, auscultation

16

Answer the next four questions on the basis of the following information.

You respond to a 19-year-old female who is twenty-five weeks pregnant and is complaining of a severe headache and _____ vision. Upon initial assessment, you notice that she has substantial _____, especially in her feet and hands. She states that she has not been under the regular care of a physician during this pregnancy.

What _____ would you expect to see in this patient's vital signs? Hypertension.*

This is toxaemia, a _____ disorder of pregnancy.

This patient is most likely suffering from the condition known as preeclampsia.*

Treatment for this patient includes rapid transport without light and sirens, an IV of normal saline or Ringer's lactate, and oxygen. It may also call for the administration of magnesium sulphate.*

Magnesium sulphate is the appropriate medication for the suppression of seizures in a _____ patient. Valium may help control seizures, but magnesium suppresses them.

If left untreated, this patient's condition may worsen, and she may begin to experience grand mal seizures.*

Seizures indicate that the patient's condition has worsened. The condition is then called

_____.

> oedema, blurred, hypertensive, eclampsia, abnormality, preeclampsia

17

Your patient is a 35-year-old woman who is eight months pregnant. You note that her blood pressure is 140/90 and oedema is present all over her body. The patient is _____ and complains of seeing spots and having a

_____.

From this information, what condition should you suspect is present? Preeclampsia.*

The patient shows symptoms and signs of preeclampsia (or _____ of pregnancy) and should be transported to the hospital. The distinction between eclampsia and preeclampsia is the presence of _____ and/or

____.

coma, anxious, seizures, toxaemia, headache

18

Which of the following signs and symptoms would be present in a pregnant patient with preeclampsia? High blood pressure, headaches, oedema, and visual disturbances.*

Patients with preeclampsia (or toxaemia of pregnancy) _____ all the signs and symptoms of the hypertensive disorders of pregnancy except _____. Once the patient begins to _____ seizures, the condition has

changed from preeclampsia to eclampsia.

manifest, seizures, experience

19

Causes of third-trimester bleeding include _____ placentae, placenta _____, and _____ rupture.

praevia,* abruptio,* uterine*

20

Your patient is a 29-year-old woman who is nine months pregnant with her third child. She reports the onset of painless _____ ___ vaginal bleeding in the last half hour.

How should you treat this patient? Treat her for signs and symptoms of shock and transport immediately.*

Bright red bleeding in late pregnancy is assumed to be _____ praevia, which is a true _____ _____ that is life-threatening to both mother and baby. Treat the mother for shock and transport _____.

immediately, medical emergency, placenta, bright red

Vocabulary 17
at /ət/ **stake** /steɪk/ být v sázce
attain /əˈteɪn/ získat, dosáhnout, docílit
block /blɒk/ blokovat, zatarasit
breech /briːtʃ/ zadeček, zadnice
clot /klɒt/ sraženina, chuchvalec, srážet se
clump /klʌmp/ shluk, skupina, dupat
dangerous /ˈdeɪn.dʒər.əs/ nebezpečný
dilution /daɪˈluː.ʃən/ oslabení, zředěný roztok
distinction /dɪˈstɪŋk.ʃən/ rozdíl, odlišnost
grade /greɪd/ stupeň
heart /hɑːt/ **rate** /reɪt/ srdeční frekvence
implant /ɪmˈplɑːnt/ uhnízdit se, usadit, implantát
in addition /əˈdɪʃ.ən/ navíc k čemu, kromě
intense /ɪnˈtens/ intenzivní, silný, ostrý
land /lænd/ dopadnout na zem, přistát
life-saving /ˈlaɪfˌseɪ.vɪŋ/ život zachraňující, první pomoc
miscarriage /ˈmɪsˌkær.ɪdʒ/ potrat (samovolný)
murmur /ˈmɜː.mər/ šelest, šeptat
os /ɒs/ ossa kost
physician /fɪˈzɪʃ.ən/ lékař, doktor
PID, Pelvic /ˈpel.vɪk/ **Inflammatory** /ɪnˈflæm.ə.tər.i/ **Disease** /dɪˈziːz/ zánětlivé onemocnění pánve
proceed /prəˈsiːd/ pokračovat, postupovat

restricted /rɪˈstrɪk.tɪd/ omezený, nepřístupný
retain /rɪˈteɪn/ udržet si, ponechat, zachovat, uchovat, zadržet, uvíznout
somewhat /ˈsʌm.wɒt/ trochu, poněkud
substantial /səbˈstæn.ʃəl/ podstatný, značný, velký
support /səˈpɔːt/ podporovat, podepřít
suppression /səˈpreʃ.ən/ potlačení, potlačování
tear /tɪər/ roztrhnout se, protrhnout se
tend /tend/ **to the needs of sb** zajišťovat potřeby někoho
tone /təʊn/ napětí svalu nebo cévní stěny, nervové napětí
toxaemia /tɒkˈsiː.mi.ə/ toxemie, otrava krve
trimester /trɪˈmes.tər/ trimestr
undetected /ˌʌn.dɪˈtekt.əd/ nezjištěný, neobjevený
Valium /ˈvæl.i.əm/ diazepam (benzodiazepinové anxiolytikum, antiepileptikum, uvolňuje svalové napětí)
violently /ˈvaɪə.lənt.li/ násilně, agresivně
vital /ˈvaɪ.təl/ **signs** /saɪnz/ životní znaky

Unit 18

1

A pregnant patient complains of painful, irregular _____ _____. The patient states that she is thirty-seven weeks pregnant and her _____ membranes ruptured two days ago.

Based on this information, you would _____ immediate transport.*

Immediate transport is _____ for this patient's condition.

Without the intact protective amniotic sac, the foetus is at risk of being _____.

indicated, amniotic, infected, labour contraction, initiate

2

The use of PASG/MAST is indicated to _____ lower-extremity _____ in a hypotensive patient.*

Third-trimester pregnancy, impaled objects, and dyspnoea are all _____ for use of the PASG/MAST.

In addition, the PASG/MAST is contraindicated with any _____ bleeding occurring above the site of the garment.

contraindications, uncontrolled, stabilize, fractures

3

What is the cause of the supine hypotensive syndrome in the pregnant patient? _____ of the uterus on the inferior vena cava.*

Supine hypotensive syndrome, a normal _____ during late pregnancy, is caused by the pressure of the pregnant uterus on the inferior vena cava when the patient is _____.

supine, occurrence, Pressure

4

You arrive at the scene of an _____ delivery in the field.

The first _____, who called for _____, reports that the patient is a 32-year-old female who is G4 P3.

What does this mean? The patient has been pregnant four times and _____ three live children.*

What does it mean if a woman is described as _____? She has delivered more than one live baby.*

responder, assistance, delivered, imminent, multipara

5

Which of the following signs most likely indicates _____ birth?

- painful uterine contraction
- urge to have a bowel movement*

- ruptured membranes
- dilation of the cervix

When the foetus is close to the _____ of the birth canal, the head presses down on the internal _____ _____, resulting in the urge to have a _____ _____. Painful uterine contractions can start well in advance of _____ delivery.

> imminent, bowel movement, anal sphincter, physical, entrance

6

When should you examine a woman who is about to give birth for crowning? During _____.*
Look for _____, or the appearance of the baby's head at the _____ of the vagina, only during a contraction.

> crowning, opening, contraction

7

During delivery a loop of umbilical cord presents from the _____ _____.
You should _____ the cord with a moist and sterile dressing.*
Covering the exposed cord will _____ drying of the cord. Additionally, you should try to _____ two fingers into the birth canal and try to keep pressure from the baby's ____ away from the cord.

> birth canal, minimize, insert, head, cover

8

During a normal delivery, you would tell the mother to stop _____ when what occurs? The head is _____.*
To avoid a _____ delivery, tell the mother to ____ pushing after the head is delivered.

> pushing, stop, precipitous, delivered

9

Answer the next four questions on the basis of the following information.
You are called to the home of a 21-year-old female in _____ labour. She is two weeks from her _____ ___ date and is having contractions of 1.5 minutes _____, which are 3 minutes apart. This is her second pregnancy. Her first child was delivered vaginally at ____ ____.
What is your first course of action for this patient? Place her on the _____ in a high Fowler's or a comfortable position and examine her for crowning.*
In this situation, the first step would be to _____ the patient for _____ to determine if you need to assist with delivery on the scene or if you can attempt to transport her.

Your patient suddenly tells you she feels something slippery between her legs. Upon visual examination, you notice a 2-inch (5 cm) segment of the umbilical cord _____ from the vagina. What is this condition called? Prolapsed cord.*

What are appropriate treatment options for this patient? Provide high-flow oxygen and rapidly transport the mother in a ____-_____ position, take pressure off the cord by placing your fingers into the vagina and gently _____ the infant, _____ the cord in a moist sterile dressing, provide supplemental oxygen, and transport quickly.*

If you opt to position the patient for transport, you should place her in the left lateral _____ position to _____ uterine blood flow and return.

You are ready to transport this patient.

If the umbilical cord is still exposed, how can you use it to evaluate the infant's perfusion? Gently feel the cord for _____ to determine the infant's _____ ____.*

The umbilical vein, found within the umbilical cord, provides _____ blood to the infant. The vein is large enough for you to feel the pulsations as blood flows from the placenta to the _____.

duration, full term, examine, oxygenated, active, crowning, expected due, stretcher, knee-chest, heart rate, protruding, lifting, wrap, recumbent, improve, pulsations, foetus

10

A patient who is thirty-seven weeks pregnant is having contractions and states that her _____ _____ about 20 minutes ago. The vaginal exam _____ that the baby's foot is present in the birth canal.

Your next action would be to ____ the patient to the cot and initiate rapid transport.*

A single-limb presentation is considered _____ vaginally and requires rapid caesarean section to successfully deliver the infant. Rapid transport is indicated.

reveals, move, water broke, nondeliverable

11

What are the blood vessels in the _____ ____? Two arteries and one vein.*

The umbilical cord contains two _____ and one vein; only

the umbilical ____ is used for

_____ ____.

arteries, vascular access, vein, umbilical cord

12

What does the term *effacement* refer to? _____ of the cervix during the first stage of _____.*
Effacement refers to the stretching and thinning of the _____, which occurs during the _____ stage of normal labour.

labour, cervix, Thinning, first

13

What does the presence of meconium on the _____ or in the _____ _____ indicate? The infant may have been distressed.*
The presence of meconium indicates that the foetus may have been _____ before birth.

amniotic fluid, distressed, neonate

14

When does the _____ stage of labour begin? Immediately ____ the birth of the baby.*
The third stage of labour _____ with the birth of the foetus and ____ with the delivery of the placenta.

begins, third, ends, upon

15

What is the appropriate treatment for a prolapsed cord? Place two fingers to _____ the presenting part of the _____ off the cord, place the mother in the ____-_____ position, _____ oxygen, and transport.*
A _____ cord should be treated by placing two fingers of a gloved hand into the vagina to raise the presenting part of the foetus off the ____, then placing the mother in the Trendelenburg or knee-chest position, administering high-flow oxygen, and _____ immediately.

knee-chest, foetus, administer, transporting, prolapsed, cord, raise

16

Regarding a single-limb presentation during an emergency delivery, this statement is true: this is a nondeliverable presentation and requires immediate transport to an appropriate receiving facility.*
A ____ presentation during delivery requires a _____ _____ to _____ the delivery. Provide high-flow oxygen and ____ to the mother during transport.

limb, care, complete, caesarean section

17

What is the order of care for a newborn born with evidence of meconium staining? Suction with the ____ _____ first, then remove remaining meconium under direct _____.*
Do not resuscitate or stimulate further until the meconium is _____ ____ the respiratory tree by direct visualization of the cords.

bulb syringe, cleared from, visualization

18

What is the correct _____ for cutting the umbilical cord after the birth of the baby? Clamp the cord in two places 5 cm _____ and cut it between the clamps.*
Generally, you want to _____ the first clamp 5-7 inches (13-18 cm) away from the _____.

apart, place, procedure, infant

19

Immediately after delivery, how should you _____ a neonate?
At the _____ of the mother's vagina, with its head slightly _____ than the body.*
Position the neonate at the level of the mother's vagina, with his or her head slightly lower than the body to _____ drainage of _____.

secretions, level, lower, position, facilitate

20

You would perform chest compressions on any newborn whose heart is less than 60 beats per minute.*
____ _____ are required when a newborn's heart rate is ____ than 60 or between 60 and 80 after 30 seconds of positive-pressure _____.
Remember to perform each _____ for approximately 30 seconds, then _____ for the need to continue resuscitation.
The appropriate range for the heart rate of a healthy neonate immediately after birth is 150-180 beats per minute.*

intervention, ventilation, less, reassess, chest compressions

Vocabulary 18
apart /əˈpɑːt/ vzdálený, oddělený
bulb /bʌlb/ kulovité rozšíření cylindrické struktury či orgánu
cervix /ˈsɜː.vɪks/ pl **cervices** /-vɪs. iːz/ hrdlo děložní
distressed /dɪˈstrest/ sklíčený, zdeptaný
duration /djʊəˈreɪ.ʃən/ délka, doba trvání

effacement /ɪˈfeɪs.mənt/ správné rozšíření děložních cest při normálním porodu

Fowler's /fowˈler/ **position** /pəˈzɪʃ.ən/ Fowlerova poloha, poloha v polosedě, při které má nemocný hlavu a trup zvednutý 45-90°

in advance /ədˈvɑːns/ před čím dříve

inch /ɪntʃ/ palec, 2,5 cm

internal /ɪnˈtɜː.nəl/ interní, vnitřní

lift /lɪft/ pozvednout, zdvih

multipara /mʌl.tiˈpær.ə/ vícerodička, žena, která vícekrát rodila

nondeliverable /ˌnɒn.dɪˈlɪv.ər.ə.bl̩/ neporoditelný

precipitous /prɪˈsɪp.ɪ.təs/ prudký, překotný

pulsation /pʌlˈseɪ.ʃən/ pulzace, tepot

responder /rɪˈspɒnd.ər/ reagující osoba

slippery /ˈslɪp.ər.i/ kluzký, klouzavý

Trendelenburg position /pəˈzɪʃ.ən/ Trendelenburgova poloha, poloha při níž pacient leží na zádech a jeho pánev je uložena výše než hlava

Unit 19

1

What is the _____ for administering positive-pressure ventilations to a Central newborn? Cyanosis _____ while oxygen is given.*

Apnoea and tachycardia may _____ be present in the newborn, but once they are corrected, you do not need to _____ to progress further inverted into the pyramid.

persists, initially, criterion, continue

2

_____ and drugs are most often delivered to a newborn through the use of which circulatory _____? Umbilical vein.*

The _____ _____, located in the umbilical cord, is used for this purpose. If the cord is left untreated at the hospital, it may be cannulated for a week or even longer. It enters immediately into the _____ _____.

hepatic circulation, umbilical vein, vessel, Medications

3

You are assessing a neonate who has a pink body and blue _____, a pulse rate of 90, positive grimace response, active _____, and _____ respiratory efforts.

What is the Apgar score for this infant? 6.*

The score would consist of one point each for appearance, pulse rate, grimace, and respiratory _____ and two points for activity.

motion, extremities, effort, irregular

4

During an _____ delivery, the newborn's head presents in the canal.

After suctioning, how can you _____ with the delivery of the anterior shoulder? Gently guide the infant's head downward*

The head will ____ ___ drop down as the shoulders begin to pass through the birth canal. The paramedic can gently _____ the head to help with the process.

assist, tend to, guide, emergency

5

During a normal delivery, you would _____ the infant's mouth and nose just _____:
- the head is out of the vagina*
- the entire infant is delivered
- the head and chest are delivered
- you clamp the cord

Suction the infant's mouth and nose immediately after the head is delivered, and you can _____ the mouth and nose. Suctioning of the infant's mouth and nose should be performed after the head has been _____.
Remember to suction the mouth first, ____ the nose.

after, access, then, suction, delivered

6

You are assisting in a delivery __ ___ _____. As the baby's head is born, you realize that the umbilical cord is _____ around the baby's neck.
What is your first step in the _____ of this problem?
Attempt to ____ the cord ____ the baby's head.*
First, attempt to slip the cord over the baby's head. If this is impossible you should _____ the cord in two places and carefully ___ it between the clamps, then _____ with the delivery.

slip over, cut, management, wrapped, continue, clamp, in the field

7

What is the appropriate _____ for the heart rate of a healthy neonate _____ after birth?
150-180 beats ___ _____.*

Heart rate at birth is normally 150-180 beats per minute, _____ to 130-140 within a few minutes.

slowing, immediately, range, per minute

8

The first step in the _____ of a distressed neonate is to ventilate with 100% oxygen for 15-30 seconds.*
_____ with 100% oxygen and then _____ the heart rate and initiate _____ compressions if necessary.

Ventilate, chest, evaluate, resuscitation

9

You have just delivered a baby girl. _____ reveals that the infant _____ loudly and has a heart rate of 140, her ____ is pink but the extremities are blue, and she is actively moving all extremities.
Her APGAR score is 9.*
With the exception of the blue extremities, the infant scores a 2 on _____, _____, _____, and _____. Her appearance scores as a 1.

Evaluation, body, cries, activity, pulse, grimace, respirations

10

All of the following statements about supplying supplemental oxygen to a neonate are correct:

- Do not withhold oxygen from a neonate in the _____ setting.*
- Administer _____ oxygen by blowing it across the neonate's face.*
- Oxygen should be _____ if possible prior to administration.*

Oxygen _____ occurs only if oxygen is administered for several days.

> toxicity, supplemental, warmed, prehospital

11

Children of what age are in the greatest danger from airway _____ caused by aspirated _____ objects? 1-3 years.*
Children between 1 and 3, who tend to ___ things into their mouths, are in greatest danger of _____ of foreign objects.

> aspiration, foreign, obstruction, put

12

You should _____ to remove foreign material from a patient's airway with forceps only in what situation? You are able to visualize the obstruction directly.*
To prevent tissue _____, you should attempt to physically _____ foreign material only if you can actually see the obstruction with a _____.

> laryngoscope, remove, damage, attempt

13

Until ruled out by a physician, documented fever in an infant younger than 3 months old is always considered to _____ ____ meningitis.*
Fever in a child younger than _____ months old is considered to be _____ unless proven otherwise; transport all infants with fever _____.

> meningitis, 3, promptly, result from

14

What volume of fluid bolus should be given initially to severely dehydrated child? 20 ml/kg.*
Give a _____ dehydrated child an _____ bolus of 20 cc/ kg of normal _____ or Ringer's solution. Reassess for _____ and repeat with 10 or 20 cc/ kg boluses as long as the child continues to _____ and you do not detect any signs of fluid _____.

initial, severely, response,
overload, improve, saline

15

The best place to assess for
cyanosis in an infant or child is
the oral mucosa.*
The best place to assess for
_____ in an infant or child is
the ____ _____, lips, or tongue.
Nail beds of an infant may not be
an _____ indicator of central
circulation _____even when they
appear cyanotic.

accurate, oral mucosa, status,
cyanosis

16

This statement _____ febrile
seizures is true: febrile seizures
occur because of a rapid rise in
skin temperature.*
_____ _____ occur in
children because of a _____
rise in temperature and not
necessarily the _____ of the
fever itself.
All paediatric patients who
have had seizures should be
transported to a hospital for
evaluation.*
The cause of seizure activity
can be determined only in the
hospital.

rapid, severity, Febrile seizures,
regarding

17

Unilateral wheezing in a
14-month-old child is suggestive
of aspiration of a foreign body.*
Wheezing localized into one lung
only minimizes the _____
of asthma or other _____
disease. If a foreign body is small
enough to pass through the
glottic _____ and carina, it will
eventually lodge somewhere in
either the ____ _____ or the
bronchioles.
If the obstruction is not complete,
air moving past the restricted lung
passage will _____ a wheeze.

main bronchi, pulmonary,
opening, produce, likelihood

18

A 2-year-old female presents
with lethargy and poor feeding.
The parent states that the patient
has had a _____ fever for the
past seven days, with _____,
nausea, and vomiting for the past
four days.
She presents with pale, cool
skin, a pulse rate of 180, and a
respiratory rate of 40. She cries
weakly when a painful stimulus __
_____. The ECG shows a rapid
narrow complex dysrhythmia.
Based upon this information, what
is the patient's _____ problem?
- respiratory distress
- respiratory failure
- hypoperfusion*

• dysrhythmia

The history of diarrhoea, nausea, and vomiting indicates a strong _____ situation resulting in the tachycardia and dyspnoea.

moderate, is applied, dehydration, primary, diarrhoea

19

A 3-year-old female is unresponsive and not breathing. Parents state that she was eating grapes when she suddenly made a high-pitched whistling noise and turned blue.

Your immediate action would be to start _____ resuscitation.*

The high-pitched whistling _____ and cyanosis _____ the patient is suffering from an airway obstruction.

Back blows and chest thrusts are performed only on infants. Since the patient is _____, your immediate step should be to start CPR.

Abdominal thrusts are performed only on conscious _____ victims. For unresponsive victims suspected of having an airway obstruction, you should begin CPR, but look in the mouth to see if you visualise the object _____ __ each ventilation attempt.

unresponsive, cardiopulmonary, indicates, prior to, choking, noise

20

Answer the next three questions on the basis of the following information.

You respond to a 4-year-old female who has taken an _____ quantity of children's aspirin. Upon arrival, you find the patient conscious, crying, and lethargic. Her mother states that she found the child playing in the bathroom. A flavoured children's aspirin bottle was found nearby with only a few tablets in it.

In this situation, you should make the _____ that the aspirin bottle was full and treat accordingly.*

Unless you know otherwise, always assume a medication bottle was full. There is nothing in this situation to indicate child abuse.

Although today the quantity of pills packaged has been reduced in order to lessen the likelihood of _____ by accidental ingestion, this child's _____ LOC (level of consciousness) suggests there is a serious overdose situation here.

Children's aspirin is in which class of medications? Salicylates.*

Correct treatment for this patient may include IV, oxygen, ECG, and activated _____.*

The appropriate treatment is IV, oxygen, ECG, and activated charcoal. Be prepared to treat dysrhythmias and to provide a fluid challenge if ordered. Sodium bicarbonate may also be ordered by medical direction.

> unknown, overdose, decreasing, charcoal, assumption

21
Tertiary injuries from a blast include:
* Extremity _____
* _____ lacerations
* Impaled objects
* Lung injuries*

Tertiary blast injuries are caused by the victim being _____ _____ from the blast and into objects on the ground. Injuries from this are _____ __ those sustained from ejection from an automobile.

Primary blast injuries result from the compression of hollow organs such as the lungs.

Secondary blast injuries are caused by flying debris propelled by the force of the _____.

> similar to, blast, fractures, Organ, propelled away

Vocabulary 19
accordingly /əˈkɔː.dɪŋ.li/ podle toho, v souladu, přiměřeně
Apgar /ˈæpgɑː/ **score** /skɔːr/ Apgar skóre, hodnocení zdravotního stavu novorozence krátce po porodu

assumption /əˈsʌmp.ʃən/ převzetí, předpoklad, domněnka
blowing /ˈbləʊ.ɪŋ/ foukání
cardiopulmonary /ˌkɑː.di.əʊˈpʊl.mə.nə.ri/ kardiopulmonární, týkající se srdce a plic
criterion /kraɪˈtɪə.ri.ən/ kriterium, měřítko
dehydration /ˌdiː.haɪˈdreɪ.ʃən/ odvodnění, vysychání
downward /ˈdaʊn.wəd/ dolů směřující, sestupný
ejection /ɪˈdʒekt.ʃən/ vyhození, katapultování
flavoured /fleɪ.vəd/ ochucený, s příchutí
grape /greɪp/ hroznové víno
grimace /ˈgrɪ.məs/ grimasa, úšklebek
inverted/ ɪnˈvɜː.tɪd/ obrácený, převrácený
laryngoscope /ˌlærɪŋˈgɒ.skəʊp/ laryngoskop, přístroj k zrakovému vyšetření hrtanu
lip /lɪp/ ret, okraj
loudly /ˈlaʊd.li/ hlasitě, důrazně
mucosa /mjuːˈkəʊ.sə/ mukóza, sliznice
nail /neɪl/ **bed** /bed/ nehtové lůžko
nausea /ˈnɔː.zi.ə/ nevolnost, nutkání ke zvracení
passage /ˈpæsɪdʒ/ průchod, trubice, kanálek
Salicylates /səˈlɪs.ɪˌleɪts/ salicitáty (aspirin, anopirin, superpirin)
warmed /ˌwɔːmd/ zahřátý, teplý
weakly /ˈwiːk.li/ slabě

Unit 20

1

Your patient is a 4-year-old girl who _____ in the middle of the night with a cough that her mother describes as sounding like a seal barking. The patient feels more comfortable _____ __. Vital signs are as follows: respiration, 26/min; pulse, 100; temperature, 101 °F (38.3 °C). On the _____ ____, you hear stridor on inspiration.

From this scenario, you should suspect what condition? Croup.* The signs, symptoms, and assessment _____ of croup are described. The seal-bark cough is a classic presentation with croup.

> awoke, physical exam, findings, sitting up

2

Your patient is a 6-year-old child who is conscious but not breathing because of an airway obstruction.

What is the first thing you should do for this patient? Perform subdiaphragmatic abdominal thrusts.*

The first step in treating a _____ child of this age with a complete airway obstruction is to perform the Heimlich _____ (i.e. subdiaphragmatic abdominal thrusts). Continue until the

obstruction is _____ or the child becomes unconscious.

> manoeuvre, relieved, conscious

3

Your patient is a 10-year-old boy who ___ _____ off his bicycle. What should you do when obtaining the history of the _____? Obtain as much information as possible from the child.*

With a child of this age, obtain as much information as possible from the patient him- or herself; this will allow the child to feel respected and _____. The adult _____ can fill in relevant details.

> has fallen, caretaker, mature, accident

4

Answer the next three questions on the basis of the following information.

You respond to a 12-year-old male who is wheezing and having difficulty breathing. The patient has a long history of asthma and states that he used his _____ but that it didn't help much. Upon examination, you _____ that the patient is tachycardic and tachypnoeic with a ___-_____ cough.

What is the primary _____ in treating this patient? Correct hypoxia, _____ bronchospasms, and decrease inflammation.*
This patient's condition might have been triggered by any of the following: allergens, exercise, and medications.
Cold air is also a common _____ for asthma.*
Treatment for this patient includes the following medications: albuterol, terbutaline, and steroids.*

> inhaler, goal, non-productive, reverse, trigger, discover

5
A 12-year-old unconscious male is being brought to the edge of the pool by two lifeguards. He is apnoeic.
How would you establish his airway? Manual _____ _____ precautions, modified jaw thrust.*
Since no information is presented about the exact nature of the patient's condition, one assumes that there is a _____ _____ involved and manual precautions must be taken. A modified jaw thrust can open an airway without disturbing the in-line _____ of the cervical spine.

> trauma mechanism, alignment, cervical spine

6
Myocardial infarction may go unrecognized in elderly patients. Why is this true? They lack _____ symptoms such as frequent chest pain or discomfort.*
More than half of all elderly patients who suffer MI do not complain of _____ _____; therefore, their AMI often goes _____. In the presence of _____ _____ such as diabetes, neuropathy prevents them from sensing pain as unaffected individuals would.

> chronic diseases, unrecognized, chest pain, typical

7
Which of the following statements regarding falls among the elderly is most accurate?
- The elderly have the highest incidence of falls.
- Fall-related injuries represent the _____ _____ of accidental death among the elderly.*
- Falls account for the highest percentage of _____ department visits among the elderly.
- A majority of falls are _____ related to infrapatellar bursitis.

Falls kill more elderly people annually than any other trauma. It is important to carefully _____ and manage these patients.

> leading cause, evaluate, primarily, emergency

8

These are typically characteristics of an abused elderly person:

- multiple physical and mental _____, such as dementia*
- incontinent, _____ _____, and over the age of 65*
- _____ handicapped, over the age of 75, and frail*

The typical abused elder is generally poor and _____ on the abuser.

> dependent, impairments, physically, mentally handicapped

9

Drug dosages are lower in elderly patients than in young adults primarily because elderly patients have a slower rate of elimination of drugs.*

The _____ of many common _____ is up to 50% lower in elderly adults primarily because of a decreased rate of _____

of the drug by the liver and kidneys.

> elimination, medications, dosage

10

Which of the following statements regarding the treatment for the care of a patient who is suffering from complications of dialysis is correct?

- If possible, obtain a blood pressure reading on the arm on which the shunt is located.
- Watch for narrow complex tachycardia to develop as the patient becomes hypoxic.
- Monitoring for dysrhythmias is frequently unnecessary in a haemodialysis patient.
- To prevent exacerbation of the problem, start an IV only if ordered by medical control.*

Fluid administration in dialysis patients should be under the _____ _____ of medical control. Dysrhythmias are _____ and, if present, are generally caused by electrolyte _____. To prevent accidental damage to the shunt, a BP should never be assessed on the arm with the _____.

> imbalances, direct authority, common, shunt

11

What is the leading cause of death among the elderly?

- metastatic _____
- _____ disease
- _____ and falls
- cardiac disease*

Because cardiac disease is so common, you should administer medications commonly prescribed for other types of emergencies with extreme _____.

> caution, respiratory, accidents, cancer

12

An elderly man is complaining of a _____ _____ of severe pain on his right leg. The _____ extremity is cool to the touch and pale. The temperature and pulse in the patient's left leg is normal. You suspect arterial occlusion.*
A sudden loss of _____ _____ to the leg within the arterial bed would account for the sudden _____ in skin colour and temperature.

> blood flow, change, affected, sudden onset

13

What does *ascites* refer to?

- _____ alcoholism
- fluid in the abdomen*
- _____ abdominal pain

- a ruptured aortic aneurysm

_____ refers to an _____ of fluid in the abdomen.

> Ascites, accumulation, chronic, severe

14

Answer the next two questions on the basis of the following information.

You arrive on the scene and find an elderly male complaining of severe abdominal and back pain. Upon further questioning, he states that the pain is all over the left side. __ _____, you feel a pulsating mass in the abdomen.
This patient is most likely suffering from abdominal aortic aneurysm.*
This patient is exhibiting the classic signs and symptoms of an _____ _____ _____.
Further palpation may cause the aneurysm to rupture, so be very careful in assessing this patient.
This patient's vital signs have been _____ steadily throughout the time he has been under your care.
Treatment for this patient should include cardiac monitoring.*
_____ _____ should always be performed when you suspect an aneurysm is present.

Cardiac monitoring, worsening,
On palpation, abdominal aortic
aneurysm

15

You are called to the home of
an elderly female who is having
difficulty breathing. She has _
_____ of chronic congestive
heart failure (CHF).
Which _____ ____ pattern is most
likely for this patient?
- shallow, rapid
  _____; decreased
  pulse rate; cool, clammy
  skin
- deep, laboured
  respirations; decreased
  _____ ____; hot, dry skin
- shallow, rapid respirations;
  increased pulse rate; cool,
  clammy skin*
- increased respiratory rate;
  decreased pulse rate;
  flushed, dry ____

What are _____ _____
associated with patients
with chronic CHF? Diuretics,
potassium, and digoxin.*

a history, respirations, pulse
rate, vital sign, skin, common
medications

16

Which of the following areas of
physical examination of an elderly
patient is often the most difficult to
accurately perform?

- _____ of the
  abdomen
- _____ of the lungs
- blood pressure _____
- examination of mental
  status*

Assessing the _____ _____ of an
elderly patient is often difficult. It is
often necessary to enlist the help of
family and caregivers to accurately
_____ if a patient's mental
status is different from the norm.

measurement, Auscultation,
mental status, Examination,
determine

17

Your patient is a 60-year-old
woman who has fallen down
her front steps and has possibly
_____ her ankle.
Which assessment finding may
be considered _____ in this
patient? Altered mental status.*
Altered mental status is an
abnormal finding in _____
_____ patients. The pulse rate
does decrease somewhat with
age but should _____ within
the normal range of 60-100.
Blood pressure often _____
with age, and respiration rates
increase slightly as patients use
less of their lung tissues.

fractured, abnormal, healthy
elderly, increases, remain

18

Your patient is a 66-year-old man who is extremely thin but has a noticeably distorted barrel-shaped chest. He reports a history of dyspnoea that has recently got worse. You note that he purses his lips when breathing, but hypoxia is ___ _____.
In addition to monitoring vital signs, breath sounds, and the ECG, starting an IV, and transporting the patient, what other _____ should you give to this patient? _____ low-flow oxygen and a bronchodilator.*
The patient is showing signs and symptoms of _____.
Administer low-flow oxygen to _____ his hypoxic drive.

> treatments, preserve, Administer, not apparent, emphysema

19

Your patient is a 67-year-old female who complains of increasing leg pain and tenderness. The skin over the affected area is ____ ___ ___, and Homan's sign is positive. Vital signs are _____.
How should you treat this patient? Elevate the leg and transport the patient for further evaluation.*
The _____ _____ suggests deep venous thrombosis. The correct action is __ _____ the leg and transport the patient for further evaluation. Do not massage the area or allow the patient to walk since pulmonary emboli may be _____.

> to elevate, unremarkable, clinical picture, warm and red, provoked

20

Dopamine can be used to:
- decrease _____ demand
- increase cardiac output*
- reduce blood pressure
- _____ dysrhythmias

_____ is a potent sympathomimetic agent, and in cases of _____ _____, it may be used to increase cardiac output.

> oxygen, Dopamine, cardiogenic shock, prevent

21

A patient is covered with _____-_____ material after an accidental spill.
An adequate level of shielding would be a cloth uniform.*
Alpha particles carry very little energy. _ _____ is adequate protection against such a _____.

> contaminant, A uniform, alpha-radioactive

Vocabulary 20

abuser /əˈbjuː.zər/ zneužívající osoba, trýznitel

account /əˈkaʊnt/ záznam, zpráva, konto, brát v úvahu, uvážit

accumulation /əˌkjuː.mjuˈleɪ.ʃən/ akumulace, nahromadění, nárůst

alpha /ˈæl.fə/ alfa

awoke /əˈwəʊk/ vzhůru, probuzený, probrat se

bursitis /bɜːˈsaɪ.tɪs/ burzitida, zánět váčku (zejm. mezi svalem nebo šlachou

caretaker /ˈkeəˌteɪ.kər/ pečovatel, opatrovatel

caution /ˈkɔː.ʃən/ opatrnost, varování, pozor

CHF, Congestive /kənˈdʒes.tɪv/ **Heart** /hɑːt/ **Failure** /ˈfeɪ.ljər/ městnavé srdeční selhání, k městnavému srdečnímu selhání dochází, když srdce selže jako pumpa a krev se hromadí před pravou komorou v pravé síni a žilním systému nebo před levou komorou v levé síni a plicním oběhu

dementia /dɪˈmen.ʃə/ demence, slabomyslnost

dependent /dɪˈpen.dənt/ závislý, odkázaný, podmíněný

dialysis /daɪˈæl.ə.sɪs/ dialýza

digoxin /dɪdʒ.ɒ k.sɪn/ digoxin, přípravek se používá k léčbě chronické srdeční nedostatečnosti

discover /dɪˈskʌv.ər/ objevit, zjistit

distorted /dɪˈstɔː.tɪd/ překroucený, pokroucený

disturb /dɪˈstɜːb/ vyrušit, rozrušit

dosage /ˈdəʊ.sɪdʒ/ dávky, dávkování

edge /edʒ/ okraj, břeh

enlist /ɪnˈlɪst/ získat, nabrat

flushed /flʌʃt/ zrudlý, červený

frail /freɪl/ křehký, slabý

haemodialysis /ˌhiː.mə.daɪˈælɪsɪs/ hemodyalýza, mimotělní očisťovací krevní metoda

handicapped /ˈhæn.dɪ.kæpt/ postižený

Homans' /ˈhəʊ.mænz/ **sign** /saɪn/ Homansovo znamení, orientační klinický test používaný k vyšetřování hluboké flebotrombózy dolní končetiny

impairment /ɪmˈpeər.mənt/ zhoršení, poškození

infrapatellar /ˌɪn.frə.pəˈtel.ər/ infrapatelární, podčéškový

majority /məˈdʒɒr.ə.ti/ většina

mature /məˈtjʊər/ dospělý, zralý

measurement /ˈmeʒ.ə.mənt/ měření, míra, velikost

modify /ˈmɒdɪˌfaɪ/ modifikovat, pozměnit

neuropathy /ˌnjʊəˈrɒp.ə.θi/ neuropatie, onemocnění nervů

non-productive /ˌnɒn.prəˈdʌk.tɪv/ neproduktivní, suchý (kašel)

noticeably /ˈnəʊ.tɪ.sə.bli/ zjevně, znatelně

occlusion /əˈkluː.ʒən/ okluze, uzavření

particle /ˈpɑː.tɪ.kl̩/ částice, částečka

provoke /prəˈvəʊk/ vyprovokovat, vyvolat

pulsate /pʌlˈseɪ.t/ pulzovat, tepat, bušit

purse /pɜːs/ našpulit rty

shaped /ʃeɪpt/ tvarovaný, ve tvaru, formovaný

shield /ʃiːld/ ochrana, štít, zastínit

subdiaphragmatic /ˌsʌbˌdaɪə.fræɡˈmæt.ɪk/ subdiafragmatický, ležící pod bránicí

sympathomimetic /ˌsɪm.pə.θə.mɪˈmet.ɪk/ **syndrome** /ˈsɪn.drəʊm/ sympatomimetický syndrom, soubor příznaků způsobený otravou látkami se sympatomimetickými účinky např. kofein, theofylin, kokain, amfetamin, efedrin

throughout /θruːˈaʊt/ po celém, ve všech částech

unaffected /ˌʌn.əˈfek.tɪd/ nedotčený, nezasažený

unrecognized /ʌnˈrek.əɡ.naɪzd/ nerozpoznaný, bez povšimnutí

Unit 21

1

Your patient is a 67-year-old male who is complaining of chest pain. The chest pain _____ after two doses of nitroglycerin. He reports a history of _____ and says that all his _____ _____ have been relieved by nitroglycerin.
How should you treat this patient? Treat the patient as though he is having an AMI and transport rapidly.*
A patient with angina whose pain does not respond to nitroglycerin is most likely suffering from MI and should be transported _____ _____.

angina, without delay, continues, previous attacks

2

Your patient is a 68-year-old male with a history of two _____ AMIs. Your assessment findings include a pulse rate of 124, peripheral oedema, and jugular vein distension. The patient _____ any chest pain or breathing difficulty.
What condition should you _____? Right ventricular failure.*
The patient's _____, _____, ___ _____ suggest right ventricular failure.

history, signs and symptoms, denies, suspect, prior

3

Your patient is a 70-year-old male. He complains of chest pain that _____ while he was raking leaves. You perform an _____ assessment and a focused history and _____ _____ and administer oxygen and nitroglycerin. The patient then states that he feels much better. What is he most likely _____ ____? Stable angina.*
The pain of stable angina is brought on __ _____ and _____ by rest, oxygen, and nitroglycerin.

by exertion, suffering from, relieved, began, initial, physical examination

4

A 72-year-old male is found unconscious in his front yard after working in the yard for five hours without a break. He is tachycardic, with hot, dry skin and shallow respirations.
Management should include what procedure? Administer high-flow oxygen.*
This patient is experiencing a ____ _____ and possible _____. It is important for him to receive _____, high _____ of oxygen, and

active _____ _____ to reduce his body temperature.

concentration, heatstroke, fluid, cooling measures, dehydration

5
Your patient is an obese 77-year-old woman who has called ___ complaining of a _____ _____ __ dyspnoea, coughing, haemoptysis, and diaphoresis. __ _____, you note tachypnoea and tachycardia, crackles and localized wheezing, and distended neck veins and varicose veins.
You should suspect pulmonary embolism.*
This patient displays many of the risk factors for pulmonary embolism; her signs and symptoms also fit. The rapid onset of the problem should lead you to hypothesize acute _____ _____.

pulmonary embolism, EMS, sudden onset of, On examination

6
You are caring for a 77-year-old female who is in moderate respiratory distress. She is sitting in a tripod position with ___-____ _____. She has a recent cold with increasing dyspnoea and a _____ _____ with yellow sputum. She denies chest pain.

She has been smoking cigarettes for the past forty years.
Vital signs are as follows: BP, 150/80; pulse, 100; respirations, 36 and laboured.
Her skin is _____, and she has _____ _____ in the legs. You hear expiratory wheezing upon auscultation of the lungs.
Her pedal oedema is most likely caused by cor pulmonale.*
Patients with COPD maintain chronic high levels of CO_2, which may result in _____ _____ and lead to right-side heart failure, or cor pulmonale.

productive cough, cyanotic, pitting oedema, pulmonary hypertension, two-word dyspnoea

7
Your patient is a 78-year-old woman who is complaining of diffuse abdominal pain, nausea, and vomiting. Physical examination reveals abdominal distension and absent bowel sounds.
You should suspect she has bowel obstruction.*
_____ signs and symptoms of myocardial infarction that are _____ ____ in elderly patients include all of the following: _____ ___ _____, syncope, and ____ pain.

There are many atypical signs and symptoms of MI in elderly patients. A tearing sensation in the chest generally _____ that a dissecting aneurysm is occurring.

Atypical, confusion and fatigue, indicates, commonly seen, neck

8

Your patient is an 82-year-old female with a suspected MI. While __ _____ to the hospital, you note that her systolic blood pressure, which had been stable, has started __ ____ and that she is becoming _____. At the same time, her ____ _____ converts to sinus tachycardia.

What should you suspect is happening? She is developing cardiogenic shock.*

Signs of cardiogenic shock include a sudden drop in _____ blood pressure and increasing confusion.

to drop, confused, systolic, en route, heart rhythm

9

Your patient is a 67-year-old male who reports a forty-five-pack-a-year smoking history, _____ respiratory infections, and a _____ cough. He is overweight and has peripheral _____.

Auscultation of the chest reveals rhonchi. There is also noticeable jugular vein distension.

What disease process should you suspect? Chronic bronchitis.*

The patient's history, signs, and symptoms are consistent with _____ _____. The 'blue bloater' frequently has peripheral oedema, cyanosis, and JVD due to right-side _____ _____ in addition to the respiratory problems.

Emphysema patients present with barrel chest and signs of wasting of the extremities.

heart failure, chronic bronchitis, chronic, frequent, cyanosis

10

A 72-year-old man trips and falls while walking to his bathroom. Physical findings include a lateral _____ of the left foot and knee. The patient has _____ and a protrusion in the left groin area. You suspect anterior dislocation of the hip.*

The outward rotation of the left extremity along with the _____ in the groin area points to an _____ _____ _____.

anterior dislocation injury, deformity, tenderness, rotation

11

Answer the next two questions on the basis of the following information.

You arrive to find a 65-year-old male in acute respiratory distress. You hear wheezes from across the room, and you note _____ accessory muscle use. The patient has assumed a tripod _____ and is breathing through pursed lips. Your physical exam reveals a barrel chest and stained _____.

Vital signs are as follows: blood pressure, 160/90; pulse, 100, strong and irregular with atrial fibrillation on the cardiac monitor; and respiratory rate, 40, with shallow and _____ breathing. Auscultation of the chest reveals wheezes and _____ lung sounds throughout all fields. What is this patient most likely suffering from? Emphysema.*

Why is this patient breathing through pursed lips? To provide positive pressure to inflate the alveoli.*

Breathing through _____ _____ is a common compensatory mechanism COPD patients use to provide positive end-expiratory pressure, which forces more alveoli to inflate.

position, fingernails, laboured, diminished, pursed lips, extreme

12

Under what _____ could the pulse oximetry reading show a elevated reading in a patient? When the patient is exposed to carbon monoxide.*

Carbon monoxide _____ can cause _ _____ high pulse oximetry reading.

a falsely, poisoning, circumstance

13

Your patient is a 67-year-old male who smokes cigarettes and has a history of previous MI. He complains of sudden-onset severe pain in his right leg. He also relates numbness and diminished _____ _____ in the right leg.

Other assessment findings are diminished pulse, pallor, and lowered skin temperature in the right leg.

You should suspect which of the following?

- femoral artery aneurysm
- occlusion of the femoral artery*
- ____ _____ _____
- hypertensive encephalopathy

The patient is displaying signs and symptoms of _____ occlusion of the femoral artery.

Aneurysms generally do not occur in the femoral artery. If an aneurysm were present, the

signs and symptoms would be
_____ ____ those presented.
Deep-vein thrombosis would
_____ __ vascular pooling
distal to the site of occlusion,
and oedema would be present
or developing in the extremity,
but arterial circulation would be

_____.

> deep venous thrombosis, acute,
> result in, different from, motor
> function, unaffected

14
Answer the next two questions
on the basis of the following
information.
You are called to the home of
a 68-year-old female who is
complaining of severe dyspnoea.
She states that it started about
45 minutes ago and has been
_____ progressively _____.
She has a _____ _____ but
denies chest pain at this time.
Her breathing is very congested.
During your assessment you
notice accessory muscle use and
rales bilaterally.
Which of the following conditions
is this patient most likely suffering
from?
- pulmonary embolism
- acute pulmonary oedema*
- pneumonia
- lung cancer

Rapid onset, rales, _____
_____ use, and dyspnoea are

classic symptoms of a patient with
acute pulmonary oedema.
In addition to oxygen, this patient
should also be treated with which
medication? Morphine sulphate.*
Morphine sulphate would be an
appropriate treatment for acute
pulmonary oedema. It increases
peripheral venous capacitance
and decreases venous return,
_____ _____ and
decreasing myocardial oxygen
demand.

> getting worse, improving
> ventilation, accessory muscle,
> cardiac history

15
You have arrived on the scene
to find a 75-year-old female
in respiratory distress. Your
assessment reveals the following:
BP, 138/90; pulse, 136/minute;
and RR, 34.
Upon auscultation, you note
diffused _____ _____ in the
apices and diminished _____
_____ in the bases. Pulse
oximetry is 82% on room air, and
the patient appears fatigued.
What treatment guidelines should
you follow for this patient?
- _____ an IV at a KVO
  rate*
- If possible, _____ via
  BVM at a rate of 24/min.
  to maximize oxygenation*

- _____ orotracheal or nasotracheal intubation*

Because the patient appears _____, respiratory failure is imminent. Inadequate tidal volume may not permit good gas exchange without manual support.

```
bilateral wheezes, breath sounds,
Attempt, ventilate, fatigued,
Establish
```

16

Your patient is a 75-year-old man. His wife called EMS because he has a terrible headache and is very confused. Vital signs are as follows: respirations, 26; pulse, 78; and blood pressure, 200/120. The _____ _____ you must address is most likely which of the following?

- hypertensive emergency*
- senile dementia
- cardiac tamponade
- cerebrovascular accident

Although the chief complaint was _____ ___ _____, it is likely that the primary problem to address is _____ _____. Senile dementia of new onset could have a variety of causes, but in this case, it may be connected to the hypertensive crisis. There is not enough information to determine if elder abuse or cardiac tamponade is present, but it is unlikely in this scenario.

Another possibility for this patient is a stroke. If _____ is occurring, prompt management of the hypertensive crisis can reduce _____.

```
stroke, primary problem,
morbidity, headache and
confusion, hypertensive crisis
```

17

You respond to a 'shortness of breath' call. Upon arrival you find the first responders placing a 70-year-old male on a nonrebreather mask. Family members state that the patient came back from the store approximately 45 minutes ago, complaining of moderate respiratory distress.

He has a history of some sort of lung disease for which he uses an inhaler.

The family does not know what type of medication the patient is taking. There is no history of fever or recent illness.

You observe that the patient is cyanotic. The oxygen reservoir on the mask does not appear to collapse, even though the litre flow is set correctly. Although he is sitting on the edge of the bed, his eyes are closed and he does not respond to verbal commands.

There is accessory muscle use evident, with intercostal muscle retractions. His breath sounds are diminished in all fields and absent in both bases. Faint expiratory wheezing is auscultated at only the apices.

His heart rate is 140; respiratory rate, 42; and BP, 106/72. The pulse oximeter registers an SpO_2 of 75%. The rest of his physical exam is unremarkable.

Based on the information given, what might be a suspected assessment? Emphysema.*

The timing of the onset, medical history, and physical findings point to emphysema as the

_____ _____.

What would be your initial priority in managing this patient's condition? Instruct the first responders to assist the patient's ventilations with a BVM and 100% oxygen.*

This patient has begun to _____ in terms of his ability to ventilate adequately as evidenced by the decreased mental status and very poor skin signs. This patient will require aggressive _____ _____ in order to be ventilated.

What airway adjunct(s) might you consider first for this patient? Bag-valve mask.*

The most immediate piece of ventilation equipment to use would be a CPAP.

CPAP eliminates the need for _____. If CPAP is not available, a BVM would be the next choice. The patient will need _____ before any attempt of intubation. In addition, as implied by the patient's presenting position, he will likely have an intact gag reflex, making the _____ of an OPA difficult, if not impossible.

What medication may be used in the management of this patient's condition? Albuterol.*

A beta agonist like albuterol is indicated in this situation. Morphine sulphate may worsen the patient's condition by potentially depressing _____ _____. Adenosine is a cardiac medication used to control supraventricular tachycardia. Epinephrine has significant cardiac ____ _____, especially in older patients.

---

primary suspect, decompensate, airway management, intubation, preoxygenation, insertion, respiratory drive, side effects

---

18

You are called to the home of a 78-year-old male who is having difficulty breathing. The patient is sitting upright in a tripod position, and you note _____ accessory muscle use. His skin is pale, cool, and clammy. _____ _____ are as follows: blood pressure, 180/72; heart rate, 90; and respiratory rate, 40. Breathing is _____ ___ _____ with a coarse rattling sound during expiration. Auscultation reveals coarse rales to the _____ ____ with no air movement in the bases. The patient can speak only in one- or two-word _____.

Family members inform you that the patient was sleeping when this episode began and that this has happened several times since his ___ one year ago. He has mild pedal oedema, and neck veins are nondistended. His family first noticed the patient having dyspnoea about 25-30 minutes ago.

This patient is exhibiting the signs and symptoms of Congestive heart failure.*

Which medication should be used for this patient? Morphine sulfate.*

Prior to an acute onset, a patient with the symptoms and history described may _____ paroxysmal nocturnal dyspnoea.* Paroxysmal nocturnal dyspnoea (PND), dyspnoea upon exertion, and increased dyspnoea are all signs of worsening CHF.

_____ for the management of this patient include all of the following: increasing venous return to the heart, decreasing myocardial oxygen demand, and improving oxygenation and ventilation.*

This patient would mostly _____ ____ giving him intermittent positive-pressure ventilation.* Increased ventilatory pressures _____ in driving off some of the pulmonary oedema.

If this patient were experiencing right-side heart failure, you would expect to find all of the following: tachycardia, profound peripheral oedema, and jugular venous _____.*

```
profound, benefit from,
distension, shallow and
laboured, nipple line, Vital
signs, sentences, exhibit, AMI,
Priorities, assist
```

19

Answer the next six questions on the basis of the following information.

You are called to a nursing home and find a bedridden 78-year-old male with insulin-dependent diabetes who is in acute respiratory distress. The staff reports that the patient has been ill for the last few days and has had a persistent productive cough with thick yellow sputum.

His blood pressure is 168/72. His respiratory rate is 40 and laboured with coarse rhonchi upon auscultation of lung sounds. Lung sounds are absent in the lower third of his lung fields. The patient is also febrile with ___, ___ ___ _____ ___.

This patient is most likely suffering from what condition? Pneumonia.*
This patient shows signs and symptoms of pneumonia.
The fever is the symptom that provides the differential diagnosis between the various choices.
Treatment of this patient should include oxygen.*
In addition to oxygen, this patient needs _____.

What common infectious disease does this patient's clinical presentation mimic?
- meningitis
- HIV/AIDS
- tuberculosis*
- hepatitis B

_____ _____ presents with fever, flu-like symptoms, and productive cough. Meningitis presents with high fever and _____ _____ but does not have respiratory involvement. HIV may not have any symptoms, although AIDS can present as a _____ __ diseases, depending upon which opportunistic disease has caused infection. _____ _ will present primarily with GI problems (nausea, vomiting, pain) and upper right quadrant abdominal pain.

What is most likely the cause of his decreased lung sounds? Atelectasis from inactivity.*
Diabetic patients heal more slowly from pneumonia when it occurs, but it is not a common disease for them. CHF and pulmonary hypertension would certainly contribute to worsening his signs and symptoms, but the most likely cause of absent or decreased ____ _____ in the lower lobes of a sick elderly patient is incomplete expansion and shallow respiration ___ __ _____.

If this patient required tracheal suctioning, what step should be followed? Sterile technique is required for suctioning this patient.*
Because _____ _____ will be performed on this patient, _____ _____ is required. Suction should be performed only upon withdrawal of the _____. For protection of the _____, gloves, eye protection, and face mask should be worn during the procedure. If the patient is being _____, you should hyperventilate before and after suctioning.
How should this patient be positioned for transport? High Fowler's position.*
Position of comfort is always the _____ transport position for nontraumatic patients when the patient is _____ ___ _____.

To _____ _____ and maximize efforts, the best position for this patient would be high Fowler's position.

---

hot, dry, and flushed skin, rescuer, antibiotics, due to inactivity, optimal, facilitate breathing, tracheal suctioning, lung sounds, sterile technique, Hepatitis B, conscious and oriented, flulike symptoms, Active tuberculosis, variety of, catheter, ventilated

---

20

Your patient is an 84-year-old man with extreme difficulty breathing, apprehension, cyanosis, and diaphoresis. Assessment findings include elevated pulse and blood pressure. Rales and rhonchi are heard on auscultation. There is no chest pain.

What condition should this patient be treated for? Left-side failure secondary to MI.*

The patient is displaying signs and symptoms of left ventricular failure, which most often occurs secondary to __.

Hypertension and tachycardia is due in part to increased left atrial pressure that is transmitted to the _____ _____.

Rales and rhonchi indicate that pulmonary _____ is present.

Right-side failure can lead to left-side failure, but such a patient generally has dry lungs and dependent oedema (usually pedal) as the presenting sign.

A dissecting aneurysm will present with pain, syncope, stroke, _____ __ _____ pulses, heart failure, pericardial tamponade, and signs of AMI.

If the ventricular failure worsens, _____ _____ may develop. You will see the systolic pressure drop dramatically (often to less than 80 mmHg) when this occurs.

---

absent or reduced, MI, pulmonary vessels, cardiogenic shock, oedema

---

21

Signs and symptoms of radiation sickness include ____ ____.

Hair loss, nausea, and vomiting are _____ signs and symptoms of _____ _____.

---

radiation sickness, common, hair loss*

Vocabulary 21

bedridden /'bed.rɪ.dən/ upoutaný na lůžko

blue bloater /'bləʊ.tər/ osoba trpící pokročilou COPD, charakteristická je cyanóza (zhoršený průchod vzduchu) a otok (zadržování tekutin)

call /kɔːl/ volat, hovor, požadavek, výzva

cerebrovascular/ ˌser.ɪ.brə'væskjʊlə/ cerebrovaskulární, týkající se mozkových cév

chief /tʃiːf/ hlavní

coarse /kɔːs/ hrubý, drsný

convert /kən'vɜːt/ přeměnit se, proměnit se

CPAP, Continuous / kən'tɪn.ju.əs/ **Positive** /'pɒz.ə.tɪv/ **Airway** / 'eə.weɪ/ **Pressure** /'preʃ.ər/ ventilační režim, druh neinvazivní mechanické ventilace u spontánně dýchajícího pacienta, která se uskutečňuje pomocí obličejové nebo nazální masky

expiratory /ɪk'spɪr.ə.tər.i/ expirační, výdechový

faint /feɪnt/ slabý, tlumený, malátný, na omdlení

falsely /'fɒls.li/ nesprávně, nepravdivě

fibrillation /ˌfaɪ.brɪ'leɪ.ʃən/ fibrilace, míhání, velmi rychlé a nepravidelné stahy, např. srdce

fingernail /'fɪŋ.gə.neɪl/ nehet na ruce

flulike /fluː.laɪk/ podobný chřipce

groin /grɔɪn/ slabiny, třísla, rozkrok

hypothesize /haɪ'pɒθ.ə.saɪz/ předpokládat, vyslovit hypotézu

inactivity /ˌɪn.æk'tɪv.ɪ.ti/ nečinnost

leaf /liːf/ pl leaves list

nonrebreather /ˌnɒn.rəbrə.ðər/

mask / mɑːsk/ dýchací maska, dýchací systém s jednocestnou klapkou, vydechovaný oxid

uhličitý je vyloučen ze systému a není znovu vdechován

nursing /'nɜː.sɪŋ/ ošetřování, péče, kojení, krmení

OPA, Oropharyngeal /'ɔː.rə .fə'rɪn. dʒi.əl/ **Airway** /'eə.weɪ/ zařízení používané k udržení otevřených horních dýchacích cest

overweight /ˌəʊ.və'weɪt/ nadváha, mít nadváhu

productive /prə'dʌk.tɪv/ produktivní, vlhký kašel

protrusion /prə'truː.ʒən/ výčnělek, výrůstek

radiation /ˌreɪ.di'eɪ.ʃən/ **sickness** / 'sɪk.nəs/ nemoc z ozáření

rake /reɪk/ hrabat, hrábě

relate /rɪ'leɪt/ týkat se, vztahovat se, souviset

senile /'siː.naɪl/ senilní

trip /trɪp/ zakopnout, klopýtnout

use /juːz/ užít, použít, použití

varicose vein /ˌvær.ɪ.kəʊs'veɪn/ křečová žíla

venous /'viː.nəs/ **capacitance** / kə'pæs.ɪ.tənts/ žilní kapacitance (rozdíl objemu prázdné a krví naplněné žíly po nafouknutí tlakové manžety)

waste /weɪst/ chřadnout, ochabovat, vyčerpat se

yard /jɑːd/ dvůr, zahrada

Unit 22

I

You respond to a 63-year-old male who is complaining of sudden onset of extreme substernal chest pain that he says 'feels like my insides are tearing'. The patient states that the pain _____ to the middle of his back between his shoulder blades. What condition is this patient most likely suffering from? Dissecting aortic aneurysm.*

This patient is exhibiting classic signs and symptoms of a

_____ _____ _____.

The tearing sensation occurs as the intimal linings of the aorta are separated as blood collects between the tissues.

What is a predisposing factor for this patient's condition? Hypertension.*

_____ is present in 75-85% of dissecting aortic aneurysm cases.

What medication may be ordered by medical control to treat this patient? Morphine sulfate.*

Morphine sulfate is the appropriate medication for this patient. Medications that increase cardiac rate, output, function, or contractile force are _____ while the dissection is occurring.

Progression of this condition may cause stroke, pericardial tamponade, and acute myocardial infarction.*

These are all consequences of further dissection. Other _____ also include syncope, heart failure, and absent or reduced pulses and death.

Hypertension, radiates, conditions, contraindicated, dissecting aortic aneurysm

2

A 63-year-old male is complaining of substernal chest pain _____ to his left arm and jaw. He is _____ and cool to the touch. The cardiac monitor shows sinus tachycardia. The patient's vital signs are as follows: BP = 136/70, P = 118, and RR = 16. You have administered oxygen and established an IV.

What should you do now? Administer _____ nitroglycerin and evaluate the patient's response to the mediaction.*

The patient's heart rate is not fast enough to be the primary source of the chest pain. Therefore, administration of nitroglycerin may resolve the chief _____, which in turn may slow the heart rate down.

sublingual, complaint, radiating, diaphoretic

3

Which of the following conditions indicates the need for rapid transport?

a) Isolated _____ trauma by a knife in the upper forearm

b) A pedestrian struck by a motor vehicle travelling about 10 mph (16 km per hour)

c) First-degree and second-degree _____ to the anterior chest

d) A pulse rate, 130; blood pressure, 90/60; and respiratory rate, 36/min*

The vital signs listed in choice *d* indicate the _____ __ _____. An isolated injury of penetrating trauma to the upper arm is not generally _____ _____. A 10-mile-per-hour _____ to a pedestrian is not generally a significant MOI. Burns to the entire chest cover a body surface area of approximately 9%; this would not in itself require rapid transport unless other problems existed.

impact, presence of shock, life-threatening, penetrating, burns

4

These activities are performed by the EMT/ paramedic in the field:

- maintaining and _____ of emergency care equipment and supplies*
- directing and coordinating patient transport by _____ the best methods*
- assigning _____ of emergency treatment*
- initiating and continuing _____ _____*

All of the activities are related to the practice of the paramedic.

emergency treatment, priorities, preparing, selecting

5

What is the _____ of a safety officer at a multicasualty incident?

- to teach the unit members to work together
- to decide when a scene is safe enough to enter*
- to stand in for the transportation officer as necessary
- to ensure patient safety before BLS unit arrives

The function of the safety officer is to _____ the scene and make the 'go/no go' _____ for the operation. The safety officer is also responsible for continuing to monitor _____ _____ during the operation.

evaluate, scene safety, decision, function

6

A tiered response system is one that dispatches responders at various levels, depending on the incident.*

In _ _____ _____, responders are _____ to calls depending upon the nature of the _____ as stated by the 112 caller and _____ by the dispatcher.

> a tiered system, incident, evaluated, dispatched

7

In a motor vehicle _____, which of the following would be most important to understand in relation to the _____ __ _____ and the potential for injury?

- speed and time of impact*
- weight of the vehicle
- road conditions at the scene
- condition of the vehicle's tyres

_____ plays a greater role in the force changes during a motor vehicle crash. While the other items are important when evaluating an _____ _____, speed has the greatest influence on the potential for _____ ___ _____.

> Speed, damage and injury, force of collision, crash, accident scene

8

Which statement about motorcycle crashes is correct?

- They seldom result in severe trauma, unless the motorcycle is operated at high speeds.
- Helmet use can reduce the incidence and severity of head injury.
- Helmet use can reduce the incidence and severity of spinal injury.*
- Leather clothing cannot protect the rider against soft-tissue injury.

Use of a _____ can protect the rider against head injury but not against _____ _____. Leather clothing is helpful in reducing the amount of ____ _____ injury. Because the energy of the accident is mostly absorbed into the rider, _____ _____ is noted even in low-speed crashes.

> severe trauma, helmet, soft tissue, spinal injury

9

Asymmetrical movement during respiration typically suggests which condition?

- COPD
- flail chest*
- _____ damage
- haemothorax

_____ movement during respiration typically suggests injury to the _____ ____.

chest wall, Asymmetrical, brain

10

Which patient is likely to need rapid transport to a trauma centre rather than assessment and stabilization on the scene?
   a) Male, age 56, ejected from a crashed vehicle with a flail chest*
   b) Female, age 60, burns to 10% BSI on her chest and abdomen
   c) Male, age 28, fell 10 feet (3 m) from a _____ onto a pile of mulch
   d) Female, age 46, _____ by car travelling 10 mph (16 km/hr), no _____ injuries.
Choice a is correct. All the others do not have _____ mechanisms, so they should not receive _____ transportation.

penetrating, critical, platform, struck, rapid

11

This statement describes a tiered EMS system: _____ _____ of resources are dispatched to calls, depending on the nature of the incident.*

A tiered EMS system is one in which varying levels of _____ are dispatched to calls depending upon the _____ of the incident as determined by the 112 _____.

resources, Varying levels, dispatcher, nature

12

A critically traumatized 18-year-old male is _____. It will be at least 15 minutes before he is freed. The community hospital is 20 minutes away by ground. A medical helicopter can be on the scene in eight minutes. A Level I trauma centre is one hour away by ground. Given the situation, which is the best mode of transport for this patient? Fly the patient from the scene to the Level I trauma centre.* _____ _____ offers the advantage of rapid transport to specialized facilities such as the Level I trauma centre. The amount of time needed to _____ the patient, coupled with the time to transport the patient to either the closest hospital or the trauma centre by ground, is too much. Flying the patient directly to the trauma centre is _____ _____.

most appropriate, Aeromedical transport, extricate, entrapped

13

Starting an IV on an _____ _____ who refuses one could result in your being held liable for which of the following?

- assault
- battery*
- libel
- slander

_____ is the unlawful touching of an individual without consent. _____ is the threat of bodily harm. _____ is saying something that is not true.

> Libel, Assault, Battery, alert patient

14

A 5-year-old male has multiple injuries in various stages of healing, including _____ ____ and a new suspected broken leg. On questioning, his mother states that he fell out of his bunk bed, but his sister, age 9, says, 'Daddy beat him.'
The mother insists that her husband will take the child to the hospital when he gets home from work.
How should you _____?
Document your findings, _____ the mother that transport to the hospital is necessary, and report your _____ of child abuse.* In cases of suspected child abuse, your responsibility is to ensure that the patient _____

_____ ____ immediately and to report your findings.

> proceed, convince, raccoon eyes, suspicions, receives necessary care

15

What should you do in order to preserve _____ _____ in cases of suspected sexual assault? Avoid cleaning wounds and handling clothing.*
To preserve physical evidence, avoid _____ clothing and cleaning or bandaging wounds, unless there is haemorrhage.
__ ___ _____ the victim to bathe, comb her hair, or change her clothing. Do not subject the patient to any _____ physical examinations.

> unnecessary, Do not allow, handling, physical evidence

16

With whom does the ultimate responsibility for patient care in the field always rest? The medical control physician.*
No matter who is actually _____ care or giving _____ to the responder, the ultimate responsibility always rests with the _____ _____ physician.

> medical control, directions, providing

17

What situation represents expressed consent? The patient says, 'Help me, my chest hurts.'*
_____ consent means that the patient gives you _____ to treat him or her, either _____ or in writing.

verbally, permission, Expressed

18

Your radio report to the hospital about the patient's medical condition should include which of the following?

- the complete medical history
- name, age, race, sex, and weight
- the chief complaint*
- estimated time of arrival on the scene

Although some details of the medical history, such as allergies, surgeries, and _____, are _____, a detailed history is not. Do not say the patient's name over the _____.

Estimated _____ at the hospital is important, but the time of your arrival on the scene is generally not important.

radio, arrival, relevant, medications

19

A person with a serious illness can delegate the right to make medical decisions to someone else by enacting which of the following legal documents?

a) living will
b) durable power of attorney for health care*
c) Do Not Resuscitate order
d) Right to Die order

A durable power of attorney for health-care _____ the right to make medical _____ to someone else in the event that the patient becomes _____ __

_____.

Choices a, b, and c are all examples of advanced directives, stating one's ____ regarding medical interventions.

delegates, disabled or incompetent, will, decisions

20

What is the legal term for an _____ deviation from the accepted _____ of care that results in harm to a patient?

- negligence*
- liability
- res ipsa loquitur
- _____

standard, abandonment, intentional

21

The ideal helicopter landing zone should:

- contain a slope of no more than 15°
- be an area of at least 100 feet by 100 feet*
- be an area of at least 90 feet by 90 feet
- be in a fenced area for safety against onlookers

The ideal helicopter _____ ____ should be at least 100 feet by 100 feet square. Larger helicopters may require more room, so consult local air medical services if you are unsure of the size of _____ used in your area. The _____ ____ should be no more than 10°, and the area should be clear of debris, fences, wires, or other _____.

---

landing zone, obstructions, ground slope, aircraft

Vocabulary 22

abandonment /əˈbæn.dən.mənt/ opuštění

accepted /əkˈsep.tɪd/ přijímaný, uznaný

advanced /ədˈvɑːnst/ **directive** / daɪˈrek.tɪv/ pokyn pro péči, kterou si pacient přeje v případě, že sám nebude schopen za sebe hovořit

aeromedical /ˌeə.rəˈmed.ɪ.kəl/ **service** /sɜːvɪs/ letecká záchranná služba

beat /biːt/ tlouci, úder

BLS, Basic /ˈbeɪ.sɪk/ **Life Support** / ˈlaɪf.səˌpɔːt/ základní podpora života, soubor znalostí a dovedností potřebný pro zajištění a udržení volných dýchacích cest a podpory cirkulace a dechu

bunk /bʌŋk/ **bed** /bed/ palanda

by ground /graʊnd/ po zemi (cesta)

comb /koʊm/ učesat, hřeben

consult /kənˈsʌlt/ poradit se, zeptat se

convince /kənˈvɪns/ přesvědčit koho o čem

decision /dɪˈsɪʒ.ən/ rozhodnutí

disabled /dɪˈseɪbld/ invalidní, neschopný

EMT, Emergency /ɪˈmɜː.dʒənt .si/ **Medical** /ˈmed.ɪ.kəl/ **Technician** / tekˈnɪʃən/ zdravotník rychlé záchranné služby

enact /ɪˈnækt/ schválit, uzákonit

extricate /ˈek.strɪ.keɪt/ vyprostit, vymanit

fence /fens/ plot, ohrada

generally /ˈdʒen.ə r.əl.i/ celkově, obvykle, obyčejně

in writing /ˈraɪ.tɪŋ/ písemně

incompetent /ɪnˈkɒm.pɪ.tənt/ neschopný, nezpůsobilý

individual /ˌɪn.dɪˈvɪd.ju.əl/ jednotlivec

leather /ˈleð.ər/ kůže zvířecí, kožené oblečení

liability /ˌlaɪ.əˈbɪl.ɪ.ti/ odpovědnost, závazky, povinnosti, ručení

liable /ˈlaɪ.ə.bl̩/ podléhající, vystavený čemu

MO, Medical /ˈmed.ɪ.kəl/ **Officer** / ˈɒf.ɪ.sər/ zdravotnický důstojník

mode /məʊd/ způsob, styl, režim
mulch /mʌltʃ/ mulč
multi /mʌl.ti-/ více, mnoha
onlooker /ˈɒnˌlʊk.ər/ přihlížející, divák
paramedic /ˌpærəˈmedɪk/ zdravotnický záchranář, člen RZP
pedestrian /pɪˈdestrɪən/ chodec
permission /pəˈmɪʃ.ən/ povolení, dovolení
pile /paɪl/ hromada
power /ˈpaʊə/ pravomoc, kompetence
reduce /rɪˈdjuːs/ snížit, omezit, zmenšit
relation /rɪˈleɪ.ʃən/ vztah, souvislost
Res ipsa loquitur lat. věc mluví sama za sebe (za vše)
rider /ˈraɪ.dər/ jezdec, cyklista, řidič motocyklu
seldom /ˈsel.dəm/ zřídka, málokdy

shoulder /ˈʃəʊl.dər/ **blade** /bleɪd/ ramenní lopatka
slope /sləʊp/ sklon, svah
speed /spiːd/ rychlost, řítit se
stand /stænd/ **in** zastoupit, zaskočit
substernal /sʌbˈstɜː.nəl/ substernální, ležící pod hrudní kostí
tiered /tɪəd/ víceúrovňový
tyre /taɪər/ pneumatika
ultimate /ˈʌl.tɪ.mət/ konečný, závěrečný, poslední
vary /ˈveə.ri/ lišit se, měnit se, kolísat
weight /weɪt/ váha

Unit 23

1

You have responded to a home for an unknown _____. Your patient, a 74-year-old male named George Evans, has been found at home with rigor mortis with dependent lividity.

The best thing to tell his family initially is 'I'm sorry to tell you that Mr Evans has died'.*

Inform the family that the patient ____ ____ in plain, simple language. This avoids any _____ and prevents any false hopes that may arise from a misunderstanding. Always deliver this news with _____ and respect.

> has died, compassion, misunderstanding, emergency

2

You are acting under the doctrine of implied consent when you treat which of the following patients?

- a person who is ____ and refuses treatment
- a _____ elderly man whose adult child is with him
- a small child whose parent is not present*
- a person who is _____ and mentally distraught

_____ consent covers situations in which the patient is not capable of consenting to treatment but a reasonable person would do so.

> Implied, confused, upset, drunk

3

At what age is a person considered capable of giving consent to treatment? 18.*

In most states, _____ for treatment must be obtained from all patients who are 18 years old or older. This can be _____ in situations of extenuating _____, such as when an underage minor is pregnant or has ____ _____ of a minor child in his or her care.

In general, the court deems an emancipated minor to be one who is _____, is economically_____, maintains a separate home, or is in the _____.*

> circumstances, consent, independent, legal custody, modified, married, military

4

What should you do when confronted with a patient whom you suspect to be a victim of elder abuse? Report your suspicions to the appropriate authority.*

Report your suspicions promptly. Many states have ____ requiring you to report any suspicions

of _____ _____, _____ _____,
or_____ _____.

> domestic violence, laws, child
> abuse, elder abuse

5
An EMS crew attempts to resuscitate a 50-year-old male in cardiac arrest and is not successful. The family sues the EMS organization for _____. The crew will need to prove that its _____ during the resuscitation were similar to the actions a reasonably prudent person would do under _____ circumstances.*
The 'reasonable person' standard sets a minimum guideline for what similarly trained _____ would do under similar circumstances, in this case, a cardiac arrest. As long as the crew could _____ that its actions were _____ and expected to be done by other _____-____ providers in a similar situation, this would avoid a negligence allegation.

> actions, personnel, negligence,
> prehospital-care, demonstrate,
> similar, reasonable

6
Which situation would constitute a moral dilemma for a paramedic?
  a) a female rape victim who insists on being cared for only by a female paramedic or EMT
  b) a patient who has sustained a potentially serious head injury but refuses care or transport*
  c) a patient who signed a Do Not Resuscitate order who is now unconscious and dying
  d) a patient who is found unconscious with no family member present to authorize care

This *b* situation constitutes a dilemma because the paramedic would have to choose between the duty to _____ ____ and the duty to _____ _____. If a patient has a signed DNR order, you should honour his or her _____. When a patient is unconscious, you treat him or her under the doctrine of _____ consent. The rape victim is simply requesting an all-female crew, and you should try to _____ her wishes.

> implied, obtain consent, provide
> care, order, accommodate

7
You are called to a physician's office to care for a patient who is _____ symptoms of a myocardial infarction. The physician tells you that she will _____ the patient herself and that she is assuming

_____ for care. She does, however, wish for you to transport the patient to the hospital.
How should you proceed? Defer to the on-scene physician and take her to the hospital with you.*
The _____ should defer to a physician who is present on the scene provided this individual is assuming responsibility for the continued care of this patient. Make sure you know the rules and regulations for your jurisdiction regarding __-_____ physicians.

paramedic, responsibility, on-scene, experiencing, stabilize

8
What do you call a legal document that specifies what type of treatment a patient does and does not want to receive? An advanced directive.*
The living will and DNR order are both examples of _____ _____ called advanced directives. They specify the kind of _____ ____ a person does and does not want to receive in the event of their

_____ _____.

legal documents, health care, imminent death

9
Your patient is a 28-year-old man who is suffering a seizure.

You monitor his condition during the seizure and throughout the postictal period, but when the patient recovers, he refuses transport or further treatment.
What should you do next?
Consult with medical control, explain the risks of refusing care, and document the patient's refusal.*
If a _____ _____ patient refuses treatment and transport, you should _____ with medical control, explain to the patient the risks of refusal in detail, _____ the informed refusal, and, if possible, have the refusal _____ by someone who is not an EMS employee.

competent adult, document, witnessed, consult

10
What is included in the management of a patient in a _____ state? Placing the patient in a recumbent position and _____ supplemental oxygen.*
Place the patient in the lateral recumbent position to prevent _____ and administer supplemental oxygen as needed; provide _____ and transport.

administering, aspiration, privacy, postictal

II

Your patient is age 7 and has a suspected broken arm and numerous bruises. The mother states that the child was hurt when he fell off his bike in the morning.
What finding would lead you to suspect that the mother's account of the injuries is not true? Purplish, yellowish, and greenish bruises.*
Although children are often uncoordinated and subject to frequent falls, the presence of bruises in _____ _____ of healing would lead you to suspect that this child had been injured on more than one _____. Carefully note the _____ the child is living in and report your _____ of abuse or neglect to the proper _____.

environment, suspicions, occasion, various stages, authorities

12

What is the paramedic's primary goal in cases of suspected child _____? Make sure that the child receives necessary treatment.*
In many states, medical personnel are _____ required to report all cases of suspected abuse and _____, but a paramedic's first _____ is to ensure that the child is transported to the hospital to _____ necessary treatment.

receive, abuse, legally, responsibility, neglect

13

You respond to a 56-year-old male who appears to be intoxicated. He is belligerent and disoriented and has a laceration on his forehead. You have made several attempts to convince him of the need for treatment, but he refuses treatment or transport. Given this situation, you should call medical direction for advice and guidance.*
Medical direction should be sought, if at all possible, for any suspected _____-_____ patient refusing _____ __ _____. Because you are required to be an advocate for the patient, it is never advisable to simply transport someone against his or her ____, even if you _____ _____ due to drug or alcohol use.
It is also not advisable to allow him or her to ____ _ _____ ____ when it is obvious that they are in need of medical attention.
Treating the patient, then leaving the scene without transport, leaves you open to legal liability and a possible charge of _____.

The patient continues to insist he does not need medical attention. In this situation, most important is to properly _____ your advice to the patient and his continued refusal.*
Documentation should include the steps you took to convince him to seek medical attention, the potential _____ of his refusal, and your assessment findings.

consequences, substance-abuse, suspect impairment, treatment or transport, sign a refusal form, will, document,* abandonment*

14

Which _____ can cause users to behave violently and aggressively? PCP.*
PCP can cause _____
_____ as well as violent and uncontrollable _____.

bizarre delusions, behaviour, drug

15

In case a patient has been violently beaten, statements made by the patient should __ _____ in the report.*
Managing the patient's injury is the _____ _____ of the EMS provider. Any statements made by the patient should be recorded as possible _____ __ ___ _____.

Regardless of any of the options considered in the previous question, the patient continues to insist he does not need medical attention.
What is most important in this situation? Properly _____ your advice to the patient and his continued refusal.*
It is important in this situation to make a complete documentation of the patient's _____ __ _____ treatment. Documentation should include the steps you took to _____ him to seek medical attention, the potential _____ of his refusal, and your assessment findings.

evidence of the crime, be reported, first priority, document, refusal to accept, convince, consequences

16

An intoxicated person refuses treatment or transport. How should you proceed? Try to _____ the person to accept your assistance.*
If a person who needs help refuses to _____ __, you should try to persuade the person to accept aid and explain the _____ of refusing it. Only after doing so should you accept and document the _____ of care.

consequences, accept it, persuade, refusal

17

Which patient may be legally placed in protective custody by the police if he or she refuses treatment? A patient who is drunk and disorderly and who refuses treatment for a head wound.*

_____ _____ is used legally in cases of patients who are drunk, ____ __ _____, or a _____ to themselves and others when it is obvious that their condition is _____ their judgement.

> Protective custody, impairing, danger, high on drugs

18

You are the first paramedic unit to arrive on the scene of a _____-_____ bus crash.
What is your first responsibility? Assume command of the incident and give _____ _____ to dispatch.*
The first paramedic unit to arrive at the scene of a mass-casualty incident would immediately _____ _____ and transmit a report to dispatch, alerting them to the need for more _____. As other units begin to arrive, they may be detailed to perform _____ or some other duty.

> preliminary report, assume command, units, multi-injury, triage

19

You respond to reports of a bus collision. Upon arrival, it appears that you have approximately thirty-five patients.
What is your first priority?
Separate the _____ _____ from the more severely injured.*
Using START triage, separating out the walking wounded from the ____ _____ injured patients is the first step in triaging large numbers of patients.
The first parameter to assess when using the START triage algorithm should be: breathing/airway.*

_____/_____ is the first parameter that should be assessed, followed by pulse and mental status.

A male patient is found to have a respiratory rate of 38. This would place him in which of the following categories?
- Delayed
- Immediate*
- Nonsalvageable
- Critical

The ____ _____ acronym dictates that patients with respiratory rates above 30 be classified as immediate.

Another male patient is found to have a respiratory rate of 28 and a radial pulse of 84. He is confused about the incident. This

patient would be placed in which of the following categories?
- Delayed
- Immediate*
- Nonsalvageable
- Critical

The _____ level of consciousness places the patient in the immediate category. Once he is moved to the _____ ____, he may be monitored for a while or transported quickly.

A female patient is found to have no spontaneous respirations. What should you do next? Reposition the airway and check her again ___ _____.* Reposition the head and _____ ___ spontaneous respirations. If they are immediately present, _____ the patient as immediate. If they are absent, categorize the patient as ____/_____ and move on to the next patient.

> examine for, categorize, dead/ unsalvageable, for respirations, decreased, START triage, walking wounded, treatment area, more severely, Breathing/ airway

20
Your patient ___ _____ a vehicle rollover in which another passenger in the vehicle died. He is _____ and not complaining of pain. His vital signs are as follows: pulse, 100; systolic BP, 90; respirations, 28. What _____ procedures are required prior to initiating transport? Quickly immobilize him using the long backboard as a splint and then transport.* Even though the patient's condition appears to be _____, the mechanism of injury indicates that _____ _____ injuries, such as internal bleeding, may be present. _____ him quickly using the long board as a full-body splint. _____ immediately in this case. You can perform additional assessments or treatments while en route.

> serious underlying, stable, has survived, alert, Transport, additional

21
Your unit is the first to arrive at the scene of a bombing at a large office building.
The purpose of your initial size-up of the incident is to determine what _____ _____ will be needed.*
The purpose of the initial scene ____-__ at a mass-casualty incident is to _____ what additional resources will be needed.

> determine, additional resources, size-up

Vocabulary 23

accommodate /əˈkɒm.ə.deɪt/ pomout, mít kapacitu, vyhovovat, přizpůsobit se

acronym /ˈæk.rə.nɪm/ akronym, písmenná zkratka

administer /ədˈmɪn.ɪ.stər/ podat, dát

advocate /ˈæd.və.keɪt/ obhajovat, podporovat, právní zástupce

algorithm /ˈæl.gə.rɪ.ðəm/ algoritmus

arise /əˈraɪz/ (arose, arisen) nastat, vzniknout, vyplývat

attention /əˈten.ʃən/ pozornost, péče, dávat pozor, všímat si

authorize /ˈɔː.θər.aɪz/ povolit, schválit, dát souhlas, oprávnit

beaten /ˈbiː.tən/ zmlácený, zbitý

behave /bɪˈheɪv/ chovat se, jednat

belligerent /bəˈlɪdʒ.ər.ənt/ útočný, agresivní

bike /baɪk/ jizdní kolo, motorka

bombing /ˈbɒm.ɪŋ/ bombový útok

charge /tʃɑːdʒ/ obžaloba, obvinění

consenting /kənˈsent.ɪŋ/ **adult** /əˈdʌlt/ zletilý, osoba ve věku, kdy může legálně začít sexuální život

consequence /ˈkɒn.sɪ.kwəns/ následek, důsledek

court /kɔːt/ soud, soudní dvůr

deem /diːm/ považovat co za jaké

defer /dɪˈfɜːr/ odložit, pozdržet, podrobit se

delusion /dɪˈluː.ʒən/ klam, mámení (smyslů)

dilemma /daɪˈlem.ə/ dilema, těžké rozhodování

disorderly /dɪˈsɔː.dəl.i/ chaotický, výtržnický

doctrine /ˈdɒk.trɪn/ doktrina, nauka

domestic /dəˈmes.tɪk/ domácí, rodinný

drunk /drʌŋk/ opilý, opilec

emancipate /ɪˈmænsɪˌpeɪt/ emancipovat, zrovnoprávnit

employee /ɪmˈplɔɪ.iː/ zaměstnanec

extenuating /ɪkˈsten.ju.eɪ.tɪŋ/ polehčující okolnosti

greenish /ˈgriː.nɪʃ/ nazelenalý

guidance /ˈgaɪ.dəns/ odborné vedení, poučení, rada

honour /ˈɒn.ər/ ctít, respektovat

insist /ɪnˈsɪst/ trvat na čem, vyžadovat

jurisdiction /ˌdʒʊə.rɪsˈdɪk.ʃən/ jurisdikce, soudní pravomoc

lividity /lɪˈvɪd.ə.ti/ promodralost, sinalost, smrtelná bledost

military /ˈmɪl.ɪ.tər.i/ armáda, vojenský

misunderstanding /ˌmɪs.ʌn.dəˈstæn.dɪŋ/ nedorozumění, špatné pochopení

nonsalvageable /ˌnɒnˈsæl.vɪdʒə.bl̩/ nezachranitelný

occasion /əˈkeɪ.ʒən/ příležitost, událost

PCP, phencyclidine /fɛnˈsɪklɪˌdiːn/ fencyklidin, disociativní anestetikum, zneužíván jako taneční droga, jako anestetikum se přestal používat kvůli psychickým nežádoucím účinkům

persuade /pəˈsweɪd/ přesvědčit, přimět

plain /pleɪn/ prostý, jednoduchý

prehospital /ˌpriːˈhɒs.pɪ.təl/ přednemocniční

preliminary /prɪˈlɪm.ɪ.nər.i/ předběžný, přípravný

prove /pruːv/ dokázat, prokázat

provided /prəˈvaɪ.dɪd/ pokud, za předpokladu že

prudent /ˈpruː.dənt/ prozíravý, opatrný

resource /rɪˈzɔːs/ zdroje, možnosti, prostředky

rigor mortis /ˌrɪg.əˈmɔː.tɪs/ posmrtná ztuhlost

rollover /ˈrəʊl.əʊ.vər/ převrácení (se na střechu)

seek /siːk/ (sought, sought) hledat, usilovat, požadovat

similar /ˈsɪm.ɪ.lər/ podobný

size /saɪz/ **up** /ʌp/ hodnotit, zhodnotit, posoudit, ujasnit

specify /ˈspes.ɪ.faɪ/ specifikovat, vymezit, určit

survive /səˈvaɪv/ žít, přečkat, přetrvat

trained /treɪnd/ školený, kvalifikovaný

underage /ˌʌn.dəˈreɪdʒ/ nezletilý, neplnoletý

violence /ˈvaɪə.ləns/ násilí, násilný čin

wounded /ˈwuːn.dɪd/ raněný

yellowish /ˈjel.əʊ.ɪʃ/ nažloutlý

Unit 24

I

Your patient is a 26-year-old construction worker who has fallen approximately 35 feet (10.7 m) and suffered _____ _____. The Glasgow Coma Scale score is 9, respiratory rate is 32, respiratory expansion is normal, the blood pressure is 100/70, and capillary refill is _____.

What _____ should this patient receive if you are using the Revised Trauma Score? 13.*
The score on the Glasgow Coma Scale _____ ____ 4 points on the Revised Trauma Score; the patient receives 3 points for respiratory rate, 1 point for respiratory expansion, 4 points for blood pressure, and 1 point for delayed _____ _____.

delayed, score, translates into, capillary refill, multiple injuries

2

What is the process of transmitting _____ ____ from the field to the hospital over the _____ lines called?

- modulation
- biotelemetry*
- multiplexing
- trunking

_____ physiological data over phone lines is called _____.

Transmitting, biotelemetry, physiological data, phone

3

What sort of communication system would you need to be able to carry on a ___-___ conversation with a _____ while also transmitting telemetry? Multiplex transmission system.*
A multiplex system allows for a two-way conversation and simultaneous transmission of

_____ _____.

telemetry readings, physician, two-way

4

What is the purpose of the START method? To rapidly _____ large numbers of patients quickly and _____.*
_____ stands for Simple Triage And Rapid Treatment and is designed to triage large _____ of patients as quickly as possible.

numbers, efficiently, triage, START

5

During a multicasualty incident, the first two arriving paramedics should assume the roles of medical group supervisor and triage officer.*
The medical group supervisor will need to establish overall responsibility for the _____

_____ interacting with other lead officers such as police, fire, and public works. The triage officer will need to _____ the number of severity of victims as early as possible.

_-____ is a mnemonic used to describe the components of an ICS system: command—finance, logistic, operations, planning.

medical section, C-FLOP, establish

6

At a mass-casualty incident (MCI), which sector should the incident commander establish first?

- triage sector*
- treatment sector
- supply sector
- transportation sector

Triage must be done before treatment can be properly _____. In many cases, triage and scene assessment _____ are in progress by the crew of the _____ _____ unit. If it is not ongoing, triage should be established _____.

performed, first arriving, activities, first

7

The first step in triage at an MCI is to _____ the walking wounded away from the scene.*

Regardless of the triage method utilized, the _____ ____ is to direct the walking wounded to a safe place where they can be _____ ___ and reassessed.

first step, cared for, direct

8

These are components of the START triage method: _____ assessment, _____ assessment, and mentation/level of consciousness.*

Neuromuscular function is not part of the START algorithm. START assesses respiration, pulse, and _____ _____.

circulation, mental status, respiration

9

The three primary parameters assessed when using the START triage system are:

- airway, breathing, and circulation (ABC)
- respiration, perfusion, mentation (RPM)*
- appearance, respiration, mentation (ARM)
- pulse, perfusion perspiration (PPP)

Using the START triage system, the three primary parameters _____ are respiration, perfusion, and mentation

(RPM). The parameters are a _____ ____ over or under 30 per minute, capillary refill under or over 2 seconds or presence of a _____ _____, and mentation (e.g. whether the patient is able to follow _____ _____).

> basic commands, respiratory rate, radial pulse, assessed

10

Which sector officer will coordinate with the police to _____ _____ and provide access at an MCI?
- triage officer
- transportation officer
- supply officer
- staging officer*

The staging officer's responsibilities include coordinating with _____, ensuring access for vehicles, maintaining a log of available units, and _____ requests for resources. The _____ _____ will establish the staging area if the incident commander has not already ordered one.

> coordinating, police, transportation officer, block streets

11

At a major incident response, what is the responsibility of the staging officer? Maintain _ ___ __

_____ available and an inventory of special equipment.*
The staging officer is primarily responsible for assembling all _____ _____ to make sure they are ____ ___ deployment as needed.

> a log of units, ready for, available vehicles

12

What is the major responsibility of the finance sector at a major incident? To document the number of personnel and hours worked.*
Finance is responsible for the _____ _____ of the incident and may not be needed in a small-scale incident. In addition to tracking _____, finance approves rental and purchase of any additional _____ needed for the incident. Logistics is responsible for _____ resources, planning evaluates, and command sets ____ ___ _____.

> acquiring, personnel, financial accounting, goals and objectives, equipment

13

This statement about the triage operation at a mass-casualty incident is correct: each patient's _____ and _____ _____

should take less than 60 seconds.*
START and METTAG, systems used at mass-casualty incidents, are designed to be _____ ___ very quickly by minimally trained personnel.

> carried out, initial assessment, triage

14

During a multicasualty incident, a conscious patient presents with a fractured femur, a palpable radial pulse, and a respiratory rate of 24/min.
According to START, this patient would be placed into what triad category? Delayed/yellow.*
According to START triage principles, transport of this patient to definitive care can be _____.
He is breathing _____, has a _____ _____, and is _____. The fractured femur is not factored into the evaluation of transport status.

> conscious, radial pulse, delayed, spontaneously

15

You are conducting triage using the START system at a major incident. You encounter a patient who is not breathing. After you _____ the airway, the patient begins to breathe at a rate of 6 respirations per minute. Into which category would you now triage this patient?
- dead or dying
- immediate or critical*
- delayed
- urgent or noncritical

When using the START triage system, you assess three parameters: respiration, pulse, and mental status (RPM). A patient with no respirations is considered ___ __ _____; if the rate is under 10 or over 30, the patient is _____ __ _____.
If the rate is between 10 and 30, _____ assessment is needed (so you would then assess pulse, and possibly also mental status, before deciding on a _____).

> immediate or critical, category, position, dead or dying, additional

16

You are on the scene of a vehicle crash involving a bus. As triage officer, the first patient you encounter is sitting on the ground, conscious, confused, and breathing __ _____ per minute. She states that she was _____ ___ of her seat and _____ the side of her head.
Your next action would be to classify the patient as immediate (red).*

A patient who is conscious and breathing over 30 times per minute is classified as immediate. There is no need to _____ ___ the presence or rate of the pulse. While she may need _____ _____, now is not the time to do so.

oxygen therapy, struck, 40 times, thrown out, check for

17

Using the START triage method at a multiple-casualty accident scene, you encounter a patient who is making no spontaneous respiratory effort _____ _____ at repositioning. What should you do next? ___ the patient as unsalvageable and move on.*
If a patient continues to remain _____ following a second attempt to open the airway, he or she is considered _____.

despite attempts, unsalvageable, Tag, apnoeic

18

Which of the following situations is most likely to be declared a major incident?
- an accident involving a school bus and car with five patients
- a fire at a _____ _____ during working hours*
- a _____ _____ on a state line with two people in the water
- a ____ involving an isolated single-family residence

This incident has a _____-_____ component along with the potential for lots of patients. All the other incidents may be severe but should not _____ the normal resources of the area.

overwhelm, fire, water accident, hazardous-materials, chemical plant

19

When responding to the scene of a hazardous-materials incident, the EMS crew should _____ from uphill and upwind.*
The patient should be _____ with the head elevated to enhance venous return. If congestive ____ _____ is present, the patient should be positioned at least semi-Fowler's (_____ __ at least 45°).

sitting up, supine, heart failure, approach

20

You respond to a twenty-five-patient mass-casualty incident at a store. The 112 caller stated that she smelled something

funny and then started to feel ___ ___ _____. You are the second unit on the scene. The initial unit is nowhere to be seen, and they do not answer their radios. What should you determine first in this situation? Whether this is a potential hazardous-materials incident in progress.*
This is a hazardous-materials incident until proven otherwise. Do not rush in after fallen rescuers because you may _____ _ _____, too.
After you are instructed by the _____ ____ to begin treating decontaminated patients, you should take universal _____ and wear protective _____.*
Always wear personal protective equipment to help avoid becoming personally contaminated. Unless you are trained to work in the hot zone, you should not treat anyone until they are properly _____.

> weak and nauseous, precautions, equipment, decontaminated, become a victim, hazmat team

21

All of the following are correct statements about the care of patients who are contaminated by hazardous material.
- Trained personnel should immediately _____

non-ambulatory patients from the hot zone.*
- Decontamination activities should be _____ ___ while the patient is in the warm zone.*
- Intravenous therapy and invasive procedures should begin only under specific _____ _____.*

An _____ assessment should be done while the patient is located within the hot zone. Only absolutely essential care, such as _____ ___ _____ _____ should be done in the hot zone.

> initial, remove, carried out, physician direction, ABCs and spinal immobilization

Vocabulary 24
accounting /əˈkaʊn.tɪŋ/ účtování, evidence
assemble /əˈsem.bl̩/ sestavit, smontovat, svolat
available /əˈveɪ.lə.bl̩/ dostupný, dosažitelný, k dispozici, vhodný
biotelemetry /ˌbaɪ.əʊ.təˈlem.ə.tri/ aplikace moderních metod přenosu k dálkovému sledování životních znaků pacientů
carry /ˈkær.i/ **on** pokračovat, vést dialog
carry /ˈkær.i/ **st out** /aʊt/ provést, uskutečnit
commander /kəˈmæn.dər/ velitel

coordinate /kəʊˈɔː.dɪ.neɪt/ koordinovat, sladit

deployment /dɪˈplɔɪ.mənt/ nasazení, rozmístění

enhance /ɪnˈhɑːns/ zlepšit, zvýšit, zesílit

factor /ˈfæk.tər/ faktor, činitel, prvek

funny /ˈfʌn.i/ zvláštní, podivný

interact /ˌɪn.təˈrækt/ interagovat, vzájemně se ovlivňovat, spolupracovat

line /laɪn/ čára, linie, přímka, řada, cesta, trasa, linka, spojení, vedení

log /lɒg/ záznam, protokol, zaevidovat

logistics /ləˈdʒɪs.tɪks/ logistika, systém přepravy a týlového zásobování

modulation /ˌmɒd.juˈleɪ.ʃən/ modulace, změna, úprava

multiplexing /ˈmʌltiˌpleksɪŋ/ multiplexování, více analogových signálů nebo digitálních datových toků je kombinováno do jednoho signálu, cílem je nejefektivnější využití daného přenosového média

plant /plɑːnt/ továrna

regardless /rɪˈgɑːd.ləs/ bez ohledu na co

rush /rʌʃ/ **in** unáhlit se, vřítit se dovnitř

seat /ˈsiː.t/ uložit do pozice, usadit, sedadlo

smell /smel/ čich, cítit (čichem), být cítit

unsalvageable /ʌnˈsæl.vɪdʒ.ə.bl̩/ nezachránitelný, jemuž není pomoci

urgent /ˈɜː.dʒənt/ urgentní, naléhavý, neodkladný

English-Czech dictionary

A

abandonment /ə'bæn.dən.mənt/ opuštění

abbreviation /əˌbriː.vi'eɪ.ʃən/ zkratka

abbreviation /əˌbriː.vɪ'eɪʃən/ zkratka slova

ABCs /ˌeɪ.biː.'siː/ ABC resuscitace

abdomen /'æb.də.mən/ břicho

abdominal /æb'dɒm.ɪ.nəl/ **thrust** / θrʌst/ břišní úder, první pomoc při dušení

abnormal /æb'nɔː.məl/ abnormální, neobvyklý

abortion /ə'bɔː.ʃən/ potrat, přerušení těhotenství

above /ə'bʌv/ nad, přes

abrasion /ə'breɪ.ʒən/ odřenina, oděrka

abrupt /ə'brʌpt/ náhlý, neočekávaný, prudký

abruptio placentae /æb'rʌp.ʃɪ.əʊ. plə'sen.ti:/ předčasné odloučení placenty

abruption / ə'brʌp.ʃən/ odtržení

abscess /'æb.ses/ absces

absorb /əb'zɔː.b/ absorbovat, vstřebat

abuse /ə'bju:z/ zneužívání, týrání, zneužívat

abuser /ə'bju:.zər/ zneužívající osoba, trýznitel

accelerate /ə k'sel.ə.reɪt/ zrychlit, přidat rychlost, vzrůst

acceptable /ək'sept.ə.b|/ přijatelný, vhodný

accepted /ək'sep.tɪd/ přijímaný, uznaný

access /'æk.ses/ přístup, vstup

accessory /ək'ses.ər.i/ akcesorní, přídatný

accident /'æksɪdənt/ nehoda, neštěstí

accidental /ˌæk.sɪ'den.təl/ náhodný, nepředvídaný, neúmyslný

accommodate /ə'kɒm.ə.deɪt/ pomout, mít kapacitu, vyhovovat, přizpůsobit se

accomplish /ə'kʌm.plɪʃ/ dosáhnout, provést, uskutečnit

accordance /ə'kɔː.dənt s/ v souladu, ve shodě

accordingly /ə'kɔː.dɪŋ.li/ podle toho, v souladu, přiměřeně

account /ə'kaʊnt/ záznam, zpráva, konto, brát v úvahu, uvážit

accounting /ə'kaʊn.tɪŋ/ účtování, evidence

accumulate /ə'kju:.mjʊ.leɪt/ akumulovat, nashromáždit se

accumulation /əˌkju:.mjʊ'leɪ.ʃən/ akumulace, nahromadění, nárůst

accuracy /'æk.jʊ.rə.si/ přesnost, správnost

accurate /'æk.jʊ.rət/ pečlivý, přesný

acetaminophen /əˌsi:.tə'mɪn.ə.fen/ paracetamol

achieve /ə'tʃi:v/ dosáhnout, docílit, uspět

acid /'æs.ɪd/ kyselina

acidosis /ˌæs.ɪ'dəʊ.sɪs/ acidóza, porucha acidobazické rovnováhy ve prospěch kyselin, zvýšení

kyselé reakce tělesných tekutin,
zvýšení aktivity vodíkových iontů
acidotic /əˈsɪd.ə.tɪk/ kyselý, o
aminokyselinách
acknowledge /əkˈnɒl.ɪdʒ/ přiznat,
uznat, brát na vědomí
acquire /əˈkwaɪər/ získat, nabýt
acronym /ˈæk.rə.nɪm/ akronym,
písmenná zkratka
acrylic /əˈkrɪl.ɪk/ akryl, akrylový
act /ækt/ akt, zákon
act /ækt/ jednat, činit, působit,
jednat podle, řídit se
ACTH, Adrenocorticotropic /əˌdriː.
nəʊˌkɔː.tɪ.kəʊˈtrɒf.ɪk/ **Hormone /**
ˈhɔː.məʊn/ adrenokortikotropní
hormon
activation /ˌæk.tɪˈveɪ.ʃən/ aktivace,
zapnutí
activity /ækˈtɪv.ɪ.ti/ aktivita,
činnost
actual /ˈæk.tʃu.əl/ skutečný,
opravdový, současný
acute /əˈkjuːt/ akutní
Addison's disease /ˈæd.ɪ.sənz.
dɪˌziːz/ Addisonova nemoc,
nedostatečnost kůry nadledvin
additional /əˈdɪʃ.ən.əl/ dodatečný,
další, doplňkový
address /əˈdres/ oslovit
Adenocard, adenosine /ə.denˈə.sin/
lék, s tlumivým účinkem na srdce,
vazodilátor, proti arytmii
adequacy /ˈæd.ə.kwə.si/
přiměřenost
adequate /ˈæd.ə.kwət/ dostatečný,
přiměřený
adipose /ˈæd.ɪ.pəʊs/, /-pəʊz/
tukový

adjacent /əˈdʒeɪ.sənt/ sousední,
přilehlý, vedlejší
adjoining /əˈdʒɔɪ.nɪŋ/ sousední,
vedlejší
adjunct /ˈædʒ.ʌŋkt/ dodatek,
doplněk, přidružený, pomocný
adjust /əˈdʒʌst/ přizpůsobit se,
upravit, nastavit
administer /ədˈmɪn.ɪ.stər/ podat,
dát
administration /ədˌmɪn.ɪˈstreɪ.ʃən/
podávání léků
admit /ədˈmɪt/ připustit, uznat,
hospitalizovat
adult /ˈæd.ʌlt/,/əˈdʌlt/ dospělý,
zletilý
advanced /ədˈvɑːnst/ **directive /**
daɪˈrek.tɪv/ pokyn pro péči, kterou
si pacient přeje v případě, že sám
nebude schopen za sebe hovořit
advanced /ədˈvɑːnst/ provedený
předem, před, pokročilý
advantage /ədˈvɑː.tɪdʒ/ výhoda,
přednost
adventitious /ˌæd.vənˈtɪʃ.əs/
nahodilý, vyskytující se na
nesprávném místě
advice /ədˈvaɪs/ rada, doporučení
advisable /ədˈvaɪ.zə.bl̩/ vhodný,
záhodný
advisory /ədˈvaɪ.zər.i/ poradenský,
poradní
advocate /ˈæd.və.keɪt/ obhajovat,
podporovat, právní zástupce
AED, Automated /ˈɔː.tə.meɪ.tɪd/
External /ɪkˈstɜː.nəl/ **Defibrillator**
/ˌdiːˈfɪb.rɪ.leɪ.tər/ automatický
externí defibrilátor

aeromedical /ˌeə.rəˈmed.ɪ.kəl/ **service** /sɜːvɪs/ letecká záchranná služba

affect /əˈfekt/ ovlivnit, působit, postihnout, zasáhnout

afterload /ˈɑːf.tər.ˈləʊd/ afterload, dotížení, napětí vyvinuté ve stěně srdeční komory během systoly, vysoký a. zatěžuje srdeční sval, zvyšuje spotřebu kyslíku, zhoršuje prokrvení myokardu a může přispívat k srdečnímu selhání

age /eɪdʒ/ věk, stárnutí, stárnout

aggravate /ˈæg.rə.veɪt/ ztížit, zhoršit

aggressively /əˈgres.ɪv.li/ agresivně, útočně

agitated /ˈædʒ.ɪ.teɪ.tɪd/ rozrušený, nervózní

agitation /ˌædʒ.ɪˈteɪ.ʃən/ nervozita, rozrušení, vzrušení, znepokojení

agonal /ˈəg.əʊ.nəl/ agonální, týkající se agónie

aim /eɪm/ **at** /ət/ zaměřit se, snažit se, mít v úmyslu, chtít

air /ˈeər/ **embolism** /ˈem.bə.lɪ.zəm/ vzduchová embolie

air bag, **airbag** /ˈeə.bæg/ airbag, bezpečnostní nafukovací vak

airborne /ˈeəˌbɔːn/ přenášený vzduchem

airflow /ˈeə.fləʊ/ proud vzduchu

airway /ˈeə.weɪ/ dýchací cesty

alarm /əˈlɑːm/ poplach, znepokojení

alcoholism /ˈæl.kə.hɒl.ɪ.zəm/ alkoholismus

aldosterone /ˈɔː.l.dəs.tər.əʊn/ aldosteron, mineralokortikoidní hormon vylučovaný nadledvinami

alert /əˈlɜːt/ bdělý, čilý, zvýšená ostražitost, stav pohotovosti, varovat

algorithm /ˈæl.gə.rɪ.ðəm/ algoritmus

align /əˈlaɪn/ sblížit se, spojit se, připojit se

alignment /əˈlaɪn.mənt/ podpora, postavení, pozice, poloha

alive /əˈlaɪv/ živý, naživu

alkali /ˈæl.kə.laɪ/ alkálie, zásada

alkalize /ˈælkəˌlaɪz/ alkalizovatt

alkalosis /ˌælkəˈləʊ.sɪs/ alkalóza, zvýšený výskyt zásaditých látek v těle

all-terrain vehicle /ˌɔːl.tə.reɪnˈviː.ɪ.kl/ terénní vůz

allegation /ˌæl.əˈgeɪ.ʃən/ nařčení, obvinění (nepodložené)

allegiance /əˈliː.dʒəns/ věrnost, loajalita

alleviate /əˈliː.vi.eɪt/ zmírnit, zmenšit

alley /ˈæl.i/ ulička, průchod

allow /əˈlaʊ/ dovolit, poskytnout, umožnit

alpha /ˈæl.fə/ alfa

alteration /ˌɒl.təˈreɪ.ʃən/ změna

altercation /ˌɔːltəˈkeɪʃən/ ostrý spor, prudká hádka

altered /ˈɔːltəd/ změněný

alternating /ˈɒl.tə.neɪ.tɪŋ/ střídavý, střídající se

alveolar /ˌæl.viˈəʊ.lər/ alveolární, sklípkový

alveolus alveoli /ˌæl.viˈəʊ.ləs/ plicní sklípek

ambient /ˈæm.bi.ənt/ okolní, prostředí se týkající

ambulance /ˈæm.bjʊ.ləns/ sanitka, záchranka

ambulation /ˈæm.bjʊ.lən.ʃən/ chůze

ambulatory /ˌæm.bjəˈleɪ.tər.i/ chodící

amenorrhoea /ˌeɪ.men.əˈriː.ə/ amenorea, vynechávání menstruačního krvácení

AMI, Acute /əˈkjuːt/ Myocardial /ˌmaɪ.əˈkɑː.di.əl/ Infarction /ɪnˈfɑːk.ʃən/ akutní infarkt myokardu

amniotic /ˌæm.niˈɒt.ɪk/ amniotický, týkající se zárodečné blány

amniotic /ˌæm.niˈɒt.ɪk/ sac /sæk/ plodový vak

amniotic fluid /ˌæm.ni.ɒt.ɪkˈfluː.ɪd/ plodová voda

amount /əˈmaʊnt/ množství, objem, částka

amputate /ˈæm.pjʊ.teɪt/ amputovat

amputation /ˌæm.pjʊˈteɪ.ʃən/ amputace

amputee /ˌæm.pjʊˈtiː/ osoba, která se podrobila amputaci

anaemia /əˈniːmɪə/ anémie, chudokrevnost

anaesthetic /ˌæn.əsˈθet.ɪk/ anestetický, anestetikum

anal /ˈeɪ.nəl/ anální, řitní

anaphylactic /ˌæn.ə.fɪˈlæk.tɪk/ anafylaktický, vztahující se k anafylaxi

anaphylaxis /ˌæn.ə.fɪˈlæk.sɪs/ anafylaxe, druh alergie,

přecitlivělosti na cizorodou bílkovinu

aneurysm /ˌæn.jʊə.rɪ.zəm/ aneuryzma, výduť, místní abnormální rozšíření krevních cév, zvláště arterií, vrozený defekt cévní stěny

angina /ænˌdʒaɪ.nə/ angína, silná svíravá bolest

anginal /ænˌdʒaɪ.nəl/ anginální, silná, svíravá bolest

angle /ˈæŋɡəl/ úhel, hrana, šikmý, nasměrovat, natočit do jistého úhlu

angry /ˈæŋ.gri/ rozzlobený

ankle /ˈæŋ.kl̩/ kotník

anniversary /ˌæn.ɪˈvɜː.sər.i/ oslava výročí, jubileum

anorexia nervosa /æn.əˌrek.si.ə.nəˈvəʊ.sə/ mentální anorexie

antagonism /ænˈtæg.ə.nɪ.zəm/ antagonismus, protiklad, rozpor

anterior /ænˈtɪə.ri.ər/ přední, předchozí

anti-emetic /ˌæn.tɪ.ɪˈmet.ɪk/ antiemetický, antiemetikum, lék proti nevolnosti a zvracení

antibody /ˈæn.ti.bɒd.i/ protilátka, vlastní, v těle

anticonvulsant /ˌæn.tɪ.kən.ˈvʌl.sənt/ antikonvulzivní, protikřečový

antidepressant /ˌæn.ti.dɪˈpres.ənt/ antidepresivum, lék

antidote /ˈæn.tɪ.dəʊt/ protijed, protilátka, protilék

antigen /ˈæn.tɪ.dʒən/ antigen

anxiety /æŋˈzaɪ.ə.ti/ úzkost, strach, obava

anxious /'æŋk.ʃəs/ úzkostlivý, zneklidněný

aorta /eɪ'ɔ:.tə/ aorta, srdečnice

aortic /eɪ'ɔ:.tɪk/ **aneurism** /ˌæn.jʊə.rɪ.zəm/ výduť srdečnice

apart /ə'pɑ:t/ vzdálený, oddělený

Apgar /'æpgɑ:/ **score** /skɔ:r/ Apgar skóre, hodnocení zdravotního stavu novorozence krátce po porodu

apical /'eɪ.pɪ.kəl/ apikální, ležící v okolí hrotu

apnoea /'æp.ni.ə/ apnoe, zástava dechu

apnoeic /æp'ni:.ɪk/ apnoický, bez dechu

apparent /ə'pær.ənt/ zřejmý, patrný, jasný

appear /ə'pɪər/ zdát se, jevit se, vypadat, objevit se

appearance /ə'pɪə.rənt s/ vzhled, zjev, zevnějšek, objevení se

appendicitis /əˌpen.dɪ'saɪ.tɪs/ zánět slepého střeva

appendix /ə'pen.dɪks/ apendix, červovitý přívěsek slepého střeva

applicable /ə'plɪk.ə.bl̩/ platný, použitelný

application /ˌæp.lɪ'keɪ.ʃən/ aplikace, použití, využití

apply / ə'plaɪ/ aplikovat, požádat, platit, použít

appointment /ə'pɔɪnt.mənt/ funkce, místo, schůzka, jednání

apprehension /æp.rɪ'hen.ʃən/ obava, strach, předtucha

apprehensive /ˌæp.rɪ'hen.sɪv/ znepokojený

approach /ə'prəʊtʃ/ blížit se, přiblížit se, přistoupit, přístup, cesta, kontakt, snaha o kontakt postoj

appropriate / ə'prəʊ.pri.ət/ náležitý, patřičný, odpovídající, přiměřený, příslušný, vhodný

appropriately /ə'prəʊ.pri.ət.li/ vhodně, náležitě, přiměřeně

approximately /ə'prɒksɪmətlɪ/ přibližně, asi

argue /'ɑ:g.ju:/ hádat se, přít se, argumentovat

arise /ə'raɪz/ (arose, arisen) nastat, vzniknout, vyplývat

arouse /ə'raʊz/ vzbudit, probudit

arrest /ə'rest/ zástava

arrhythmia /ə'rɪð.mi.ə/ arytmie, nepravidelný rytmus

arrow /'ær.əʊ/ šipka, ukazatel

arsenic /'ɑ:.sən.ɪk/ arzén

arteria /a:'tiə.riə/ **dorsalis** /dɔr.sə.lɪs/ **pedis** /ped.ɪs/ *lat.* hřbetní tepna nohy, je pokračováním a. tibialis anterior

arterial /ɑ:'tɪə.ri.əl/ arteriální, tepenný

arterionecrosis /ɑ:ˌtɪə.rɪə.ne'krəʊ.sɪs/ arterionekróza, nekróza arterií

arteriosclerosis /ɑ:ˌtɪə.ri.əʊ.sklə'rəʊ.sɪs/ arterioskleróza, tvrdnutí tepen

arteriosum /ɑ:ˌtiə.ri'ɒs.əm/ ligamentum arteriosum, lat. vazivový pruh, na který se po svém uzavření mění ductus arteriosus, Botallova dučej

artery /'ɑ:tərɪ/ tepna

arthritis /ɑːˈθraɪ.tɪs/ artritida, zánět kloubů

articulation /ɑːˌtɪk.juˈleɪ.ʃən/ kloub, skloubení

artificial /ˌɑː.tɪˈfɪʃ.əl/ **ventilation** /ˌven.tɪˈleɪ.ʃən/ umělé dýchání

ascent /əˈsent/ stoupání, výstup

ascertain /ˌæs.əˈteɪn/ zjistit, dopátrat se

ascites /æˈsaɪ.tɪːz/ ascites, abnormální hromadění tekutiny v břišní dutině

asleep /əˈsliːp/ spící, usnout

asphyxia /æsˈfɪksɪə/ asfyxie, zadušení

aspirate /ˈæs.pɪ.rət/ aspirovat, vdechnout, odsát, odsávat

aspiration /ˌæspɪˈreɪʃən/ aspirace, dýchání

aspirator /æs.pə.reɪ.tər/ aspirátor, přístroj na odsávání

assault /əˈsɒlt/ útok, napadení, přepadnout

assemble /əˈsem.bl̩/ sestavit, smontovat, svolat

assessment /əˈses.mənt/ hodnocení, ohodnocení, posudek, posouzení, stanovení, určení

assign /əˈsaɪn/ zadat, přidělit

assist /əˈsɪst/ asistovat, pomáhat

assistance /əˈsɪs.tənt s/ asistence, pomoc, podpora

associated /əˈsəʊ.si.eɪ.tɪd/ spojený, související

assume /əˈsjuːm/ domnívat se, převzít, vzít na sebe odpovědnost, zaujmout

assumption /əˈsʌmp.ʃən/ převzetí, předpoklad, domněnka

assurance /əˈʃɔː.rəns/ jistota, zajištění, pojištění

assure /əˈʃɔːr/ ujistit, zajistit, ubezpečit

asthma /ˈæs.mə/ astma

asymmetrical /ˌeɪ.sɪˈmet.rɪk.əl/ asymetrický, nesouměrný

asymptomatic /əˌsɪmp.təˈmæt.ɪk/ asymptomatický, bezpříznakový

asynchronous /eɪˈsɪŋ.krə.nəs/ asynchronní, nesoudobý, nesoučasný

asystole /ə.sɪs.tə.lɪ/ asystola, asystolie, uvolnění srdeční svaloviny, zástava srdeční činnosti

at /ət/ **least** /liːst/ při nejmenším, alespoň

at /ət/ **rest** /rest/ v klidu, bez pohybu

at /ət/ **stake** /steɪk/ být v sázce

ataxia /əˈtæk.si.ə/ ataxie, ztráta kontroly volních pohybů

ataxic /əˈtæk.sɪk/ ataktický, nesouladný, nekoordinovaný pohyb

atelectasis /ˌætəˈlek.tə.sɪs/ atelektáza, neúplné roztažení části plic, spojené se ztrátou jejich vzdušnosti

atherosclerosis /ˌæθ.ə.rəʊ.skləˈrəʊ.sɪs/ ateroskleróza, arterioskleróza, kornatění tepen

atmosphere /ˈæt.mə.sfɪər/ atmosféra, ovzduší, prostředí

atrial /ˈeɪ.tri.əl/ **fibrillation** /ˌfaɪ.brɪˈleɪ.ʃən/ fibrilace srdečních předsíní, porucha srdečního rytmu

atrial /'eɪ.tri.əl/ síňový, týkající se předsíně

atrium pl atria /'eɪ.tri.əm/ atrium, srdeční předsíň

atropine /'æt.rə.pɪn/ **sulfate** /'sʌl.feɪt/ atropin-sulfát, lék

attach /ə'tætʃ/ připojit, přilepit se, nalepit se

attack /ə'tæk/ útok, napadení, záchvat

attain /ə'teɪn/ získat, dosáhnout, docílit

attempt /ə'temp t/ pokus, pokoušet se, snažit

attend /ə'tend/ účastnit se, věnovat se, pečovat, starat se

attention /ə'ten.ʃən/ pozornost, péče, dávat pozor, všímat si

attentive /ə'ten.tɪv/ pozorný, věnující pozornost

attitude /'æt.ɪ.tjuːd/ postoj, stanovisko, přístup

attribute /'æt.rɪ.bjuːt/ přičítat, přisuzovat, symbol

atypical /ˌeɪ'tɪp.ɪ.kəl/ netypický, neobvyklý

audible /'ɔː.dɪ.bl̩/ slyšitelný

auditory /ˈɔːdɪtərɪ/ auditivní, sluchový

aura /'ɔː.rə/ aura, předzvěst, bezprostřední známky blížícího se záchvatu

auscultation /ˌɔː.skəl'teɪ.ʃən/ auskultace, vyšetření poslechem

authority /ɔː'θɒr.ɪ.ti/ oprávnění, pravomoc, úřad, správní orgán, úřední činitelé

authorize /'ɔː.θər.aɪz/ povolit, schválit, dát souhlas, oprávnit

automacity /ɔː'tɒm.ə.sɪt.i/ automacie, stereotypní, někdy periodicky se opakující děj

available /ə'veɪ.lə.bl̩/ dostupný, dosažitelný, k dispozici, vhodný

average /'æv.ər.ɪdʒ/ průměr, činit v průměru

awake /ə'weɪk/ probudit se, probrat se, být vzhůru, bdělý

aware /ə'weər/ bdělý, vnímající, uvědomovat si

awareness /ə'weə.nəs/ povědomí, vědomí, vnímavost, uvědomování si

away /ə'weɪ/ pryč, daleko

awoke /ə'wəʊk/ vzhůru, probuzený, probrat se

B

back /bæk/ **and forth** /fɔːθ/ pohyb sem a tam

back /bæk/ **out** /aʊt/ vycouvat

back /bæk/ záda, páteř

back-up /'bæk.ʌp/ podpořit, podložit, záloha

backboard /'bæk.bɔːd/ páteřní deska

backflow /'bæk.fləʊ/ zpětný tok

backpressure /ˌbæk'preʃ.ər/ zpětný tlak

backward /'bæk.wəd/ zpět, zpětný, dozadu

backyard /ˌbæk'jɑːd/ dvorek, zahrada za domem

bag /bæg/ **mask** /mɑːsk/ dýchací maska, ambuvak, resuscitační vak, samorozpínatelný vak s maskou

bag / bæg/ pytel, dát do pytle

bag /bæg/ **valve** /vælv/ dýchací vak, ruční zařízení, poskytnutí ventilace pozitivním tlakem pacientovi, který nedýchá, nebo dýchá nedostatečně

bag-valve mask /mɑːsk/ dýchací maska

balance /'bæl.əns/ vyrovnávat, rovnováha

ballistics /bə'lɪs.tɪks/ balistika

balloon /bə'luːn/ balonek

band /bænd/ páska, pásek

bandage /'bæn.dɪdʒ/ obvaz, obinadlo, bandáž, obvázat

bark /bɑːk/ štěkat

barky /'bɑː.ki/ štěkavý

barrel /'bær.əl/ sud, barel

barrier /'bær.i.ər/ překážka, zábrana

basal /beɪsəl/ bazální, spodní

base /beɪs/ spodina, základ, základna

based /beɪst/ založený, vycházející z, působící

basic /'beɪ.sɪk/ základ, základní

basilar /'bæz.ɪ.lər/ basilární, základnový

bathe /beɪð/ koupat, omýt, vymýt ránu

battery /'bæt.ər.i/ útok, ublížení na zdraví

Battle's /'bætəl/ **sign** /saɪn/ Battleův příznak, modravé zabarvení kůže nad výběžkem spánkové kosti, naznačuje frakturu lební baze

be /biː/ **in charge** /tʃɑːdʒ/ **of** být zodpovědný za, mít na starost

be /biː/ **over** /'əʊ.vər/ být skončený

be /biː/ **trapped** /træpd/ být uvězněný, chycený

bear /beər/ **down** /daʊn/ tlačit, rodit, vyřítit se, ležet svou vahou na

beat /biːt/ tlouci, úder

beaten /'biː.tən/ zmlácený, zbitý

Beck's triad /'traɪ.æd/ Beckova triáda, nízký arteriální tlak, vysoký venózní tlak, chybějící tep na srdečním hrotu při srdeční tamponádě spolu s oslabenými ozvami

bed /bed/ lůžko (anat.)

bedridden /'bed.rɪ.dən/ upoutaný na lůžko

bee /biː/ včela

behave /bɪ'heɪv/ chovat se, jednat

behaviour /bɪ'heɪ.vjə/ chování, jednání, reakce

belligerent /bə'lɪdʒ.ər.ənt/ útočný, agresivní

bend /bend/ (bent, bent) ohnout, sklonit, pokrčit, oblouk, ohnutí, ohyb

beneficial /ˌben.ɪ'fɪʃ.əl/ prospěšný, blahodárný

benefit /'ben.ɪ.fɪt/ prospěch, užitek, mít užitek

benzodiazepines /ben'zɒ.dɪ.az'e.piːnz/ benzodiazepiny

beta-2 /'biː.tə.tuː/ **agonists** /'æg.ə.nɪsts/ beta-2 agonisté, uvolňují a otevírají dýchací cesty, které se během astmatického záchvatu zužují, astma „uvolňovače" nebo bronchodilatátory

bicuspid valve /baɪˈkʌs.pɪdˌvælv/ dvojcípá chlopeň

bike /baɪk/ jizdní kolo, motorka

bilateral /baɪˈlæt.ər.əl/ bilaterální, dvoustranný

bilaterally /ˌbaɪˈlæt.ər.ə.li/ bilaterálně, dvoustranně

bilirubin /ˌbɪl.ɪˈruː.bɪn/ bilirubin, žlučové barvivo

bin /bɪn/ zásobník, nádoba

bind /baɪnd/ (bound, bound) spojit, vázat, vazba

binge eating /bɪndʒˌiː.tɪŋ/ záchvatovité přejídání

biotelemetry /ˌbaɪ.əʊ.təˈlem.ə.tri/ aplikace moderních metod přenosu k dálkovému sledování životních znaků pacientů

bipolar disorder /baɪˈpəʊ.lə.dɪˌsɔː.dər/ bipolární afektivní porucha, psychická porucha, která se projevuje nadměrnými změnami nálad, vitality a psychických funkcí

birth /bɜːθ/ **canal** /kəˈnæl/ porodní cesta

birth /bɜːθ/ **control** /kənˈtrəʊl/ **pill** /pɪl/ antikoncepční pilulka

bite /baɪt/ kousnout, uštknout, kousnutí

bitterly /ˈbɪt.ə.li/ prudce, ostře

bizarre /bɪˈzɑːr/ bizarní, divný, podivný

black out /ˈblæk.aʊt/ ztratit vědomí, omdlít

bladder /ˈblæd.ər/ měchýř

blade /bleɪd/ čepel, lopatka

blast /blɑːst/ výbuch, výstřel, rána, poryv

bleach /bliːtʃ/ odbarvit, bělicí prostředek

bleb /bleb/ puchýřek

bleed /bliːd/ krvácet, krvácení

blind /blaɪnd/ slepý

blindly /ˈblaɪnd.li/ slepě, naslepo

blister /ˈblɪs.tər/ puchýř

blistering /ˈblɪs.tər.ɪŋ/ vytváření puchýřů

bloating /ˈbləʊ.tɪŋ/ otok, nadýmání

block /blɒk/ blokovat, zatarasit

blockage /ˈblɒk.ɪdʒ/ ucpání, neprůchodnost

blood /blʌd/ **loss** /lɒs/ krevní ztráta

blood /blʌd/ **pressure** /ˈpreʃ.ər/ krevní tlak

blood /blʌd/ **sample** /ˈsɑːm.pl̩/ vzorek krve

blood /blʌd/ **vessel** /ˈves.əl/ krevní céva

blood-borne /bɔːn/ nesený krví

bloodshot /ˈblʌd.ʃɒt/ krví podlitý (oči)

blow /bləʊ/ (blew, blown) foukat, vyfouknout, vanout, vyletět

blowing /ˌbləʊ.ɪŋ/ foukání

BLS, Basic /ˈbeɪ.sɪk/ **Life Support** /ˈlaɪf.səˌpɔːt/ základní podpora života, soubor znalostí a dovedností potřebný pro zajištění a udržení volných dýchacích cest a podpory cirkulace a dechu

blue bloater /ˈbləʊ.tər/ osoba trpící pokročilou COPD, charakteristická je cyanóza (zhoršený průchod vzduchu) a otok (zadržování tekutin)

blunt /blʌnt/ tupý, oblý, přímý

blurred /blɜːd/ neostrý, nejasný, zastřený, rozmazaný

board /bɔːd/ deska

boardlike /bɔːd.laɪk/ podobný desce

bob /bɒb/ pohodit hlavou, pohupovat se, poskakovat

bodily /ˈbɒd.ɪ.li/ tělesný

bolus /bəʊ.ləs/ jednorázově podaná dávka léku

bombing /ˈbɒm.ɪŋ/ bombový útok

bone /bəʊn/ **marrow** /ˈmær.əʊ/ kostní dřeň

border /bɔː.dər/ okraj, hranice

borderline /ˈbɔː.də.laɪn/ hranice, mezní, hraniční

bound /baʊnd/ skákat, běžet

bowel /ˈbaʊ.əl/ **movement** /ˈmuːv.mənt/ vyprázdnění stolice:

bowel /ˈbaʊ.əl/ střevo, útroby

bradycardia /ˌbræd.ɪˈkaːdi.ə/ bradycardie, zpomalená srdeční činnost

bradypnoea /ˌbræd.ɪ.ˈpni.ə/ bradypnoe, zpomalené dýchání

brain /breɪn/ mozek

brainstem /ˈbreɪn.stem/ mozkový kmen

breach /briːtʃ/ porušení, nedodržení

break /breɪk/ (broke broken) prasknout, zlomit, rozbít

break /breɪk/ **down** /daʊn/ porucha, porušení, havárie, defekt, zhroutit se, nevydržet

breath /breθ/ dech, dýchání

breathing /ˈbriː.ðɪŋ/ dýchání, dýchací

breech /briːtʃ/ **presentation** /ˌprez.ənˈteɪ.ʃən/ poloha koncem pánevním

breech /briːtʃ/ zadeček, zadnice

brief /briːf/ krátký, stručný

bright /braɪt/ jasný, světlý, zářivý

bring /brɪŋ/ **about** /əˈbaʊt/ způsobit, vyvolat

bronchial /ˈbrɒŋ.ki.əl/ **tree** /triː/ průduškový strom

bronchiole /ˈbrɒŋ.ki.əʊl/ průdušinka

bronchiolitis /ˈbrɒŋ.ki.əˈla.ɪ.tɪs/ bronchiolitida, zánět průdušinek

bronchitis /brɒŋˈkaɪ.tɪs/ bronchitida, zánět průdušek

bronchoconstriction /ˌbrɒŋ.kəʊ.kənˈstrɪk.ʃən/ zúžení průdušek

bronchodilation /ˌbrɒŋ.kəʊ.ˈdɪleɪʃən/ dilatace, rozšíření průdušek

bronchospasm /ˌbrɒŋ.kəʊ.ˈspæz.əm/ bronchospasmus, křeč průdušek

bronchus /ˈbrɒŋ.kəs/ **bronchi** /-kaɪ/ průduška

Brown-Sequard's /braʊn-sei.kahr/ **syndrome** /ˈsɪn.drəʊm/ Brown-Sequardův syndrom, soubor příznaků, které se vyvinou po hemisekci míchy, protětí její levé nebo pravé poloviny či při útlaku její poloviny, pacient trpí stejnostrannou poruchou hybnosti a vibračního a diskriminačního čití a poruchou citlivosti pro bolest, teplo a chlad na straně opačné

brownie /ˈbraʊ.ni/ sušenka

bruise /bruːz/ modřina, podlitina

bruising /'bruː.zɪŋ/ pohmožděniny, podlitiny
bruit /bruːt/ šum, šelest
brush /brʌʃ/ vyčistit kartáčkem, otřít
BSA, Body /'bɒd.i/ **Surface** /'sɜː.fɪs/ **Area** /'eərɪə/ oblast povrchu těla
BSI, British /'brɪt.ɪʃ/ **Standards** / 'stæn.dədz/ **Institution** / ˌɪnstɪ'tjuːʃən/ Britský úřad pro standardizaci
bubble /'bʌb.l/ bublat, být plný čeho
bucket /bʌkɪt/ kbelík, vědro
build /bɪld/ (built, built) posílit, upevnit, vybudovat
buildup /'bɪld.ʌp/ vytvořit, narůstat, hromadit se, nárůst, hromadění, zvětšení objemu
bulb /bʌlb/ baňka, kulovité rozšíření cylindrické struktury či orgánu, žárovka
bulge / bʌldʒ/ naběhnout, zduřet, vyboulit se, vyklenutí, vydutí, vyboulenina
bulimia /buˌlɪm.i.ə/ bulimie, porucha příjmu potravy
bulky /'bʌl.ki/ objemný velký, rozměrný, tlustý
bullet /'bʊl.ɪt/ kulka, střela
bundle /'bʌn.dl/ svazek
bunk /bʌŋk/ **bed** /bed/ palanda
bunkroom /bʌŋk.rʊm/ lůžko, nocovat
burn /bɜːn/ popálenina, hořet
burnout /'bɜːnaʊt/ vyhoření, naprosté vyčerpání

bursitis /bɜː'saɪ.tɪs/ burzitida, zánět váčku (zejm. mezi svalem nebo šlachou
bury /'ber.i/ zahrabat, pohřbít
buttock /'bʌt.ək/ hýždě, zadek
BVM, Bag Valve Mask, Ambu bag, manual resuscitator, self-inflating bag dýchací maska s ventilem
by ground /graʊnd/ po zemi (cesta)
bystander /'baɪˌstæn.dər/ náhodný divák, přihlížející, svědek

C
C-spine, cervical /sə'vaɪ.kəl/ **spine** / spaɪn/ krční páteř
caesarean section /sɪˌzeə.ri.ən'sek.ʃən/ císařský řez
cafeteria /ˌkæf.ə'tɪə.ri.ə/ jídelna, restaurace
caffeinated /'kæf.ɪ.neɪ.tɪd/ s kofeinem (nápoj)
caffeine /'kæf.iːn/ kofein
calcaneus /kæl'keɪ.niəs/ kost patní
calcium /'kæl.si.əm/ vápník, kalcium
calculate /'kælkjʊˌleɪt/ vypočítat, spočítat, spoléhat na co
calf /kɑːf/ lýtko
call /kɔːl/ volat, hovor, požadavek, výzva
calm (sb) /kɑːm/ **down** /daʊn/ uklidnit, utišit, upokojit
campus /'kæm.pəs/ areál univerzity
canal / kə'næl/ kanálek
cancer /'kænt .sər/ rakovina
cancerous /'kæn.sər.əs/ rakovinný

IRENA BAUMRUKOVÁ

cannula /ˈkæn.jʊl.ə/ kanyla, dutá jehla, trubička
capable /ˈkeɪ.pə.bļ/ schopný, způsobilý, zdatný
capacity /kəˈpæs.ə.ti/ objem, schopnost, výkonnost
capillary /kəˈpɪl.ər.i/ bed /bed/ místo propojení kapilár tepének a žilek
capillary /kəˈpɪl.ər.i/ kapilára, vlásečnice, kapilární
capillary /kəˈpɪl.ər.i/ refill /ˈriː.fɪl/ zpětné plnění kapilár
capnometer /kæpˈɒm.ɪ.tər/ kapnometr, analyzátor respiračních plynů jednotlivých dechů pro kontrolu intubace
capnometry /kæpˈnɒm.ə.tri/ měření koncentrace oxidu uhličitého ve vzduchu
capture /ˈkæp.tʃər/ zajmout, získat
carbamate /ˈkɑː.bəˌmeɪt/ sůl nebo ester kyseliny karbamové (karbamová kyselina – H₂N–COOH, kyselina, která se okamžitě rozpadá na oxid uhličitý a amoniak; její soli jsou karbamáty, otrava, stažení zorniček, svalový třes, salivace, ataxie, dyspnoe
carbohydrate /ˌkɑː.bəʊˈhaɪ.dreɪt/ uhlovodan
carbon /ˈkɑː.bən/ dioxide /daɪˈɒk.saɪd/ oxid uhličitý
carbon /ˈkɑː.bən/ uhlík
carbon monoxide /ˌkɑː.bən.məˈnɒk.saɪd/ oxid uhelnatý
cardiac /ˈkɑː.di.æk/ srdeční

cardiac /ˈkɑːdɪˌæk/ output /ˈaʊtˌpʊt/ minutový objem krve vypuzené srdcem
cardiac arrest /ˈkɑr.di.æk əˈrest/ zástava srdce
cardiogenic /ˈkɑː.di.ə.ˈdʒen.ɪk/ shock /ʃɒk/ kardiogenní šok, způsobený těžkou poruchou srdeční funkce, komplikace rozsáhlého či opakovaného infarktu myokardu
cardiopulmonary /ˌkɑː.di.əʊˈpʊl.mə.nə.ri/ kardiopulmonární, týkající se srdce a plic
cardioversion /ˌkɑː.di.əˈvɜː.ʃən/ kardioverze, elektrický výboj použitý při léčbě srdečních arytmií
care /keə/ for /fɔː/ starat se, mít zájem, ošetřovat
care /keə/ péče, starost, dohled, pozornost, pečovat, starat se
care /keə/ provider /prəˈvaɪ.dər/ ošetřovatel, pečovatel
careful /ˈkeə.fəl/ opatrný, pečlivý, důkladný
caregiver /ˈkeəˌgɪv.ər/ pečovatel, opatrovatel
caretaker /ˈkeəˌteɪ.kər/ pečovatel, opatrovatel
carina /kəˈraɪn.ə/ člunek, výběžek
caring /ˈkeə.rɪŋ/ starostlivý, pečující
carotid artery /kəˌrɒt.ɪdˈɑː.tər.i/ karotida, krkavice, krční tepna
carpopedal /ˌkɑː.pəˈpiː.d.əl/ karpopedální, týkající se zápěstí a nohy
carry /ˈkær.i/ nést, vézt

carry /'kær.i/ **on** pokračovat, vést dialog

carry /'kær.i/ **st out** /aʊt/ provést, uskutečnit

cartilage /'kɑː.təl.ɪdʒ/ chrupavka

cartilage /'kɑː.təl.ɪdʒ/ **ring** /rɪŋ/ chrupavčitý prstenec

case /keɪs/ případ, daná situace, pouzdro, obal

catastrophic /ˌkæt.ə'strɒf.ɪk/ katastrofální, tragický

catching /'kætʃ.ɪŋ/ nakažlivý, přenosný

catecholamine /kat.ə.kəl.am.in/ katecholamin, nejběžnější jsou epinefrin (adrenaline), norepinefrin (noradrenalin) a dopamin

catheter /'kæθɪtə/ katétr, cévka

Caucasian /kɔː'keɪ.ʒən/ běloch

causative /'kɔː.zə.tɪv/ kauzativní, příčinný, způsobující

cause /kɔːz/ příčina, záležitost, věc, důvod, přimět, způsobit

caution /'kɔː.ʃən/ opatrnost, varování, pozor

cautiously /'kɔː.ʃəs.li/ opatrně, ostražitě

cavitation /ˌkæv.ɪ'teɪ.ʃən/ kavitace, vytváření dutin

cavity /'kæv.ɪ.ti/ dutina

cease /siːs/ přestat, ustat, zastavit se

cell /sel/ buňka

cell, cellular /'sel.jʊ.lər / telephone /'telɪˌfəʊn/ mobilní telefon

cellular /'sel.jʊ.lər/ buněčný

center /'sen.tər/ střed, centrum, středisko

central /'sen.trəl/ centrální, středový

cerebral /'ser.ɪ.brəl/ mozkový

cerebrospinal /ˌser.ɪ.brə'spaɪ.nəl/ cerebrospinální, mozkomíšní

cerebrovascular /ˌser.ɪ.brə'væskjʊlə/ cerebrovaskulární, týkající se mozkových cév

cerebrum /sɪ'riː.brəm/ cerebrum, velký mozek

cervical /'sɜː.vɪkəl/ **spine** /spaɪn/ krční páteř

cervical /sə'vaɪ.kəl/ krční, krčkový

cervix /'sɜː.vɪks/ **cervices** /-vɪs.iːz/ hrdlo děložní

cessation /ses'eɪ.ʃən/ skončení, zastavení, ustání

chain /tʃeɪn/ řetěz, řetězec

challenge /'tʃæl.ɪndʒ/ čelendž, provokační injekce, vyvolání odezvy

chamber /'tʃeɪm.bə/ komora

charcoal /'tʃɑːr.koʊl/ dřevěné uhlí, živočišné uhlí

charge /tʃɑːdʒ/ obžaloba, obvinění

charred /tʃɑːd/ ohořelý, spálený

chart /tʃɑːt/ graf, diagram, schéma, nákres

check /tʃek/ kontrolovat, zkontrolovat, kontrola

chemical /'kem.ɪ.kəl/ chemický, chemická látka

chemistry /'kem.ɪ.stri/ chemické pochody složení, vlastnosti, procesy

chest /tʃest/ hrudník, prsa

chest /tʃest/ wall /wɔːl/ hrudní stěna

CHF, Congestive /kənˈdʒes.tɪv/ Heart /hɑːt/ Failure /ˈfeɪ.ljər/ městnavé srdeční selhání, k městnavému srdečnímu selhání dochází, když srdce selže jako pumpa a krev se hromadí před pravou komorou v pravé síní a žilním systému nebo před levou komorou v levé síní a plicním oběhu

chickenpox /ˈtʃɪk.ɪn.pɒks/ varicela, plané neštovice

chief /tʃiːf/ hlavní

childbearing /ˈtʃaɪldˌbeə.rɪŋ/ rození dětí

childbirth /ˈtʃaɪld.bɜːθ/ porod, narození dítěte

chill /tʃɪl/ vychladit, zimnice

chin /tʃɪn/ brada

chin-lift /tʃɪn/, /lɪft/ zvednutí brady

chlamydia /kləm.iˈde.ə/ Chlamydia, lat. rod mikroorganismů schopných množení jen v buňce, obligátní intracelulární paraziti

choice /tʃɔɪs/ výběr, volba

choke /tʃəʊk/ dusit se

cholecystitis /ˌkəʊ.lɪ.sɪˈstaɪ.tɪs/ cholecystitida, zánět žlučníku

cholinergic /kɒ.lɪn.ə.dʒɪk/ cholinergický

chronic /ˈkrɒn.ɪk/ chronický

circle /ˈsɜː.kl̩/ kruh, vrátit se zpět

circulate /ˈsɜː.kjʊ.leɪt/ cirkulovat, obíhat, šířit se

circulation /ˌsɜː.kjʊˈleɪ.ʃən/ cirkulace, oběh

circumstance /ˈsɜː.kəm.stɑːnt s/ okolnost, poměry

claim /kleɪm/ požadavek, nárok

clammy /ˈklæm.i/ studeně vlhký, lepkavý

clamp /klæmp/ svorka, upevnit svorkou, spona, sepnout

classify /ˈklæs.ɪ.faɪ/ klasifikovat, třídit

clavicle /ˈklævɪkəl/ klavikula, klíční kost

clavicular /kləˈvɪkjʊlə/ klavikulární, klíční

clear /klɪər/ čistý, jasný, průzračný, očistit, vyprázdnit

clearly /ˈklɪə.li/ jasně

closure /ˈkləʊ.ʒə/ zavření, uzavírka

clot /klɒt/ sraženina, chuchvalec, srážet se

clubbing /ˈklʌb.ɪŋ/ paličkovité prsty

clump /klʌmp/ shluk, skupina, dupat

cluster /ˈklʌs.tər/ shluk, hlouček, skupinka, trs, hrozen

coach /kəʊtʃ/ vést, učit, trenér

coarse /kɔːs/ hrubý, drsný

cocaine /kəʊˈkeɪn/ kokain

coccyx /ˈkɒk.sɪks/ kostrč, kostrční kost

coexist /ˌkoʊ·ɪgˈzɪst/ koexistovat, žít vedle sebe

cognitive /ˈkɑg.nə.tɪv/ kognitivní, poznávací

cold /kəʊld/ nachlazení, rýma

cold /kəʊld/ sore /sɔːr/ opar na rtu, v nose

colicky /ˈkɒl.ɪ.ki/ trpící kolikou, kolikový

colitis /kə.lɪ.tɪs/ kolitida, zánět tlustého střeva

collapse /kəˈlæps/ zhroutit se, kolaps

collar /ˈkɑl.ər/ límec

collection /kəˈlekʃən/ nahromadění, soubor, sbírání, sbírka

collectively /kəˈlek.tɪv.li/ společně, celkově, dohromady

collision /kəˈlɪʒ.ən/ srážka, kolize

colon /ˈkoʊ.lən/ trakčník

coma /ˈkəʊ.mə/ kóma, hluboké bezvědomí

comb /koʊm/ učesat, hřeben

Combi tube /komˈbi.tju:b/ trubice s dvěma průsvity k ventilaci průdušnice při vložení naslepo

comfort /ˈkʌm.fət/ pohodlí, uklidnění, utěšit, poskytnout útěchu

comfortable /ˈkʌmf.tər.bəl/ pohodlný, příjemný

command /kəˈmɑːnd/ příkaz, ovládnutí, kontrola, velení

commander /kəˈmæn.dər/ velitel

commercial /kəˈmɜːʃəl/ obchodní, komerční, průmyslově vyráběný

commit /kəˈmɪt/ spáchat, dopustit se

common /ˈkɒmən/ běžný, obvyklý, častý, společný

commonly /ˈkɒm.ən.lɪ/ obvykle, běžný

communicable /kəˈmjuː.nɪ.kə.bĺ/ nakažlivý, přenosný

communicate /kəˈmjuː.nɪ.keɪt/ komunikovat, být spojen

company /ˈkʌm.pə.ni/ společnost, firma

compare /kəmˈpeər/ porovnat, srovnat

comparison /kəmˈpærɪsən/ srovnání, porovnání

compartment /kəmˈpɑːt.mənt/ oddělení, prostor, vymezený prostor

compartment /kəmˈpɑːt.mənt/ **syndrome** /ˈsɪn.drəʊm/ kompartmentový syndrom, imobolizace nervu nebo šlachy v určitém prostoru

compensate /ˈkɒm.pən.seɪt/ kompenzovat, vyvážit, vyrovnat, vyrovnat se

compensatory /ˌkɒm.pən.seɪt.ə ri/ kompenzační

competency /ˈkɒmpɪtənsɪ/ schopnost, odborná způsobilost

complain /kəmˈpleɪn/ stěžovat si, naříkat si

complaint /kəmˈpleɪnt/ stížnost, nemoc, neduh, potíž

complete /kəmˈpliːt/ dokončený, hotový, úplný, doplnit, dokončit, skončit

completeness /kəmˈpliː.t.nəs/ úplnost, kompletnost

complex /kɒm.pleks/ složitý

compliance /kəmˈplaɪ.ənt s/ dodržování, soulad, kompliance, poddajnost, schopnost proměny velikosti a tvaru (např. plíce při vdechu)

component /kəmˈpəʊnənt/ složka, součást

composed /kəmˈpəʊzd/ **of** složený z

composition /ˌkɒm.pəˈzɪʃ.ən/ skladba, složená
compress /kəmˈpres/ obklad, stlačit, zmáčknout
compression /kəmˈpreʃən/ komprese, stlačení, stisknutí, slisování
compromise /ˈkɒmprəˌmaɪz/ oslabit, ohrozit, vydat v nebezpečí, zhoršit, kompromis, zhoršení
concern /kənˈsɜːn/ zájem, starost, obavy, znepokojení
concise /kənˈsaɪs/ stručný, výstižný, zkrácený
conclude /kənˈkluːd/ usoudit, dojít k závěru
conclusion /kənˈkluː.ʒən/ závěr, úsudek
concussion /kənˈkʌʃ.ən/ otřes mozku
condensation /ˌkɒn.den.ˈseɪ.ʃən/ orosení, opocení, kondenzace páry
condition /kənˈdɪʃ.ən/ stav, fyzická kondice, potíže, onemocnění, podmínka
conditioning /kənˈdɪʃ.ən.ɪŋ/ udržování kondice, cvičení, navykání si
conduct /kənˈdʌkt/ provádět, vést, řídit, chování, počínání
conduction /kənˈdʌk.ʃən/ vedení, přenos, kondukce tepla, elekrického proudu
confidential /ˌkɒn.fɪˈden.tʃəl/ důvěrný, tajný

confidentiality /ˌkɒn.fɪ.den.tʃiˈæl.ɪ.ti/ důvěrnost informací, mlčenlivost
confined /kənˈfaɪnd/ stísněný, omezený, být omezen na
confirmation /ˌkɒn.fəˈmeɪ.ʃən/ potvrzení, schválení
confirmed /kənˈfɜːmd/ potvrzený
confrontational /ˌkɒn.frʌnˈteɪ.ʃən.əl/ konfrontační
confused /kənˈfjuːzd/ zmatený, popletený
confusion /kənˈfjuː.ʒən/ zmatek, záměna
congestion /kənˈdʒes.tʃən/ ucpání, zácpa
congestive /kənˈdʒes.tɪv/ **heart** / hɑːt/ **failure** /ˈfeɪ.ljər/ městnavé srdeční selhání, k městnavému srdečnímu selhání dochází, když srdce selže jako pumpa a krev se hromadí před pravou komorou v pravé síni a žilním systému nebo před levou komorou v levé síni a plicním oběhu
congestive /kənˈdʒes.tɪv/ městnavý, působící ucpávání
conjunction /kənˈdʒʌŋk.ʃən/ spojení, kombinace
conjunctivitis /kənˌdʒʌŋk.tɪˈvaɪ.tɪs/ zánět očních spojivek
conscious /ˈkɒn.tʃəs/ při vědomí, vědomý si
consciously /ˈkɒn.ʃəs.li/ vědomě, umyslně
consciousness /ˈkɒn.ʃəs.nəs/ vědomí, povědomí
consent /kənˈsent/ souhlas, svolení

consenting /kənˈsent.ɪŋ/ **adult /**
əˈdʌlt/ zletilý, osoba ve věku, kdy
může legálně začít sexuální život

consequence /ˈkɒn.sɪ.kwəns/
následek, důsledek

consideration /kənˌsɪd.əˈreɪ.ʃən/
úvaha, zřetel, kritérium, faktor,
který je třeba brát
v úvahu

considered /kənˈsɪd.əd/
považovaný, uvážený

consist /kənˈsɪst/ skládat se, být
složen z čeho

consistent /kənˈsɪs.tənt/ **with** /wɪð/
shodný, odpovídající, v souladu

consolidation /kənˌsɒl.ɪˈdeɪ.ʃən/
upevnění, konsolidace, sloučení

constant /ˈkɒn.stənt/ neustálý,
nepřetržitý

constantly /ˈkɒn.stənt.li/ neustále,
nepřetržitě

constitute /ˈkɒn.stɪ.tjuːt/
znamenat, představovat

constricted /kənˈstrɪkt.ɪd/ zúžený,
stáhnutý

constriction /kənˈstrɪk.ʃən/ stažení,
zúžení

consult /kənˈsʌlt/ poradit se, zeptat
se

consumption /kənˈsʌmp.ʃən/
spotřeba, konzumace

contain /kənˈteɪn/ obsahovat,
zahrnovat

container /kənˈteɪ.nər/ nádoba

containment /kənˈteɪn.mənt/
uzavření, omezení

contaminant /kənˈtæm.ɪ.nənt/
znečisťující látka

contamination /kənˌtæm.ɪˈneɪ.ʃən/
kontaminace, zamoření

content /kənˈtent/ obsah, náplň

continue /kənˈtɪn.juː/ pokračovat,
zůstat

continuous /kənˈtɪn.ju.əs/
nepřetržitý, neustálý, pravidelný

continuously /kənˈtɪn.ju.əs.li/
nepřetržitě, neustále

contract /kənˈtrækt/ stáhnout,
zúžit se

contractile /kənˈtræk.taɪl/
kontraktilní, stažitelný

contractility /ˌkən.trækˈtɪ.lə.ti/
kontraktilita, stažitelnost

contraction /kənˈtræk.ʃən/ stah,
stažení, smrštění

contraindicate /ˌkɒn.trəˈɪn.dɪ.keɪt/
kontraindikovat

contraindication /ˌkɒn.trəˌɪn.
dɪˈkeɪ.ʃən/ kontraindikace, příčiny
vylučující užití určitých léků nebo
léčebných postupů

contrecoup /ˈkɒn.trə.kuːp/ zpětný
odraz, zpětná síla (vyvolávající
např. pohmoždění na opačné
straně)

contribute /kənˈtrɪb.juːt/ přispět,
přispívat, darovat, podílet

contusion /kənˈtjuː.ʒən/
pohmožděnina, zhmožděnina

convert /kənˈvɜːt/ přeměnit se,
proměnit se

convince /kənˈvɪns/ přesvědčit
koho o čem

cool /kuːl/ chladný, studený

cooling /ˈkuː.lɪŋ/ ochlazování

cooperate /kəʊˈɒp.ər.eɪt/
kooperovat, spolupracovat

cooperative /kəʊˈɒp.ər.ə.tɪv/ spolupracující, vstřícný

coordinate /kəʊˈɔː.dɪ.neɪt/ koordinovat, sladit

COPD, Chronic /ˈkrɒnɪk/ **Obstructive** /əbˈstrʌk.tɪv/ **Pulmonary** /ˈpʊl.mə.nə.ri/ **Disease** /dɪˈziːz/ chronické obstruktivní onemocnění plic

cope /kəʊp/ **with** /wɪð/ zvládnout, poradit si, vypořádat se, snášet, vyrovnat se, vydržet

copious /ˈkəʊ.pi.əs/ hojný, bohatý

copper /ˈkɒp.ər/ měď

copperhead /ˈkɒp.ər.hed/ jedovatý had, jed ničí červené krvinky

cor /kɔːr/ **pulmonale** /ˈpʊl.mə.nə.l/ lat. plicní srdce, chorobné zvětšení pravé srdeční komory

coral /ˈkɒr.əl/ **snake** /sneɪk/ korálovec

cord /kɔːd/ šňůra, pupečník

core /kɔːr/ střed, jádro, střed těla

corneal /kɔːˈni.əl/ korneální, týkající se rohovky

corner /ˈkɔː.nər/ koutek

coronary /ˈkɒr.ən.ər.i/ koronární, věnčitý

correct /kəˈrekt/ správný, přesný, napravit

corrective /kəˈrek.tɪv/ korekční, nápravný

correlate /ˈkɒrɪˌleɪt/ souviset, být ve vzájemném vztahu

correlation /ˌkɒr.əˈleɪ.ʃən/ korelace, vzájemná souvislost

corresponding /ˌkɒr.ɪˈspɒn.dɪŋ/ odpovídající

cortisol /ˈkɔː.tɪ.sɒl/ kortizol, glukokortikoidní hormon vylučovaný nadledvinami

costal /ˈkɒsˌtəl/ žeberní

cotton /ˈkɒt.ən/ bavlna, vata

cottonmouth /ˈkɒt.ən.maʊθ/ ploskolebec vodní, druh jedovatého hada

cough /kɒf/ kašel, kašlat

count /kaʊnt/ **for** hrát roli, znamenat

count /kaʊnt/ počítat

counteract /ˌkaʊn.tərˈækt/ působit proti, potlačovat

counterproductive /ˌkaʊn.tə.prəˈdʌk.tɪv/ kontraproduktivní, mající opačný účinek

countertraction /ˌkaʊn.tərˈtræk.ʃən/ protitah, repozice zlomeniny tahem ze dvou opačných stran

coup /kap/ mrtvice, záchvat

couple /ˈkʌp.l/ spojovat dohromady

courageous /kəˈreɪ.dʒəs/ odvážný, statečný

course /kɔːs/ průběh, kúra (léčebná), postup

court /kɔːt/ soud, soudní dvůr

covering /ˈkʌv.ər.ɪŋ/ pokrývající

CPAP, Continuous /kənˈtɪn.ju.əs/ **Positive** /ˈpɒz.ə.tɪv/ **Airway** /ˈeə.weɪ/ **Pressure** /ˈpreʃ.ər/ ventilační režim, druh neinvazivní mechanické ventilace u spontánně dýchajícího pacienta, která se uskutečňuje pomocí obličejové nebo nazální masky

CPR, Cardiopulmonary /ˌkɑː.di.əʊˈpʊl.mə.nə.ri/ **Resuscitation** /

rɪˌsʌs.ɪˈteɪ.ʃən/ kardiopulmonární resuscitace

crack /kræk/ čistý kokain (hovor. název)

crackle /ˈkræk.|/ praskot, praskání, šustění

cramp /kræmp/ křeč

cranial /ˈkreɪ.ni.əl/ kraniální, lebeční

crash /kræʃ/ havárie, nehoda, zhroucení, srážka, nabourat

craving /ˈkreɪ.vɪŋ/ bažení, chuť na co

create /kriˈeɪt/ vytvořit, stvořit, vyvolat

crepitus /ˈkrep.ɪ.təs/ krepitus, praskot

crew /kruː/ posádka

crib /krɪb/ (dětská) postýlka

cricoid /ˈkraɪ.kɔɪd/ cartilage /ˈkɑː.təl.ɪdʒ/ chrupavka prstencová, nejspodnější chrupavka hltanová

cricoid /ˈkraɪ.kɔɪd/ prstenčitý

cricothyreotomy /ˈkraɪ.kəˌθaɪəˈrɒ.tə.mɪ/ krikotyreotomie, chirurg. rozdělení chrupavky prstencové a štítné

crime /kraɪm/ zločin, trestný čin

criterion /kraɪˈtɪə.ri.ən/ kriterium, měřítko

critical /ˈkrɪt.ɪ.kəl/ kritický, zlomový, rozhodující, nebezpečný

Crohn's disease /ˈkrəʊnz.dɪˌziːz/ Crohnova nemoc, regionální enteritida

crop /krɒp/ úroda, sklizeň

crossing /ˈkrɒs.ɪŋ/ přejezd, přechod, křížení

crouch /kraʊtʃ/ skrčit se, přikrčit se, dřepnout si

croup /kruːp/ difterický krup, dětský zánět hrtanu, štěkavý kašel, hrtanová křeč

crow /krəʊ/ kokrhat (kohout)

crowning /ˈkraʊ.nɪŋ/ stadium porodu, kdy se hlava plodu objeví v rodidlech

crush /krʌʃ/ drtit, rozdrtit, rozmačkat, rozmáčknout

crush /krʌʃ/ syndrome /ˈsɪn.drəʊm/ těžký stav vzniklý rozsáhlým rozdrcením kosterního svalstva např. při zavalení, následek dlouhého tlaku na svalstvo, zejm. paží a nohou

crushing /ˈkrʌʃ.ɪŋ/ drtivý

cuff /kʌf/ manžeta, záložka

cumulative /ˈkjuː.mjʊ.lə.tɪv/ kumulativní, hromadící se

curl /kɜːl/ natočit, stočit

current /ˈkʌr.ənt/ proud, současný, aktuální

curtain /ˈkɜː.tən/ opona

curved /kɜːvd/ zahnutý, zakřivený

custody /ˈkʌs.tə.di/ zadržení, vazba

cut st off /kʌt/ odříznout, přerušit, zastavit

CVA, Cerebrovascular/ ˌser.ɪ.brəˈvæskjʊlə/ Accident / ˈæksɪdənt/ mrtvice

cyanide /ˈsaɪə.naɪd/ kyanid

cyanosis /ˌsaɪəˈnəʊ.sɪs/ cyanóza

cycle /ˈsaɪ.k|/ cyklus

cyst /sɪst/ cysta

cystitis /sɪˈstaɪ.tɪs/ cystitida, zánět močového měchýře

D

dam /dæm/ hráz, přehrada

damage /'dæm.ɪdʒ/ poškodit, poškození, škoda

damaged /'dæm.ɪdʒd/ poškozený

danger /'deɪn.dʒər/ nebezpečí, ohrožení

dangerous /'deɪn.dʒər.əs/ nebezpečný

dangerously /'deɪn.dʒər.əs.li/ nebezpečně

dashboard /'dæʃˌbɔːd/ přístrojová deska auta

daydream /'deɪ.driːm/ být duchem nepřítomný, snění za bílého dne

dead /ded/ mrtvý

deadly /'ded.li/ smrtící, smrtelný

deal with /dɪəl/ řešit, zabývat se

debilitating /dɪ'bɪl.ɪ.teɪt.ɪŋ/ oslabující, vysilující

debrief /ˌdiː'briːf/ vyslechnout hlášení o průběhu mise apod.

debriefing /ˌdiː'briːf.ɪŋ / skupinový rozbor traumatické události, druh krizové intervence a pomoci, řízená diskuse spojená s edukací

debris /'deb.riː/, /'deɪ.briː/ trosky, úlomky, pozůstatky

deceased /dɪ'siːst/ zemřelý

deceleration /diːˌselə'reɪʃən/ zpomalení, zbrzdění

decerebrate /diˌser.ə'breɪt/ **posturing** /'pɒs.tʃər.ɪŋ/ decerebrační postavení, vnitřní rotace

decision /dɪ'sɪʒ.ən/ rozhodnutí

decode /diː'kəʊd/ dekódovat, rozluštit

decompensated /diː'kɒmpenˌseɪt.əd/ dekompenzovaný

decompensation /diːˌkɒm.pen'seɪ.ʃən/ dekompenzace, selhání kompenzačních mechanismů, udržujících určitou chorobu v přijatelných mezích, vzniká postupem nemoci, následkem přidružení jiné choroby nebo nedodržením léčby

decompress /ˌdiː.kəm'pres/ snížit tlak

decompression /ˌdiː.kəm'preʃ.ən/ dekomprese, snížení tlaku

decompression /ˌdiː.kəm'preʃ.ən/ **sickness** /'sɪk.nəs/ dekompresní nemoc

decontamination /ˌdiː.kən.tæm.ɪ'neɪ.ʃən/ dekontaminace, odmoření

decorticate /ˌdi.ko:'ti'keɪt/ **posturing** /'pɒs.tʃər.ɪŋ/ dekortikační postavení (rigidita), při zvýšeném nitrolebním tlaku, následkem ischemie mozku nebo poškození hemisfér, změny postavení končetin, flexe loktů, zápěstí a prstů a extenze dolních končetin

decrease /dɪ'kriːs/ snížit se, zmenšit, pokles

deem /diːm/ považovat co za jaké

deep /diːp/ hluboký, dlouhý

deeply /'diːp.li/ hluboce, zhluboka

defamation /ˌdefə'meɪʃən/ pomluva, hanobení

defence /dɪ'fent s/ obrana, obhajoba, ochrana

defer /dɪ'fɜ:r/ odložit, pozdržet, podrobit se

defibrillate /ˌdiːˈfɪb.rɪ.leɪt/ defibrilovat

defibrillation /diːˌfɪb.rɪˈleɪ.ʃən/ defibrilace, léčebný úkon, kterým se zruší fibrilace komor, použití elektrického výboje, který na čas „vymaže" veškerou chaotickou srdeční činnost a umožní nástup pravidelnějšího rytmu, výkon zachraňující život, fibrilace komor bez léčby vede rychle k smrti

deficiency /dɪˈfɪʃ.ənt.si/ deficit, nedostatek, nedostatečnost

deficit /ˈdef.ɪ.sɪt/ deficit, nedostatek

definitive /dɪˈfɪn.ɪ.tɪv/ definitivní, konečný

deflate /dɪˈfleɪt/ vyfouknout, splasknout

deflation /dɪˈfleɪ.ʃən/ vyfouknutí

deformity /dɪˈfɔː.mɪ.ti/ deformita, zdeformování, znetvoření

degenerative /dɪˈdʒen.ər.ə.tɪv/ degenerativní

degree /dɪˈgriː/ stupeň, míra, postupně

dehydrated /ˌdiː.haɪˈdreɪ.tɪd/ dehydratovaný, odvodněný

dehydration /ˌdiː.haɪˈdreɪ.ʃən/ odvodnění, vysychání

delay /dɪˈleɪ/ zdržet, odkládat, odložit, zpozdit, zpoždění

delayed /dɪˈleɪd/ zpožděný, odložený

delegate /ˈdel.ɪ.gət/ delegát, zástupce, pověřit

delirium tremens /dɪˌlɪr.i.əmˈtrem.ənz/ kvalitativní porucha vědomí při chronickém alkoholismu

deliver /dɪˈlɪv.ər/ předat, doručit

delivery /dɪˈlɪv.ər.i/ porod, narození, dodání

delusion /dɪˈluː.ʒən/ klam, mámení (smyslů)

delusional /dɪˈluː.ʒən.əl/ klamný

demand /dɪˈmɑːnd/ požadavek, žádat, požadovat

demented /dɪˈmen.tɪd/ dementní, vyšinutý

dementia /dɪˈmen.ʃə/ demence, slabomyslnost

demonstrate /ˈdem.ən.streɪt/ předvádět, vyložit, ukázat, dokázat, dát najevo

deny /dɪˈnaɪ/ odmítat, zapřít, popřít, popírat

department /dɪˈpɑːt.mənt/ oddělení, úsek, obor

dependence /dɪˈpen.dənt s/ závislost

dependent /dɪˈpen.dənt/ závislý, odkázaný, podmíněný

deploy /dɪˈplɔɪ/ nasadit, rozmístit

deployment /dɪˈplɔɪ.mənt/ nasazení, rozmístění

depressant /dɪˈpres.ənt/ látka s tlumivým účinkem

depression /dɪˈpreʃ.ən/ pokles, krize, deprese, stlačení

deprive /dɪˈpraɪv/ zbavit, sebrat, připravit o co

depth /depθ/ hloubka, intenzita, důkladnost

derangement /dɪˈreɪndʒd.mənt/ vyšinutí, pomatenost, porucha

dermis /ˈdɜː.mɪs/ dermis, škára, kožní vrstva

descend /dɪˈsend/ sestoupit, klesání

despite /dɪˈspaɪt/ navzdory, i přes

destination /ˌdes.tɪˈneɪ.ʃən/ destinace, místo určení, cílová stanice cíl cesty

destruction /dɪˈstrʌk.ʃən/ destrukce, zkáza, zničení

detached /dɪˈtætʃt/ oddělený, samostatně stojící

detachment /dɪˈtætʃmənt/ oddělení, odstup, odloučení

detect /dɪˈtekt/ zjistit, objevit, určit

detector /dɪˈtek.tər/ detektor, čidlo

deteriorate /dɪˈtɪə.ri.ə.reɪt/ zhoršit, zhoršovat

deterioration /dɪˌtɪə.ri.əˈreɪ.ʃən/ zhoršení kvality, úpadek

determination /dɪˌtɜː.mɪˈneɪ.ʃən/ určení, stanovení

determine /dɪˈtɜː.mɪn/ určit, stanovit, zjistit, rozhodnout

detoxify /diːˈtɒk.sɪ.faɪ/ detoxikovat

devastating /ˈdev.ə.steɪ.tɪŋ/ devastující, zničující, katastrofální

development /dɪˈvel.əp.mənt/ vývoj, vznik

deviate /ˈdiː.vi.eɪt/ odchýlit se

deviation /ˌdiː.vɪˈeɪʃən/ deviace, odchylka, úchylka, vybočení

device /dɪˈvaɪs/ zařízení, prostředek, vybavení, přístroj

dextrose /ˈdek.strəʊs/ dextróza, D-glukóza

diabetic /ˌdaɪəˈbet.ɪk/ diabetický

diabetic /ˌdaɪəˈbet.ɪk/ ketoacidosis /ˈkiː.təʊ ˌæs.ɪˈdəʊ.sɪs/ diabetická ketoacidóza, acidóza způsobená nadměrným množstvím ketolátek v krvi

diagnose /ˈdaɪəgˌnəʊz/ stanovit diagnózu

diagnosis /ˌdaɪ.əgˈnəʊ.sɪs/ diagnóza

dialysis /daɪˈæl.ə.sɪs/ dialýza

diameter /daɪˈæm.ɪ.tər/ průměr (kružnice)

diaphoresis /ˌdaɪ.ə.fəˈriː.sɪs/ diaforéza, pocení

diaphoretic /ˌdaɪ.ə.fəˈret.ɪk/ diaforetický, opocený

diaphragm /ˈdaɪ.ə.fræm/ bránice, přepážka

diarrhoea /ˌdaɪ.əˈriː.ə/ průjem

diastole /daɪˈæs.tə.li/ diastola, ochabnutí srdeční svaloviny po předchozí kontrakci (systole)

diastolic /daɪˈæs.tə.lɪk/ diastolický

differential /ˌdɪf.əˈren.t ʃəl/ různící se, rozdílový

diffuse /dɪˈfjuːz/ pronikat, rozšířit se, roztrousit (se)

diffused /dɪˈfjuːst/ rozptýlený, roztroušený, rozšířený, nejasný, neohraničený

diffusion /dɪˈfjuː.ʒən/ difuze, pronikání

digestion /daɪˈdʒes.tʃən/ trávení, zažívání

digestive /da ɪˈdʒes.tɪv/ trávicí, zažívací

digit /ˈdɪdʒ.ɪt/ prst na ruce i noze, číslice

digital /ˈdɪdʒ.ɪ.təl/ digitální

digitalis /ˌdɪdʒ.ɪˈteɪ.lɪs/ digitalis, náprstník bot.

dignity /'dɪg.nɪ.ti/ důstojnost (v chování)

digoxin /dɪdʒ.ɒ k.sɪn/ digoxin, přípravek se používá k léčbě chronické srdeční nedostatečnosti

dilatation /ˌdɪl.ə'teɪ.ʃən/ dilatace, rozšíření

dilated /daɪ'leɪtɪd/ rozšířený, dilatovaný

dilation /daɪ'leɪ.ʃən/ dilatace, rozšíření, roztažení

dilemma /daɪ'lem.ə/ dilema, těžké rozhodování

diligent /'dɪl.ɪ.dʒənt/ svědomitý, pečlivý

dilute /daɪ'lu:t/ zředit, oslabit

dilution /daɪ'lu:ʃən/ oslabení, zředěný roztok

diminish /dɪ'mɪnɪʃ/ zmenšit se, slábnout, ubývat

diphenhydramine /di.fen'hɪ.drə.mɪːn/ difenylhydramin, antihistaminikum, užívané v léčbě alergických poruch

direct /da ɪ'rekt/ nasměrovat, zamířit, řídit, dohlížet

direction /da ɪ'rek.ʃən/ směr, vedení, řízení, pokyn, instrukce

directive /daɪ'rek.tɪv/ směrnice

directly /da ɪ'rekt .li/ přímo, okamžitě

director /daɪ'rek.tər/ vedoucí, šéf

disable /dɪ'seɪbl/ zmrzačit, vyřadit z činnosti

disabled /dɪ'seɪbld/ invalidní, neschopný

disadvantage /ˌdɪs.əd'vaːn.tɪdʒ/ nevýhoda

disappear /ˌdɪs.ə'pɪər/ zmizet

disassemble /ˌdɪs.ə'sem.bl̩/ rozmontovat, rozložit

disaster /dɪ'zɑː.stər/ pohroma, neštěstí, katastrofa

disc /dɪsk/ ploténka (meziobratlová), kotouč

discharge /dɪs'tʃɑːdʒ/ výtok, odtok, sekret, výměšek, propustit, vyměšovat, vylučovat

discoloration /dɪˌskʌl.ə'reɪ.ʃən/ zabarvení, změna barvy

discomfort /dɪ'skʌmp .fət/ obtíž, mírná bolest, nepohoda, znepokojení, nepohoda

discontinuation /ˌdɪs.kənˌtɪn.ju'eɪ.ʃən/ ukončení, zastavení

discover /dɪ'skʌv.ər/ objevit, zjistit

disease /dɪ'ziːz/ onemocnění

disentanglement /ˌdɪs.ɪn'tæŋ.gl̩.mənt/ rozpletení, vyproštění

disinfection /ˌdɪs.ɪn'fek.'ʃən/ desinfekce

dislocation /ˌdɪs.lə'keɪ.ʃən/ dislokace, vykloubení, narušení

dislodge /dɪ'slɒdʒ/ uvolnit, vytlačit, vypudit

disorder /dɪ'sɔː.dər/ porucha, choroba, potíže

disorderly /dɪ'sɔː.dəl.i/ chaotický, výtržnický

dispatch /dɪ'spætʃ/ vyslat, poslat, odeslat, odeslání

dispatcher /dɪ'spætʃər/ dispečer

displace /dɪ'spleɪs/ vytlačit, nahradit

displacement /dɪ'spleɪs.mənt/ vytlačení, odsunutí

dispose of /dɪˈspəʊz/ odklidit, odstranit, zbavit se něčeho

disposition /ˌdɪs.pəˈzɪʃ.ən/ rozmístění, umístění

disrupt /dɪsˈrʌpt/ narušit, zkomplikovat, přerušit, roztrhat

disruption /dɪsˈrʌp.ʃən/ disrupce, trhlina, porušení, protržení, porucha, otevření rány

dissecting /daɪˈsekt.ɪŋ/ **aortic** /eɪˈɔː.tɪk/ **aneurysm** /ˈæn.jʊə.rɪ.zəm/ disekující aneurysma aorty

dissipate /ˈdɪs.ɪ.peɪt/ rozptýlit se

distal /ˈdɪ.stəl/ distální, vzdálený od centra, periferní

distance /ˈdɪs.tənt s/ vzdálenost

distant /ˈdɪs.tənt/ vzdálený, odměřený, nepřístupný

distend /dɪˈstend/ roztáhnout se, zduřet

distension /dɪˈsten.tʃən/ distenze, roztažení, rozepětí, rozšíření

distinct /dɪˈstɪŋkt/ odlišný, zřetelný

distinction /dɪˈstɪŋk.ʃən/ rozdíl, odlišnost

distinguish /dɪˈstɪŋ.gwɪʃ/ rozlišit, rozeznat, odlišit

distorted /dɪˈstɔː.tɪd/ překroucený, pokroucený

distraught /dɪˈstrɔːt/ silně rozrušený

distress /dɪˈstres/ nouze, tíseň, utrpení, strádání, bolest, úzkost, strach

distribute /dɪˈstrɪb.juːt/ rozdávat, distribuovat

distributive /dɪˈstrɪbjʊtɪv/ distributivní, rozdělený

disturb /dɪˈstɜːb/ vyrušit, rozrušit

disturbance /dɪˈstɜː.bənt s/ nepokoj, výtržnost, porucha

diuretic /ˌdaɪ.jʊəˈret.ɪk/ diuretický, močopudný lék

dive /daɪv/ potápět se v moři ap.

diverticulitis /ˌdaɪ.və.tɪk.jʊˈlaɪ.tɪs/ divertikulitida, zánět divertikulu

divide /dɪˈvaɪd/ rozdělit, dělit se

diving /ˈdaɪ.vɪŋ/ **reflex** /ˈriː.fleks/ reflex zahrnující kardiovaskulární a metabolické adaptace pro uchování kyslíku vyskytující se u živočichů během potápění do vody

dizziness / ˈdɪz.ɪ.nəs/ závrať, točení hlavy, mrákotný stav

Do Not Resuscitate /rɪˈsʌs.ɪ.teɪt/ **order** /ˈɔː.dər/ pokyn neoživovat

doctrine /ˈdɒk.trɪn/ doktrina, nauka

domestic /dəˈmes.tɪk/ domácí, rodinný

doom /duːm/ zkáza, zánik

dopamine /ˈdəʊ.pə.miːn/ dopamin, chemická látka, která umožňuje přenos impulsů v mozku

dosage /ˈdəʊ.sɪdʒ/ dávky, dávkování

dose /dəʊs/ porce, dávka, příděl

down /daʊn/ dole, spadnout, srazit

downhill /ˌdaʊnˈhɪl/ dolů z kopce, pod kopcem

downward /ˈdaʊn.wəd/ dolů směřující, sestupný

downwind /ˌdaʊnˈwɪnd/ po větru, ve směru větru

drain /dreɪn/ odvést, odtéct, vysušit

drainage /ˈdreɪ.nɪdʒ/ odvodnění, odtok

draw /drɔ:/ pohybovat se, táhnout, natáhnout, načerpat

drawing /ˈdrɔ:.ɪŋ/ natáhnutí

dress /dres/ ošetřit, ovázat ránu

drip /drɪp/ kapat, kapka, kapačka

drive /draɪv/ úsilí, snaha, odpal

driveway /ˈdraɪvˌweɪ/ příjezdová cesta, vjezd

drizzle /ˈdrɪz.əl/ mrholit, mžení

drool /dru:l/ slintat, sliny tekoucí z úst

droop /dru:p/ viset, klesat vysílením, sklonit hlavu

drop /drɒp/ klesnout, spadnout, pokles, kapka, upustit na zem

droplet /ˈdrɒp.lət/ kapka, kapička

drowning /ˈdraʊn.ɪŋ/ tonutí, utopení

drowsiness /ˈdraʊ.zɪ.nəs/ ospalost, mátožnost

drowsy /ˈdraʊ.zi/ ospalý, mátožný

drunk /drʌŋk/ opilý, opilec

due /dju:/ **to** /tʊ/ kvůli, následkem, v důsledku, díky

dig /dɪg/ **out** /aʊt/ vykopat, vyhrabat

dull /dʌl/ tupý, pomalý, tlumený

dullness /ˈdʌl.nəs/ tupost, netečnost, hloupost

duodenum /ˌdju:.əˈdi:.nəm/ dvanácterník

duplex /ˈdju:.pleks/ dvojitý, zdvojený

dura mater /ˌdjʊə.rəˈmeɪ.tə/ dura mater, tvrdá plena

durable /ˈdjʊərəbəl/ trvalý

duration /djʊəˈreɪ.ʃən/ délka, doba trvání

dusky /ˈdʌs.ki/ tmavý, tlumený o barvě

duty /ˈdju:tɪ/ povinnost, úkol, služba

dysphasia /disˈfeɪ.zɪə/ dysfázie, porucha řeči

dyspnoea /dɪs.pni:.ə/ dyspnoe, dušnost, porucha dýchání

dysrhythmia /dɪsˈrɪθ.mɪə/ dysrytmie, porucha rytmu

E

earlobe /ˈɪə.ləʊb/ ušní lalůček

easing /ˈi:z.ɪŋ/ zmírnění, uvolnění

eatery /ˈi:tərɪ/ veřejná jídelna

ecchymosis /ˌekiˈməʊ.sɪs/ ekchymóza, tečkovité krvácení na sliznicích

eclampsia /ɪˈklæmp.si.ə/ eklampsie, pozdní gestóza, komplikace těhotenství

ectopic pregnancy /ekˌtɒp.ɪkˈpreg.nən.si/ mimoděložní těhotenství

edge /edʒ/ okraj, břeh

effacement /ɪˈfeɪs.mənt/ správné rozšíření děložních cest při normálním porodu

effect /ɪˈfekt/ efekt, účinek, dopad

effective /ɪˈfek.tɪv/ efektivní, účinný

effectiveness /ɪˈfek.tɪv.nəs/ účinnost, efektivnost

efficiently /ɪˈfɪʃ.ənt.li/ efektivně, účinně

effort /ˈef.ət/ snaha, úsilí

eject /ɪˈdʒekt/ vyhodit, prudce vyvrhnout

ejection /ɪˈdʒekt.ʃən/ vyhození, katapultování

elasticity /ˌɪl.æsˈtɪs.ɪ.ti/ elasticita, pružnost

elder /ˈeldə/ starší člověk

elderly /ˈel.dəl.i/ postarší, starší

electrical /ɪˈlek.trɪ.kəl/ **line** /laɪn/ elektrické vedení

electrocution /ɪˌlek.trəˈkjuː.ʃən/ smrt elektickým proudem

electrolyte /ɪˈlek.trə.laɪt/ elektrolyt, roztok, který vede elektřinu

element /ˈelɪmənt/ element, prvek, součást

elevate /ˈel.ɪ.veɪt/ zvednout

elevated /ˈel.ɪ.veɪ.tɪd/ vysoký, zvýšený

elevation /ˌel.ɪˈveɪ.ʃən/ zvýšení, povýšení

eliminate /ɪˈlɪm.ɪ.neɪt/ eliminovat, odstranit

elimination /ɪˌlɪm.ɪˈneɪ.ʃən/ eliminace, vylučování, odstranění, vypouštění

emanate /ˈem.ə.neɪt/ vycházet, proudit, vyzařovat

emancipate /ɪˈmænsɪˌpeɪt/ emancipovat, zrovnoprávnit

emancipated /ɪˈmæn.sɪ.peɪ.tɪd/ emancipovaný, zletilý

embedded /ɪmˈbed.ɪd/ pevně usazený, zarytý

embolism /ˈembəˌlɪzəm/ embolie, náhlé zablokování krevní cévy

embolus emboli /ˈem.bə.ləs/ embolus, vmetek, krevní sraženina

emerge /ɪˈmɜːdʒ/ objevit se, vynořit se

emergency /ɪˈmɜː.dʒənt.si/ naléhavá nutnost, pohotovost

emesis /eˈmɪ.sɪs/ emeze, zvracení

emotional /ɪˈməʊ.ʃən.əl/ emocionální, citový

emotionally /ɪˈməʊ.ʃən.əl.i/ emočně, citově

emphysema /ˌemp.fəˈsiː.mə/ emfyzém, rozedma (plic), rozšíření tkání plynem nebo vzduchem

employee /ɪmˈplɔɪ.iː/ zaměstnanec

EMT, Emergency /ɪˈmɜː.dʒənt.si/ **Medical** /ˈmed.ɪ.kəl/ **Technician** / tekˈnɪʃən/ zdravotník rychlé záchranné služby

en route, enroute /ˌɒnˈruːt/ cestou, během cesty

enact /ɪˈnækt/ schválit, uzákonit

encephalopathy /enˌsef.əˈlɒp.ə.θi/ encefalopatie, mozkové onemocnění různého původu

enclose /ɪnˈkləʊz/ uzavřít, obklopit

encode /ɪnˈkəʊd/ zakódovat, zašifrovat

encounter /ɪnˈkaʊntə/ setkat se, setkání, zkušenost

encourage /ɪnˈkʌr.ɪdʒ/ povzbudit, vést

end /end/ **-tidal** /ˈtaɪ.d əl/ týkající se respiračního vzduchu, hodnota CO_2 na konci výdechu, $ETCO_2$

endocardium /ˌen.dəˈkɑː.di.əm/ endokard, srdeční nitroblána

endocrine /ˈen.də.krɪn/ endokrinní, s vnitřní sekrecí

endometriosis /ˌen.dəʊˌmiː.triˈəʊ.sɪs/ endometrióza, ložiska tkáně podobná děložní sliznici na neobvyklých místech

endometritis /ˌen.də.miˈtraɪ.tɪs/ endometritida, zánět děložní sliznice

endotracheal /en.dɒ.trəˈkiː.əl/ **tube** /tjuːb/ (**ET tube)** endotracheální trubice, trubice do průdušnice

enforcement /ɪnˈfɔː.smənt/ prosazování, prosazení, vymáhání, vynucení

engage /ɪnˈɡeɪdʒ/ obsadit, zaměstnávat, zapadat, zajistit

enhance /ɪnˈhɑːns/ zlepšit, zvýšit, zesílit

enlist /ɪnˈlɪst/ získat, nabrat

ensure /ɪnˈʃɔːr/ zajistit, postarat se

entire /ɪnˈtaɪə/ celý, úplný, veškerý

entrap /ɪnˈtræp/ chytit do pasti, polapit

entrapment /ɪnˈtræp.mənt/ uvíznutí, chycení do pasti

envenomation /ɪnˌven.əˈmeɪ.ʃən/ vniknutí jedu do těla při kousnutí nebo štípnutí

environment /ɪnˈvaɪ.rən.mənt/ prostředí pro činnost, životní prostředí

epidural /ˌepɪˈdjʊərəl/ epidurální, umístění nad durou

epigastric /ˌepɪˈɡæs.trɪk/ epigastrický, nadbřiškový

epigastrium /ˌepɪˈɡæs.tri.əm/ nadbřišek

epiglottis /ˌep.ɪˈɡlɒt.ɪs/ příklopka hrtanová

epiglottitis /ˌep.ɪ.ɡləˈtaɪ.tɪs/ epiglotitida, zánět příklopky hrtanové

epinephrine /ˌepɪˈnef.ri:n/ epinefrin (US), hormon vylučovaný nadledvinou, adrenalin

episode /ˈep.ɪ.səʊd/ epizoda, záchvat

equal /ˈiːkwəl/ stejný, rovnat se (čemu)

equation /ɪˈkweɪ.ʒən/ rovnice, srovnání

equilibrium /ˌiːkwɪˈlɪbriəm/ rovnováha, vyrovnanost, vyváženost

equipment /ɪˈkwɪp.mənt/ vybavení, zařízení, výstroj

equivalent /ɪˈkwɪv.əl.ənt/ ekvivalent, protějšek, obdoba, stejný, rovnající se čemu

erratic /ɪˈræt.ɪk/ nepředvídatelný, nevypočitatelný

error /ˈer.ər/ omyl, chyba

erythrocyte /ɪˈrɪθ.rəʊ.saɪt/ erytrocyt, červená krvinka

escape /ɪˈskeɪp/ únikový, utéct, uniknout, uprchnout

essential /ɪˈsen.t ʃəl/ základní, důležitý, hlavní

establish /ɪˈstæb.lɪʃ/ navázat, založit, vytvořit, ustavit, vybudovat

estimate /ˈes.tɪ.meɪt/ odhad, odhadnout

ethanol /ˈeθ.ə.nɒl/ etanol, etylalkohol

ethics /ˈeθɪk/ etika, morálka

euphoria /juːˈfɔː.ri.ə/ euforie, radostná nálada

eustress /juː.stres/ dobrý, pozitivní stres

evacuate /ɪˈvæk.ju.eɪt/ evakuovat, vyklidit

evaluate /ɪˈvæl.ju.eɪt/ zhodnotit, ocenit, stanovit

evaluation /ɪˌvæl.juˈeɪ.ʃən/ ohodnocení, ocenění, zhodnocení, vyhodnocení

event /ɪˈvent/ událost, případ, akce

evidence /ˈevɪdəns/ důkaz, známka čeho, svědčit

evident /ˈev.ɪ.dənt/ zjevný, očividný, zřejmý

evisceration /ɪˌvɪs.əˈreɪ.ʃən/ eviscerace, vynětí orgánů z těla

exacerbation /ɪɡˌzæsəˈbeɪʃən/ zhoršení, ztížení

examination /ɪɡˌzæm.ɪˈneɪ.ʃən/ lékařská prohlídka, vyšetření

examine /ɪɡˈzæm.ɪn/ prohlédnout, vyšetřit

examiner /ɪɡˈzæm.ɪ.nər/ vyšetřovatel, zkoušející

exceed /ɪkˈsiːd/ převládat, přesahovat (míru), převýšit, přesáhnout

excellent /ˈek.səl.ənt/ vynikající

excess /ekˈses/ nadměrný, přebytečný

excessive /ekˈses.ɪv/ nadměrný, přílišný, nepřiměřený

exchange /ɪksˈtʃeɪndʒ/ výměna

exclude /ɪkˈskluːd/ vyloučit, vyřadit, zabránit vniknutí

excluding /ɪkˈskluː.dɪŋ/ vyjma, kromě

excretion /ɪkˈskriː.ʃən/ exkrece, vyměšování, vylučování

excruciating /ɪkˈskruː.ʃi.eɪ.tɪŋ/ nesnesitelný, mučivý

exercise /ˈek.sə.saɪz/ cvičit, cvičení, výkon

exert /ɪɡˈzɜːt/ vyvíjet, uplatnit, vyvinout (tlak)

exertion /ɪɡˈzɜː.ʃən/ úsilí, námaha

exhalation /ˌeks.h əˈleɪ.ʃən/ vydechnutí

exhale /eksˈheɪl/ vydechnout, vydechovat

exhaustion /ɪɡˈzɔːs.tʃən/ vyčerpání, vyčerpanost

exhibit / ɪɡˈzɪb.ɪt/ ukázka, projevit, projevovat příznaky

exophthalmos /ˌeks.ɒfˈθæl.məs/ exoftalmus, vystouplé oko

expand /ɪkˈspænd/ rozšířit se, zvětšit, roztáhnout

expansion /ɪkˈspæn.tʃən/ expanze, rozpínání, roztahování, rozrůstání

expectorate /ɪkˈspek.tər.eɪt/ vykašlávat (hlen)

expedite /ˈek.spə.daɪt/ urychlit

expel /ɪkˈspel/ být vyloučen, vypudit, vyhnat

expend /ɪkˈspend/ vydat, vynaložit, spotřebovat

experience /ɪkˈspɪə.ri.ənt s/ zkušenost, prožít, zažít, prožívat, prodělat, ucítit

experienced /ɪkˈspɪə.ri.ənst/ zkušený, zběhlý

expiration /ˌek.spəˈreɪ.ʃən/ vypršení, uplynutí

expiratory /ɪkˈspɪr.ə.tər.i/ expirační, výdechový

explosion /ɪkˈspləʊ.ʒən/ exploze, výbuch (též přen.)

explosive /ɪkˈspləʊ.sɪv/ výbušnina, výbušný

explosive /ɪkˈspləʊ.sɪv/ **delivery** / dɪˈlɪv.ər.i/ překotný porod

exposed /ɪkˈspəʊzd/ exponovaný, odhalený, obnažený, nechráněný, vystavený

exposure /ɪkˈspəʊ.ʒə/ obnažení, vystavení

express /ɪkˈspres/ vyjádřit, projevit, vyslovit

expressed /ɪkˈspresd/ vyjádřený, projevený, vyslovený

expression /ɪkˈspreʃ.ən/ projev, vyjádření, výraz, výraz tváře

expulsion /ɪkˈspʌl.ʃən/ expulze, vypuzení z těla, vykašlávání, vypuzení

extension /ɪkˈsten.tʃən/ natažení, prodloužení, rozšíření

extensive /ɪkˈsten.sɪv/ rozsáhlý, značný

extenuating /ɪkˈsten.ju.eɪ.tɪŋ/ polehčující okolnosti

external /ɪkˈstɜː.nəl/ externí, vnější, zevní

extraction /ɪkˈstræk.ʃən/ extrakce, vynětí

extravasation /eksˌtræ.və'seɪ.ʃən/ extravazát, výron, únik tekutiny do okolní tkáně

extreme /ɪkˈstriːm/ extrém, krajnost, nejvyšší bod

extremely /ɪkˈstriːm.li/ extrémně, nesmírně, neobyčejně

extremity /ɪkˈstrem.ɪ.ti/ končetina

extricate /ˈek.strɪ.keɪt/ vyprostit, vymanit

extrication /ˌek.strɪˈkeɪ.ʃən/ vyproštění, vysvobodit, vyprostit

extubate /eks.tjʊ.beɪt/ extubovat

extubation /ˌeks.tjʊˈbeɪ.ʃən/ extubace

eyebrow /ˈaɪ.braʊ/ obočí

eyewear /ˈaɪweər/ oční optika

F

face /feɪs/ **down** /daʊn/ směřovat dolů

facial /ˈfeɪ.ʃəl/ obličejový, lícní

facilitate /fəˈsɪl.ɪ.teɪt/ usnadnit, ulehčit

factor /ˈfæk.tər/ faktor, činitel, prvek

faecal /ˈfiː.kəl/ fekální, týkající se stolice

faeces /ˈfiː.siːz/ fekálie, výkaly

fail /feɪl/ selhat, neuspět

failure /ˈfeɪ.ljə/ porucha, selhání, závada, výpadek, neúspěch, nezdar, neschopnost

faint /feɪnt/ slabý, tlumený, malátný, na omdlení, ztratit vědomí, omdlít

faith /feɪθ/ víra, důvěra, náboženské vyznání

fall /fɔːl/ (fell, fallen) padnout, padat k zemi, pád

fallopian tube /fəˌləʊ.pi.ənˈtjuːb/ vejcovod

false /fɒls/ **imprisonment** /ɪmˈprɪz. ən.mənt/ neoprávněné zadržení

falsely /ˈfɒls.li/ nesprávně, nepravdivě

familiar /fəˈmɪl.i.ər/ **with** /wɪð/ seznámený, dobře známý

farther /ˈfɑː.ðər/ dále

fast-moving /fɑːsˈtmuː.vɪŋ/ rychle se pohybující

fat-based /fæt.beɪst/ tukový

421

fatigue /fə'tiːg/ únava, oslabení, vysílení, vyčerpání, unavit se
favourably /'feɪ.vər.ə.bḷi/ příznivě
fear /fɪə/ strach, obava, úzkost
febrile /'fiː.braɪl/ febrilní, horečnatý
feedback /'fiːd.bæk/ zpětná vazba
feeding /ˌfiː.dɪŋ/ krmení, výživa, stravování
feeling /'fiː.lɪŋ/ pocit, mínění, citlivost
female /'fiː.meɪl/ žena
femoral /'femərəl/ femorální, stehenní
femur femora /'fiː.mər/ femur, kost stehenní
fence /fens/ plot, ohrada
fertilize /'fɜː.tɪ.laɪz/ oplodnit
fever /'fiː.vər/ horečka
fibrillate /'faɪ.brɪ.leɪt/ fibrilovat, jednotlivá vlákna srdečního svalu nebo jejich skupiny se stahují samostatně, fibrilace komor bez léčby vede rychle k smrti
fibrillation /ˌfaɪ.brɪ'leɪ.ʃən/ fibrilace, míhání, velmi rychlé a nepravidelné stahy, např. srdce, fibrilace srdečních komor
fibroserous /ˌfaɪ.brə'sɪə.rəs/ fibroserózní, týkající se vláknité a serózní blány
fibula pl -ae /'fɪb.jʊ.lə/ fibula, kost lýtková
field /fiːld/ terén
fight or flight /ˌfaɪt.ɔː.'flaɪt/ reakce na nebezpečí, zůstat a čelit situaci nebo uprchnout
fill /fɪl/ naplnit, zaplnit
final /'faɪ.nəl/ závěrečná zkouška

finding /'faɪndɪŋ/ závěr, zjištění, nález
fingernail /'fɪŋ.gə.neɪl/ nehet na ruce
fingerstick /'fɪŋ.gə.stɪk/ píchnutí do prstu
fire fighter /'faɪəˌfaɪ.tər/ hasič
fire-fighting /'faɪəˌfaɪ.tɪŋ/ protipožární zásahy
firewall /'faɪə.wɔːl/ protipožární přepážka, požární zeď
fireworks /'faɪəˌwɜːk/ rachejtle, zábavní pyrotechnika
firm /fɜːm/ pevný
firmly /'fɜːm.li/ pevně
fist /fɪst/ pěst, praštit pěstí
fit /fɪt/ odpovídat, pasovat, slučovat se, zapadat, odpovídat, v dobré kondici
fixture /'fɪks.tʃər/ příslušenství, vybavení
flaccid /'flæksɪd/ ochablý, povadlý
flail /fleɪl/ chest /tʃest/ paradoxní dýchání při zlomenině žeber
flail /fleɪl/ volně se pohybující (bez svalové kontroly)
flaming /'fleɪ.mɪŋ/ planoucí, hořící
flank /flæŋk/ bok, slabina, strana
flare /fleər/ zarudnutí, vzplanout
flash /flæʃ/ blesk, záblesk, blesknout, vznítit se, zapálit se
flat /flæt/ plochý, rovný
flavoured /fleɪ.vəd/ ochucený, s příchutí
flexion /flek.ʃən/ flexe, ohnutí, ohyb, ohýbání
flight /flaɪt/ of stairs /steərz/ rameno schodiště mezi patry
flood /flʌd/ záplava, povodeň

flotation /fləʊˈteɪ.ʃən/ **equipment** / ɪˈkwɪp.mənt/ plovací vybavení

flow /fləʊ/ tok, proud, příliv, téci, proudit

flowing /ˈfləʊ.ɪŋ/ proudící, plynoucí, tekoucí

fluid /ˈfluː.ɪd/ tekutina, kapalina

flulike /ˈfluː.laɪk/ podobný chřipce

flush /flʌʃ/ propláchnout, pročistit

flushed /flʌʃt/ zrudlý, červený

flutter /ˈflʌt.ər/ chvění, míhání, kmitání srdečních komor nebo síní

fly /flaɪ/ (flew, flown) letět

flying /ˈflaɪ.ɪŋ/ létající

focused /ˈfəʊkəst/ cílený, zaměřený, soustředěný

foetal /ˈfiː.təl/ fetální, plodový

foetus /ˈfiː.təs/ fetus, plod

fontanelle /ˌfɒn.təˈnel/ fontanela, neosifikované místo v lebce novorozeněte

food /fuːd/ **-borne** /bɔːn/ přenášený potravou

footwear /ˈfʊt.weər/ obuv

force /fɔːs/ síla, účinnost, nutit, vyvíjet tlak, přinutit, donutit, zatlačit, natlačit

forced /fɔːst/ nucený, násilný

forcefully /ˈfɔːs.fəl.i/ silně, energicky

forceps /ˈfɔː.seps/ chirurgické, lékařské kleště

forearm /ˈfɔː.rɑːm/ předloktí

forehead /ˈfɒrɪd/, /ˈfɔːˌhed/ čelo hlavy

foreign /ˈfɒr.ən/ **body** /ˈbɒd.i/ cizí tělísko

foreshadow /fɔːˈʃæd.əʊ/ naznačovat, předznamenat

form /fɔːm/ formulář

formation /fɔːˈmeɪ.ʃən/ formování, vytvoření, útvar

forward /ˈfɔː.wəd/ přední, dopředu, posunout dopředu

foul /faʊl/ odporný

found /faʊnd/ nalezený

Fowler's /ˈfowˈler/ **position** /pəˈzɪʃ. ən/ Fowlerova poloha, poloha v polosedě při které má nemocný hlavu a trup zvednutý 45 – 90°

fracture /ˈfræk.tʃə/ zlomenina

frail /freɪl/ křehký, slabý

Frank-Starlings mechanism / ˈmekəˌnɪzəm/ Frankův-Starlingův mechanismus, zákon, zvýšená náplň srdce na konci diastoly (preload) zvýší intenzitu srdečního stahu, množství krve vypuzené při následné systole – tepový objem

fraternity /frəˈtɜː.nə.ti/ bratrstvo, jednota

freak /friːk/ bizarní, neobvyklý, ztratit hlavu, šílet

free /friː/ svobodný, volný, zbavený, prostý

frequency /ˈfriː.kwən.si/ frekvence, četnost výskytu

friction /ˈfrɪk.ʃən/ frikce, tření

frostbite /ˈfrɒst.baɪt/ omrzlina

frostbitten /ˈfrɒstˌbɪt.ən/ omrzlý

froth /frɒθ/ pěna, pěnit se

frown /fraʊn/ zamračit se, zamračený pohled

fruity /ˈfruː.tɪ/ ovocný

fulcrum /ˈfʊl.krəm/ opora, podpora

full /fʊl/ plný, úplně

full-blown /ˌfʊlˈbləʊn/ zralý, plnohodnotný, rozvinutý

full-term (infant) /fʊlˈtɜːm/ plně donošené dítě, kojenec narozený mezi 38. a 41. týdnem

fundal /ˈfʌn.dəl/ týkající se fundu, dna

fundus /ˈfʌn.dəs/ pl. -di fundus, dno, f. uteri dno dělohy

fungus /ˈfʌŋ.gəs/ (pl fungi) houba, plíseň:

funny /ˈfʌn.i/ zvláštní, podivný

furosemide /fjʊr.ɔsˈæm.aɪd/ furosemid, silné diuretikum

furthermore /ˌfɜː.ðəˈmɔːr/ navíc, kromě toho

G

gag /gæg/ navalovat se, téměř zvracet

gag /gæg/ **reflex** /ˈriːfleks/ reflex zvracení

gain /geɪn/ získat, nabýt

gall bladder, gallbladder /ˈgɔːlˈblæd.ər/ žlučník

gallon /ˈgæl.ən/ galon, v Británii 4,546 l, v USA 3,785 l

garbage /ˈgɑː.bɪdʒ/ **can** /kæn/ popelnice

garbled /ˈgɑː.bl̩d/ zkomolený, překroucený

garment /ˈgɑːmənt/ oděv, oblek

gas /gæs/ plyn

gaseous /ˈgeɪ.si.əs/ plynný

gasp /gɑːsp/ lapat po dechu, zalapat po dechu

gastric /ˈgæs.trɪk/ gastrický, žaludeční

gastric /ˈgæs.trɪk/ **tube** /tjuːb/ žaludeční sonda

gastritis /gæsˈtraɪ.tɪs/ gastritida, zánět žaludku

gather /ˈgæð.ər/ shromáždit, získat, zjistit, dozvědět se

gauze /gɔːz/ gáza, mul

gear /gɪə/ rychlostní stupeň (u auta), výstroj, výzbroj, vybavení

gel /dʒel/ gel

general /ˈdʒen.ər.əl/ celkový, všeobecný

generalized /ˈdʒen.ə r.ə.laɪzd/ všeobecný

generally /ˈdʒen.ə r.əl.i/ celkově, obvykle, obyčejně

generate /ˈdʒen.ər.eɪt/ generovat, shromáždit, vytvořit, vyvolat

genital /ˈdʒen.ɪ.təl/ genitálie, pohlavní

genitourinary /ˌdʒen.ɪ.təʊˈjʊə.rɪ.nər,i/ močopohlavní

gentle /ˈdʒen.tl̩/ jemný

gently /ˈdʒent.li/ jemně, mírně

geriatric /ˌdʒer.iˈæt.rɪk/ geriatrický

gestation /dʒesˈteɪ.ʃən/ gestace, gravidita, těhotenství

get up /get.ʌp/ vstát, být vzhůru

Glasgow /ˌglɑːz.gəʊ/ **Coma** /ˈkəʊ.mə/ **Scale** /skeɪl/ Glasgowská škála kómatu

glottic /ˈglɒt.ɪk/ hlasivkový

glottis /ˈglɒt.ɪs/ **glottides** glotis, hlasivková štěrbina, nejužší část hrtanu

gloved /glʌvd/ v rukavicích

glucometer /ˌgluːkəˈm.ɪ.tər/ glukometr

glucose /'glu:.kəʊs/ glukóza, hroznový cukr
goal /gəʊl/ cíl
goblet /'gɒb.lət/ sklenka, pohárek
goggle /'gɒg‚l/ ochranné brýle
golden /'gəʊl.dən/ **rule** /ru:l/ zlaté pravidlo
gonorrhoea /‚gɒn.ə'ri:.ə/ gonorea, kapavka
goof /gu:f/ **around** /ə'raʊnd/ blbnout, dělat kraviny
govern /'gʌv.ən/ řídit, ovládat
gown /gaʊn/ plášť
grab /græb/ snažit se popadnout
grade /greɪd/ stupeň, kvalita
gradual /'græd.jʊ.əl/ postupný, pozvolný
gradually /'græd.jʊ.li/ postupně
grain /greɪn/ obilí, zrní
grand mal /‚grɑ:nd'mæl/ velký epileptický záchvat
grape /greɪp/ hroznové víno
grave /greɪv/ závažný, smrt, hrob
Graves' /greɪvz/ **disease** /dɪ'zi:z/ Gravesova-Basedowova nemoc, autoimunitní onemocnění štítné žlázy provázené její hyperfunkcí
gravida /‚græv.ɪ.də/ gravidní
gravidity /græv'ɪd.ɪ.ti/ gravidita, těhotenství
greenish /'gri:.nɪʃ/ nazelenalý
greenstick /gri:n.stɪk/ **fracture** /'fræktʃə/ nalomená kost
grimace /'grɪ.məs/ grimasa, úšklebek
groin /grɔɪn/ slabiny, třísla, rozkrok
gross /grəʊs/ hrubý, drsný

ground /graʊnd/ zem, podlaha, území, dopadnout, přistát
grounded /graʊnd.ɪd/ uzemněný
growth /grəʊθ/ růst, vývoj
grunt /grʌnt/ chrčet, chrochtat
guard /gɑ:d/ bránit, chránit se
guidance /'gaɪ.dəns/ odborné vedení, poučení, rada
guideline /'gaɪd.laɪn/ směrnice, instrukce
gunpowder /'gʌn‚paʊ.dər/ střelný prach
gunshot /'gʌn.ʃɒt/ střela, výstřel
gutter /'gʌt.ər/ okap, okapový žlab
gynaecology /‚gaɪ.nə'kɒl.ə.dʒi/ gynekologie

H
haematoma haematomata /‚hi:.mə'təʊ.mə/ hematom, krevní výron, podlitina, modřina
haematuria /‚hi:.mə.t'jʊə.ri.ə/ hematurie, krev v moči
haemodialysis /‚hi:mə.daɪ'ælɪsɪs/ hemodyalýza, mimotělní očisťovací krevní metoda
haemodynamic /‚hi:mə.daɪ'næm.ɪk/ hemodynamický, týkající se krevní cirkulace
haemopneumothorax /'hi:.mə‚nju:.mə'θo:.ræks/ hemopneumotorax, nahromadění krve a plynu v plicích
haemoptysis /hi:'mɒ.ptɪ.sɪs/ hemoptýza, vykašlávání krve
haemorrhage /'hem.ər.ɪdʒ/ krvácení, vnitřní krvácení

haemostasis /ˌhiː.məˈsteɪ.sɪs/ hemostáza, zástava krvácení, zástava krevní cirkulace

haemothorax /ˈhiː.məˈθoː.ræks/ hemotorax, nahromadění krve v dutině hrudní

hallmark /ˈhɔːl.mɑːk/ typický znak, známka

hallucination /həˌluː.sɪˈneɪ.ʃən/ halucinace, přelud

hallucinogen /həˈluː.sɪ.nə.dʒen/ halucinogen, prostředek na vyvolání halucinace

hand /hænd/ **over** /ˈəʊ.vər/ předat, odevzdat

hand-held /ˈhændheld/ přenosný, ruční

handgun /ˈhændˌgʌn/ ruční střelná zbraň, pistole ap.

handicapped /ˈhæn.dɪ.kæpt/ postižený

handle /ˈhæn.d|/ zvládnout, poradit si, ovládat, brát do ruky, manipulovat

handlebar /ˌhæn.d|.bɑː/ řídítka jízdního kola

handling /ˈhænd.lɪŋ/ manipulace

hands-on /ˌhændˈzɒn/ praktický, osobní, přímý

handwash /ˈhændˌwɒʃ/ mýt ruce

hang /hæŋ/ viset

hanging /ˈhæŋɪŋ/ zavěšení, pověšení, oběšení

hard /hɑːd/ silně, tvrdě

harden /ˈhɑː.dən/ ztvrdnout, ztuhnout

harm /hɑːm/ ublížit, zranit, poškodit, ublížení, zranění

harmful /ˈhɑːm.fəl/ škodlivý, zhoubný, zdravotně závadný

harsh /hɑːʃ/ drsný, výrazný

hazard /ˈhæz.əd/ hazard, riziko, nebezpečí

hazmat /ˈhæz.mæt/ nebezpečný materiál

head on, head-on /ˌhedˈɒn/ čelně, zepředu, zpříma

heal /hiːl/ hojit, léčit, vyléčit se, zahojit

health care, healthcare /helθ//keə/ zdravotní péče

health /helθ/ **status** /ˈsteɪ.təs/ zdravotní stav

hear /hɪər/ (heard, heard) slyšet

heart /hɑːt/ **rate** /reɪt/ srdeční frekvence

heartbeat /ˈhɑːt.biːt/ tlukot srdce

heat /hiːt/ **cramp** /kræmp/ křeč z horka

heat /hiːt/ **exhaustion** /ɪgˈzɔːs.tʃən/ vyčerpání z horka

heat /hiːt/ **stroke** /strəʊk/ úžeh, úpal

heave /hiːv/ zvedat se (žaludek), dávit

Heimlich maneuver /ˈhaɪm.lɪk. məˌnu.vər/ Heimlichův manévr, hmat určený k vypuzení předmětu, který ucpal dýchací cesty

held /held/ držený, ovládaný

helmet /ˈhel.mət/ helma

helpless /ˈhelplɪs/ bezmocný, bezradný

hemiparalysis /ˌhem.ɪ.pəˈræl.ə.sɪs/ viz hemiparesis

hemiparesis /ˌhem.ɪ.pəˈriː.sɪs/ hemiparéza, částečné ochrnutí jedné poloviny těla

hepatic /hepˈæt.ɪk/ hepatický, jaterní

hepatitis /ˌhep.əˈtaɪ.tɪs/ hepatitida, zánět jater

herniation /ˌhɜː.niˈeɪ.ʃən/ herniace, vysunutí části orgánu mimo jeho přirozené místo, vytvoření kýly

herpes /ˈhɜː.piːz/ herpes opar

herpes /ˈhɜː.piːz/ **simplex** /ˈsɪm.pleks/ opar rtu

herpes /ˈhɜː.piːz/ **zoster** /zɒ.stər/ pásový opar

herpes-virus /ˈhɜː.piːzˈvaɪ.rəs/ skupina virů způsobující opary

HHNK, Hyperosmolar /ˌhaɪ.pə.ɒz.mɒ.lər/ **Hyperglycaemic** /ˌhaɪ.pə.glaɪˈsiː.mɪk/ **Nonketotic** /ˌnɒn.ke.tɒt.ɪk/ **Coma** /ˈkəʊmə/ hyperosmolární diabetické kóma bez ketoacidózy, vysoká hladina krevního cukru, která způsobuje výraznou hyperosmolaritu se ztrátami tekutin a minerálních látek močí při výrazné polyurii, projevuje se zejm. nervovými a oběhovými příznaky až kómatem

hiatal /haɪˈeɪ.təl/ **hernia** /ˈhɜː.ni.ə/ hiátová hernie neboli hiátová kýla je vysunutí (herniace) z horní části žaludku do hrudníku přes trhliny nebo zeslabení bránice

hiatus /haɪˈeɪ.təs/ otvor, mezera

high-pitched /ˌhaɪˈpɪtʃt/ vysoký, ostrý, pronikavý zvuk

hip /hɪp/ bok, kyčel

histamine /ˈhɪs.tə.miːn/ histamin

history /ˈhɪs.tər.i/ anamnéza, příběh, historka

hit /hɪt/ (hit, hit) udeřit, narazit, vrazit, zasáhnout, trefit, narazit, udeřit, uhodit

hives /haɪvz/ kopřivka

hoarse /hɔːs/ chraplavý, ochraptělý

hoarseness /hɔːsnɪs/ ochraptění, chrapot, chraplavost

hold /həʊld/ pořádat, podržet, pojmout, obsahovat

hole /həʊl/ díra, otvor, mezera

hollow /ˈhɒl.əʊ/ prázdný, vpadlý, propadlý

Homans' /ˈhəʊ.mænz/ **sign** /saɪn/ Homansovo znamení, orientační klinický test používaný k vyšetřování hluboké flebotrombózy dolní končetiny

homeless /ˈhəʊm.ləs/ bez domova, bezdomovec

homeostasis /ˌhəʊ.mi.əʊˈsteɪ.sɪs/ homeostáza, dynamická rovnováha

honour /ˈɑn.ər/ ctít, respektovat

hopeless /ˈhəʊp.ləs/ zoufalý, beznadějný

host /həʊst/ hostitel

humerus pl -ri /ˈhjuː.mə.rəs/ humerus, kost pažní

humid /ˈhjuː.mɪd/ vlhký

humidified /hjuːˈmɪd.ɪ.faɪd/ zvlhčený

humidity /hjuːˈmɪd.ɪ.ti/ vlhkost

humoral /ˈhjuː.mər.əl/ humorální, týkající se tělesných tekutin

hunting /ˈhʌn.tɪŋ/ **knife** /naɪf/ lovecký nůž

hurt /hɜːt/ (hurt, hurt) zranit, poranit

hydration /haɪˈdreɪ.ʃən/ hydratace, zavodnění

hydrogen /ˈhaɪ.drɪ.dʒən/ vodík

hyperactivity /ˌhaɪ.pərˈæk'tɪv.ɪ.ti/ hyperaktivita

hyperadrenalism /ˌhaɪ.pər.ædˈri:. nəl.ɪzm/ hyperadrenalismus, zvýšená sekrece adrenalinu

hyperextension /ˌhaɪ.pərˈɪkˈstenʃən/ nadměrné protažení

hyperflexion /ˌhaɪ.pəˈflæk.ʃən/ hyperflexe, násilné ohnutí

hyperglycaemia /ˌhaɪ. pə.glaɪˈsiːmi.ə/ hyperglykémie, zvýšené množství glukózy v krvi

hyperglycaemic /ˌhaɪ.pə.glaɪ.ˈsiː. mɪk/ s nadměrným množstvím glukózy v krvi

hyperkalaemia /ˌhaɪ.pə.kæˈliːmi.ə/ hyperkalemie, nadbytek draslíku v krvi

hyperosmolar /ˌhaɪ.pə.ɒz.mɒ.lər/ **coma** /ˈkəʊmə/ hyperosmolární kóma, akutní komplikace cukrovky

hyperresonance /ˌhaɪ.pə.ˈrez. ən.əns/ nadměrná zvučnost

hyperresonant /ˌhaɪ.pə.ˈrez.ən.ənt/ nadměrně zvučný, rezonující

hypersensitivity /ˌhaɪ.pə.ˌsen. sɪˈtɪv.ɪ.ti/ hypersensitivita, přecitlivělost

hypertension /ˌhaɪ.pəˈten.ʃən/ hypertenze, vysoký krevní tlak

hypertensive /ˌhaɪ.pəˈten.sɪv/ hypertenzní, se zvýšeným krevním tlakem

hyperthermia /ˌhaɪ.pəˈθɜː.mɪ.ə/ hypertermie, přehřátí

hypertonia /ˌhaɪ.pəˈtəʊ.niə/ hypertonie, zvýšené napětí (svalové)

hypertrophy /haɪˈpɜː.trə.fi/ hypetrofie, zvětšení, zbytnění, zvětšení orgánu

hyperventilate /haɪ.pəˈven.tɪ.leɪt/ nadměrně rychle dýchat

hyperventilation /ˌhaɪ.pəˌven.tɪˈleɪ. ʃən/ hyperventilace, chorobně zvýšená plicní ventilace

hypervolaemia /ˌhaɪ.pəˌvoˈliːmi.ə/ hypervolemie, nadbytek cirkulující krve

hyphaema /haɪ.θe.mə/ hyféma, krev v přední komoře oční před duhovkou

hypocalcaemia /ˌhaɪ.pəʊ.kælˈsiː. mi.ə/ hypokalcemie, nedostatek vápníku v krvi

hypoglycaemia /ˌhaɪ.pəʊ.glaɪˈsiː. mi.ə/ hypoglykémie, snížená koncentrace glukózy v krvi

hypokalaemia /ˌhaɪ.pəʊ.kæˈliːmi.ə/ hypokalemie, nedostatek draslíku v krvi

hypomagnesaemia /ˌhaɪ.pəʊ.ˌmæg. nəˈsiːmi.ə/ hypomagnezemie, nedostatek hořčíku v krvi

hypoperfusion /ˌhaɪ.pəʊ.pəˈfjuː. ʒən/ nedokrvení, snížená perfuze, nedostatečné zásobování orgánů tekutinou

hypotension /ˌhaɪ.pəʊˈten.tʃən/ hypotenze, nízký tlak

hypothermia /ˌhaɪ.pəʊ'θɜː.mi.ə/ hypotermie, nízká tělesná teplota, podchlazení

hypothesize /haɪ'pɒθ.ə.saɪz/ předpokládat, vyslovit hypotézu

hypotonia /ˌhaɪpəʊ'təʊ.niə/ hypotonie, snížené svalové napětí

hypoventilation /ˌhaɪpəʊˌven.tɪ'leɪ. ʃən/ hypoventilace, omezené dýchání

hypovolaemia /ˌhaɪpəʊ.və'lː.mi.ə/ hypovolemie, nízký objem krve v těle

hypoxaemia /ˌhai.pɒk'siː.mi.ə/ hypoxemie, snížené množství kyslíku v krvi

hypoxia /haɪ'pɒk.sɪə/ hypoxie, nedostatečné zásobování tkání kyslíkem

hypoxic /haɪ'pɒk.sɪk/ **drive** /draɪv/ stimulace dýchání nízkým stavem PaO$_2$ (parciální tlak kyslíku v tepenné arteriální krvi)

I

ice /aɪs/ **pack** /pæk/ sáček s ledem, ledový obklad

ICP, Intracranial /ɪn.trə'kreɪ.ni.əl/ **Pressure** /'preʃ.ər/ nitrolebeční tlak

identifiable /aɪ'den.tɪ.faɪ.ə.bļ/ identifikovatelný, rozpoznatelný

identification /aɪˌden.tɪ.fɪ'keɪ.ʃen/ identifikace, určení, rozpoznání

identify /aɪ'den.tɪ.faɪ/ identifikovat, určit, rozeznat, rozpoznat, ztotožňovat se

idioventricular /ˌɪd.i.əʊ.ven'trɪk. jə.lər/ idioventrikulární, týkající se pouze

srdečních komor

iliac /'ɪl.i.æk/ **crest** /krest/ kyčelní hřeben

illegal /ɪ'liː.gəl/ nezákonný

illegible /ɪ'ledʒ.ə.bļ/ nečitelný

illness /'ɪl.nəs/ nemoc

image /'ɪm.ɪdʒ/ představa, obraz, dojem

imbalance /ˌɪm'bæl.ənt s/ nerovnováha, nevyrovnanost

immediate /ɪ'miː.di.ət/ bezprostřední, okamžitý

immediately /ɪ'miː.di.ət.li/ okamžitě, ihned

immerse /ɪ'mɜːs/ ponořit se, potopit

immersion /ɪ'mɜː.ʃən/ ponoření, potopení

imminent /'ɪm.ɪ.nənt/ bezprostřední, hrozící, blízký, nadcházející

immobilization /ɪˌməʊ.bəl.aɪ'zeɪ. ʃən/ imobilizace, znehybnění, fixace

immunocompromised /ˌim. jə.nəʊ'kɒm.prə.maɪzd/ s ohroženou imunitou

impact /'ɪm.pækt/ dopad, náraz, úder, účinek, vliv, výsledek, dopadat, natlačit

impair /ɪm'peər/ oslabit, poškodit, narušit, zhoršit, oslabit, omezit funkci

impaired /ɪm'peəd/ oslabený, poškození

impairment /ɪm'peər.mənt/ zhoršení, poškození

impale /ɪm'peɪl/ nabodnout, napíchnout

impending /ɪmˈpen.dɪŋ/ blížící se, bezprostředně hrozící, nastávající, budoucí

imperative /ɪmˈper.ə.tɪv/ nezbytně nutný, zcela nezbytný

implant /ɪmˈplɑːnt/ uhnízdit se, usadit, implantát

implantation /ˌɪm.plænˈteɪ.ʃən/ implantace, uhnízdění vajíčka v děloze

implied /ɪmˈplaɪd/ implicitní, nepřímo vyjádřený

impression /ɪmˈpreʃ.ən/ dojem, pocit, znak

improper /ɪmˈprɒp.ər/ nevhodný, nesprávný, nestandardní, nezákonný

improperly /ɪmˈprɒp.ər.li/ nesprávně, nevhodně

improve /ɪmˈpruːv/ zlepšit, zotavit se, uzdravit se

improvement /ɪmˈpruːv.mənt/ zlepšení, zdokonalení

impulse /ˈɪm.pʌls/ impuls, podnět

in addition /əˈdɪʃ.ən/ navíc k čemu, kromě

in advance /ədˈvɑːns/ před čím dříve

in extremis /ˌɪn.ɪkˈstriː.mɪs/ krajní, v krajním případě

in order to /ˈɔː.dər/ aby, kvůli

in writing /ˈraɪ.tɪŋ/ písemně

inability /ˌɪn.əˈbɪl.ɪ.ti/ neschopnost, nemožnost, nezpůsobilost

inaccurate /ɪˈnæk.jʊ.rət/ nepřesný

inactivity /ˌɪn.ækˈtɪv.ɪ.ti/ nečinnost

inadequate /ɪˈnæd.ɪ.kwət/ nedostatečný, neschopný

inadvertent /ˌɪn.ədˈvɜː.tənt/ neúmyslný, nepozorný, nedbalý

inappropriate /ˌɪn.əˈprəʊ.pri.ət/ nepatřičný, nevhodný, neúčelný

inappropriately /ˌɪn.əˈprəʊ.pri.ət.li/ nepatřičně, nevhodně

inattentiveness /ˌɪn.əˈten.tɪv.nəs/ nepozornost

inch /ɪntʃ/ palec, 2,5 cm

incidence /ˈɪnt.sɪ.dənt s/ výskyt, počet případů, četnost nemoci ap.

incident /ˈɪnt.sɪ.dənt/ incident, mimořádná událost, případ

incline /ɪnˈklaɪn/ sklánět se, tíhnout, mít sklon

incompatible /ˌɪn.kəmˈpæt.ɪ.bl̩/ inkompatibilní, neslučitelný

incompetent /ɪnˈkɒm.pɪ.tənt/ neschopný, nezpůsobilý

incomplete /ˌɪn.kəmˈpliːt/ neúplný, nedokončený

incomprehensible /ɪnˌkɒm.prɪˈhen.sɪ.bl̩/ nesrozumitelný

incomprehensibly /ɪnˌkɒm.prɪˈhen.sɪ.bli/ nesrozumitelně

incontinent /ɪnˈkɒn.tɪ.nənt/ inkontinentní, neschopný udržet moč, stolici

increase /ɪnˈkriːs/ zvýšit, zvýšení

increasingly /ɪnˈkriː.sɪŋ.li/ stále více, čím dál tím víc (jaký)

indicate /ˈɪn.dɪ.keɪt/ indikovat, označit, ukazovat

indication /ˌɪn.dɪˈkeɪ.ʃən/ indikace, údaj, označení, léčebný příkaz

indicator /ˈɪn.dɪ.keɪ.tər/ indikátor, ukazatel

individual /ˌɪn.dɪˈvɪd.ju.əl/ jednotlivec

indoors /ˌɪnˈdɔːz/ uvnitř, v domě

infancy /ˈɪn.fənt .si/ dětství (útlé)

infant /ˈɪnfənt/ nemluvně, kojenec, malé dítě, dítě do 1 roku

infarction /ɪnˈfɑːk.ʃən/ infarkt

infectious /ɪnˈfek.ʃəs/ nakažlivý, infekční

inferior /ɪnˈfɪə.ri.ər/ dolní

inferior /ɪnˈfɪə.ri.ər/ **vena cava** /ˌviː. nəˈkeɪ.və/ dolní dutá žíla

infiltration /ˌɪn.fɪlˈtreɪ.ʃən/ infiltrace, prosakování, prostoupení orgánů zánětlivými či nádorovými buňkami či jinými látkami

inflamed /ɪnˈfleɪmd/ zanícený

inflammation /ˌɪn.fləˈmeɪ.ʃən/ zánět

inflammatory /ɪnˈflæm.ə.tər.i/ zánětlivý

inflate /ɪnˈfleɪt/ nafouknout

inflation /ɪnˈfleɪ.ʃən/ naplnění, nafouknutí

influence /ˈɪnfluəns/ vliv, účinek

influenza /ˌɪn.fluˈen.zə/ chřipka

informed /ɪnˈfɔːmd/ informovaný, poučený

infrapatellar /ˌɪn.frə.pəˈtel.ər/ infrapatelární, podčéškový

infrastructure /ˈɪn.frəˌstrʌk.tʃər/ infrastruktura

infusion /ɪnˈfjuː.ʒən/ infuze, nalévání, nálev

ingestion /ɪnˈdʒes.tʃən/ přijímání potravy, trávení

inguinal /ˈɪŋ.gwɪ.nəl/ ingvinální, tříselný

inhalation /ˌɪn.həˈleɪ.ʃən/ vdechování, nádech

inhale /ɪnˈheɪl/ nadechovat

inhaler /ɪnˈheɪ.lər/ inhalátor, inhalační přístroj

inhibit /ɪnˈhɪb.ɪt/ zabránit, tlumit, zpomalovat, znemožnit

initial /ɪˈnɪʃ.əl/ iniciála, šifra, počáteční, výchozí

initially /ɪˈnɪʃ.əl.i/ nejprve, zpočátku, původně, na začátku

initiate /ɪˈnɪʃ.i.eɪt/ zahájit, započít

injury /ˈɪndʒərɪ/ úraz

inner /ˈɪn.ər/ vnitřní

innervate /ˈɪn.ə.veɪt/ inervovat, povzbudit (nerv nebo orgán k činnosti)

insatiable /ɪnˈseɪ.ʃə.bl̩/ nenasytný

insect /ˈɪn.sekt/ hmyz

insert /ɪnˈsɜːt/ vložit, vsunout

insertion /ɪnˈsɜː.ʃən/ zasazení, aplikace (vložka)

insist /ɪnˈsɪst/ trvat na čem, vyžadovat

insomnia /ɪnˈsɒm.ni.ə/ insomnie, nespavost

inspect /ɪnˈspekt/ prohlédnout, prozkoumat

inspection /ɪnˈspek.ʃən/ prohlédnutí, prohlídka, kontrola, vyšetřování nemocného pohledem

inspiration /ˌɪn.spɪˈreɪ.ʃən/ inspirace, vdechnutí, vdech

inspiratory /ɪnˈspaɪə.rə.tər.i/ inspirační, vdechový

instability /ˌɪn.stəˈbɪl.ɪ.ti/ nestabilita, labilita

instead /ɪnˈsted/ místo toho, raději

institute /ˈɪn.stɪ.tjuːt/ zahájit, započít

institutionalization /ˌɪnt.stɪˌtjuː.ʃən.əl.aɪˈzeɪ.ʃən/ hospitalizace, umístění do léčebného ústavu

instruct /ɪnˈstrʌkt/ instruovat, nařídít, dát pokyn

instrument /ˈɪn.strə.mənt/ nástroj, přístroj

insufficiency /ˌɪn.səˈfɪʃ.ən.si/ nedostatečnost

insulin /ˈɪn.sjʊ.lɪn/ inzulín

insult /ˈɪn.sʌlt/ poškození tělesného orgánu, tkáně, urazit, slovně napadnout

intact /ɪnˈtækt/ intaktní, netknutý, nedotčený, neporušený

intake /ˈɪn.teɪk/ příjem, přísun

integral /ˈɪn.tɪ.grəl/ nedílný, celý

integration /ˌɪn.tɪˈgreɪ.ʃən/ integrace, začlenění, včlenění

integrity /ɪnˈteg.rə.ti/ integrita, celistvost

intense /ɪnˈtens/ intenzivní, silný, ostrý

intensity /ɪnˈten.sɪ.ti/ intenzita, síla, ostrost

intentional /ɪnˈtenʃənəl/ úmyslný, záměrný

interact /ˌɪn.təˈrækt/ interagovat, vzájemně se ovlivňovat, spolupracovat

intercostal /ˌɪn.təˈkɒs.təl/ interkostální, mezižeberní

intercostals /ˌɪn.təˈkɒs.təlz/ mezižeberní svaly

interfere /ˌɪn.təˈfɪər/ interferovat, narušovat, vadit, obtěžovat

interference /ˌɪn.təˈfɪə.rəns/ interference, zasahování, rušení

interim /ˈɪn.tər.ɪm/ prozatímní, dočasný, interval, časový úsek

interior /ɪnˈtɪə.ri.ər/ interiér, vnitřek, vnitřní

intermediate /ˌɪn.təˈmiː.di.ət/ prostřední, středně pokročilý

intermittent /ˌɪn.təˈmɪt.ənt/ občasný, přerušovaný

internal /ɪnˈtɜː.nəl/ interní, vnitřní

interrupt /ˌɪn.təˈrʌpt/ přerušit, narušovat, překážet

interruption /ˌɪn.təˈrʌp.ʃən/ přerušení, přerušování, vyrušování

intervention /ˌɪn.təˈven.ʃən/ intervence, zákrok, zásah

intestine /ɪnˈtes.tɪn/ střevo, trakčník

intolerance /ɪnˈtɒl.ər.ənt s/ intolerance, nesnášenlivost

intoxication /ɪnˌtɒk.sɪˈkeɪ.ʃən/ intoxikace, otrava, opilost

intraabdominal /ɪn.trə.æbˈdɒm.ɪ.nəl/ intraabdominální, nitrobřišní

intracerebral /ˌɪn.trəˈser.ə.brəl/ intercerebrální, nitromozkový, ležící uvnitř mozku

intracranial /ˌɪn.trəˈkreɪ.ni.əl/ intrakraniální, nitrolebeční

intramuscular /ˌɪn.trəˈmʌs.kjʊ.lər/ intramuskulární, nitrosvalový

intraosseous /ˌɪn.trəˈɒs.i.əs/ intraoseální, nitrokostní

intrathoracic /ˌɪn.trə.θɔːˈræs.ɪk/ intratorakální, nitrohrudní
intravenous /ˌɪn.trəˈviː.nəs/ intravenózní, nitrožilní
intravenous /ˌɪn.trəˈviː.nəs/ **line** /laɪn/ nitrožilní linka
intravenously /ˌɪn.trəˈviː.nəs.li/ nitrožilně
introduce /ˌɪn.trəˈdjuːs/ zavést, přijít, představit
intubate /ɪnˈtjuː.beɪt/ intubovat, zavést rourku do průdušnice
intubation /ˌɪn.tjuːˈbeɪ.ʃən/ intubace, zavedení rourky do průdušnice
invasion /ɪnˈveɪ.ʒən/ narušení, vpád
invasive /ɪnˈveɪ.sɪv/ invazivní, šířící se, narušující
inverted/ ɪnˈvɜː.tɪd/ obrácený, převrácený
involuntary /ɪnˈvɒləntərɪ/ bezděčný, mimovolný, vůlí neovladatelný, nedobrovolný
involvement /ɪnˈvɒlv.mənt/ účast, zapojení se, vztah
inward /ˈɪn.wəd/ dovnitř směřující, vnitřní
ion /ˈaɪ.ɒn/ iont
ipecac /ˈɪp.ɪ.kæk/ ipecac, lék způsobující zvracení, používaný např. při otravě
iris /ˈaɪrɪs/ oční duhovka
irregular /ɪˈreg.jə.lər/ nepravidelný
irregularity /ɪˌreg.jəˈlær.ə.ti/ nepravidelnost, nesouměrnost
irreversible /ˌɪr.ɪˈvɜː.sɪ.bl̩/ nezvratný

irritability /ˌɪr.ɪ.təˈbɪl.ɪ.ti/ iritabilita, dráždivost, podráždění, podrážděnost, nedůtklivost
irritable /ˈɪr.ɪ.tə.bl̩/ iritabilní, dráždivý, podrážděný
irritant /ˈɪr.ɪ.tənt/ iritující, obtíž, dráždidlo
irritate /ˈɪr.ɪ.teɪt/ dráždit kůži, ránu
irritation /ˌɪr.ɪˈteɪ.ʃən/ podráždění
ischaemia /ɪsˈkiː.mɪ.ə/ ischémie, místní nedokrvenost tkáně
ischaemic /ɪsˈkiː.mɪk/ ischemický, nedokrvený
isolation /ˌaɪ.səlˈeɪ.ʃən/ izolace, osamění, odloučení
isotonic /ˌaɪ.səʊˈtɒn.ɪk/ izotonický, se stejným osmotickým tlakem
itching /ˈɪtʃ.ɪŋ/ svědění, svědící
itchy /ˈɪtʃ.i/ svědivý
item /ˈaɪ.təm/ položka, věc, předmět, bod, záležitost
IV, intravenous /ˌɪn.trəˈviː.nəs/ intravenózní, nitrožilní

J

jagged /ˈdʒæg.ɪd/ rozeklaný, zubatý
jaundice /ˈdʒɔː.n.dɪs/ žloutenka
jaw /dʒɔː/ čelist
jaw /dʒɔː/ **thrust** /θrʌst/ zajištění otevřených dýchacích cest, předsunutí spodní čelisti
jeopardize /ˈdʒep.ə.daɪz/ ohrozit
jerk /dʒɜːk/ trhnout, škubnout, cuknutí, trhnutí, škubnutí
judge /dʒʌdʒ/ posoudit
judgment /ˈdʒʌdʒ.mənt/ úsudek, názor, soudnost, posouzení, soud, odsouzení

jugular /ˈdʒʌɡ.jə.lər/ jugulární, hrdelní, krční, týkající se hrdla
jugular /ˈdʒʌɡ.jə.lər/ **vein** / veɪn/ jugulára, krční žíla
junction /ˈdʒʌŋk.ʃən/ uzel, křížení, spojení
junctional /ˈdʒʌŋk.ʃən.əl/ **tachycardia** /ˌtæk.ɪˈkɑː.di.ə/ tachykardie vznikající v atrioventrikulárním uzlu při srdeční frekvenci vyšší než 75 úderů za minutu
jungle /ˈdʒʌŋ.ɡl/ **gym** /dʒɪm/ prolézačka na dětském hřišti
junky- /ˈdʒʌŋ.ki/ **sounding** / ˈsaʊndɪŋ/ rachotivý
jurisdiction /ˌdʒʊə.rɪsˈdɪk.ʃən/ jurisdikce, soudní pravomoc
JVD, Jugular /ˈdʒʌɡ.jə.lər/ **Venous** / ˈviː.nəs/ **Distension** /dɪˈsten.tʃən/ roztažení krční tepny

K
Kaposi's /kæˈpəʊ.sɪz/ **sarcoma** / sɑːˈkəʊ.mə/ Kaposiho sarkom, kožní onemocnění nádorového charakteru, u nemocných s AIDS, červenofialové kožní uzly, postiženy bývají i vnitřní orgány
keep from /kiːp/ (kept, kept) ubránit, ubránit se, uchovat
ketoacidosis /ˈkiː.təʊˌæ.ɪˈdəʊ.sɪs/ ketoacidóza, acidóza, způsobená nadměrným množstvím ketolátek v krvi
ketone /ˈkiː.təʊn/ keton
kidney /ˈkɪd.ni/ **stones** /stəʊnz/ ledvinové kameny
kidney /ˈkɪd.ni/ ledvina

knee /niː/ -**chest** /tʃest/ **position** / pəˈzɪʃ.ən/ pacientka spočívá na kolenou a horní části hrudníku (při porodu)
kneecap /ˈniː.kæp/ kolenní čéška
knife /naɪf/ nůž, pobodat, říznout
knock /nɒk/ srazit, udeřit

L
label /ˌleɪ.bəl/ nálepka, označit, opatřit štítkem
labour /ˈleɪ.bər/ porodní stahy, začátek porodu
laboured /ˈleɪ.bəd/ obtížný, namáhavý
lacerate /ˈlæs.ər.eɪt/ potrhat, rozervat
laceration /ˌlæsəˈreɪʃən/ lacerace, tržná rána
lack /læk/ nedostatek, postrádat, chybět
lacrimation /ˌlæk.riˈmeɪ.ʃən/ slzení
lactate /lækˈteɪt/ laktát, mléčnan, sůl nebo ester mléčné kyseliny, tvorba l. ve velkém rozsahu způsobuje okyselení vnitřního prostředí, metabolickou acidózu
lactic /ˈlæk.tɪk/ **acid** /ˈæs.ɪd/ kyselina mléčná
ladder /ˈlæd.ər/ žebřík
land /lænd/ dopadnout na zem, přistát
landing /ˈlændɪŋ/ **zone** /zəʊn/ místo přistání, přistávací plocha
lapse /læps/ uplynulá doba, výpadek, vynechání
large /lɑːdʒ/ **bore** /bɔː/, **large-bore** jehla s velkým průměrem, velká jehla

laryngeal /lə'rɪn.dʒi.əl/ laringeální, hrtanový

laryngectomy /ˌlær.ɪn'dʒek.təm.i/ laryngektomie, odstranění hrtanu

laryngoscope /ˌlærɪŋ'gɒ.skəʊp/ laryngoskop, přístroj k zrakovému vyšetření hrtanu

laryngoscopy /ˌlærɪŋ'gɒ.skə.pi/ laryngoskopie, zrakové vyšetření hrtanu pomocí laryngoskopu

laryngospasm /læ'rɪŋ.gə.spæz.əm/ křeč hrtanu

larynx /'lær.ɪŋks/ (pl. larynges) larynx, hrtan

last /lɑːst/ trvat

lasting /'lɑːstɪŋ/ trvalý, stálý

late /leɪt/ pozdní, pokročilý, ke konci

lateral /'læt.rəl/ laterální, boční, postranní

law /lɔː/ -**enforcement** /ɪn'fɔːs. mənt/ **agency** /'eɪ.dʒən.si/ policie a bezpečnostní složky

law /lɔː/ **enforcement** /ɪn'fɔːs.mənt/ prosazování práva, prosazování zákona

law /lɔː/ právo, zákon

lawn mower /'lɔːnˌməʊ.ər/ sekačka trávy

layer / 'leɪ.ə/ vrstva, úroveň, poloha

lead /led/ olovo

lead /liːd/ svod (EKG)

lead /liːd/ zavést, řídit, vedení, vést, být v čele

leading /'liː.dɪŋ/ vedoucí

leaf /liːf/ **leaves** list

leak /liːk/ unikání, otvor, prosakovat

leakage /'liː.kɪdʒ/ únik, ucházení

leaking /liːk.ɪŋ/ výtok, vytékání

lean /liːn/ **forward** /'fɔː.wəd/ naklonit se dopředu

leather /'leð.ər/ kůže zvířecí, kožené oblečení

LeFort II fracture / 'fræk.tʃə/ poranění střední obličejové etáže (nosní kůstky, nazomaxilární komplex), hlavní linie zlomeniny se setkávají v bodu nad nosními kostmi a tvoří trojúhelníkový úsek, oddělený od lebky

legal /'liːgəl/ právní

lengthy /'leŋ.θi/ vleklý, zdlouhavý

lens /lenz/ čočka, kontaktní čočka

lesion /'liː.ʒən/ léze, rána, zranění, poranění, poškození, porucha, postižené místo

lessen /'les.ən/ zmenšit, zmírnit, zmenšit se

lethal /'liː.θəl/ smrtící, smrtonosný

lethargic /lə'θɑː.dʒɪk/ letargický, otupělý, netečný

lethargy /'leθ.ə.dʒi/ letargie, netečnost

leukocyte /'lju:.kə.saɪt/ leukocyt, bílá krvinka

levothyroxine /lev.ɒ.θaɪ'rɒk.sɪn/ levothyroxine, lék na poruchy štítné žláty

liability /ˌlaɪ.ə'bɪl.ɪ.ti/ odpovědnost, závazky, povinnosti, ručení

liable /'laɪ.ə.bl̩/ podléhající, vystavený čemu

libel /'laɪ.bəl/ pomluva, křivé nařčení

licensure /'laɪ.sən.ʃər/ udělení licence

lie /laɪ/ spočívat, ležet
life support /'laɪf.sə‚pɔ:t/ podpora života
life-saving /'laɪf‚seɪ.vɪŋ/ život zachraňující, první pomoc
life-threatening /'laɪf‚θret.ən.ɪŋ/ životu nebezpečný, život ohrožující
lifeguard /'laɪf.gɑ:d/ plavčík na plážích ap.
lift /lɪft/ pozvednout, zdvih
lifting /lɪft.ɪŋ/ zdvihání, zvedání
ligament /'lɪg.ə.mənt/ vaz mezi kostmi, kloubu ap.
ligamentum /‚lɪg.ə'men.təm/ arteriosum /ɑ:‚tiə.ri'ɒs.əm/ ligamentum arteriosum, lat. vazivový pruh, na který se po svém uzavření mění ductus arteriosus, Botallova dučej
light /laɪt/ světlo
light-headed /‚laɪt'hed.ɪd/ malátný, mající závrať, zmámený
light-headedness /‚laɪt'hed.ɪd.nəs/ malátnost
lightning /'laɪt.nɪŋ/ blesk, elektrický výboj
like /laɪk/ podobný čemu
likelihood /'laɪ.kli.hʊd/ pravděpodobnost
likely /'laɪklɪ/ pravděpodobný, vhodný
limb /lɪm/ končetina
lime /laɪm/ vápno
limit /'lɪm.ɪt/ mezní hodnota, omezení, hranice, omezit
limited /'lɪm.ɪ.tɪd/ limitovaný, omezený, malý
limp /lɪmp/ ochablý, skleslý

line / laɪn/-drive /draɪv/ odpal v basebalu, silný úder, míček letí na nebo lehce nad trajektorií
line /laɪn/ čára, linie, přímka, řada, cesta, trasa, linka, spojení, vedení
lingual /'lɪŋgwəl/ lingvální, jazykový
lip /lɪp/ ret, okraj
liquefaction /‚lɪkwɪ'fækʃən/ zkapalnění
list /lɪst/ seznam, soupis
listening /'lɪs.ən.ɪŋ / poslech, naslouchání
liver /'lɪv.ər/ játra
lividity /lɪ'vɪd.ə.ti/ promodralost, sinalost, smrtelná bledost
living /'lɪvɪŋ/ will /wɪl/ poslední vůle
load /ləʊd/ naložit, náklad, zátěž, zatížení, nálož
lobe /ləʊb/ lalok, lalůček
LOC, Level /'levəl/ of consciousness /'kɒn.ʃəs.nɪs/ hladina vědomí
LOC, Loss /lɒs/ of consciousness / 'kɒn.ʃəs.nɪs/ ztráta vědomí
localize /'ləʊ.kəl.aɪz/ lokalizovat, určit polohu
localized /'ləʊ.kəl.aɪzd/ umístěný
locate /ləʊ'keɪt/ najít, vypátrat
log /lɒg/ -roll /rəʊl/, logroll přetočit jako jeden celek
log /lɒg/ záznam, protokol, zaevidovat
logistics /lə'dʒɪs.tɪks/ logistika, systém přepravy a týlového zásobování
lone /ləʊn/ osamocený, samotný
look /lʊk/ pohled, vypadat, budit dojem

looking /lʊk.ɪŋ/ vzhled, vypadající
loop /luːp/ smyčka, obtočit
loose /luːs/ volný, uvolněný, nepřivázaný
loose /luːs/ **weight** /weɪt/ ubrat na váze
loss /lɒs/ ztráta, úbytek, úmrtí, smrt
lotion /ˈləʊ.ʃən/ pleťové mléko, pleťová voda
loudly /ˈlaʊd.li/ hlasitě, důrazně
low /ləʊ/ nízký
low-pitched /ˌləʊˈpɪtʃt/ hluboký, tlumený
lower /ˈləʊ.ə/ **airways** /ˈeə.weɪz/ dolní dýchací cesty
LPM, Liter /ˈliːtə/ **Per** /pə/ **Minute** / ˈmɪnɪt/ litrů za minutu
lumbar /ˈlʌm.bər/ lumbální, bederní
lumen /ˈluː.mən/ pl -mina lumen, průchod, průsvit
lung /lʌŋ/ plíce

M

magnesium /mæɡˈniː.zi.əm/ magnézium, hořčík
magnesium /mæɡˈniː.zi.əm/ **sulphate** /ˈsʌl.feɪt/ síran hořečnatý
main /meɪn/ hlavní, nejdůležitější
mainstem /meɪn.stəm/ **bronchus** /ˈbrɒŋ.kəs/ hlavní průduška
maintain /meɪnˈteɪn/ udržovat, uchovat, zachovat
maintenance /ˈmeɪntɪnəns/ údržba, péče, zachování, udržování
major /ˈmeɪ.dʒə/ hlavní, významný, větší, velký, důležitý, významnější, závažný, převážný

majority /məˈdʒɒr.ə.ti/ většina
malaise /mælˈeɪz/ malátnost, nevolnost
malfeasance /mælˈfiː.zəns/ trestný čin
Mallory-Weis /ˈmæl.ər.i-vaɪs/ **syndrome** /ˈsɪn.drəʊm/ Malloryho-Weissův syndrom, stav charakterizovaný krvácením z lineárních ruptur v oblasti ezofagogastrické junkce, vzniká při silném zvracení, někdy u alkoholiků, jedna z příčin hematemeze
malocclusion /mæl.əˈkluː.ʒən/ špatný skus
mammalian /məˈmeɪ.li.ən/ týkající se savců
manage /ˈmæn.ɪdʒ/ řídit, vést, organizovat, zvládnout, dokázat
management /ˈmænɪdʒmənt/ řízení, ošetření, léčba
mandate /ˈmæn.deɪt/ nařizovat
manhole /ˈmænˌhəʊl/ otvor, průlez, kanalizace
manic /ˈmæn.ɪk/ maniakální, šílený
manifest /ˈmæn.ɪ.fest/ projevit, projev
manipulation /məˌnɪp.jʊˈleɪ.ʃən/ manipulace, ovládání, zacházení
manner /ˈmæn.ər/ chování, styl, zvyk
manoeuvre /məˈnuː.və/ manévr, manipulace, řídit, vést
manual /ˈmæn.ju.əl/ ruční, návod, pokyny
margin /ˈmɑː.dʒɪn/ okraj, pokraj, lem, lemovat

mark /mɑːk/ znak, známka,
skvrna, stopa, otisk
marked /mɑːkt/ zřetelný, výrazný
markedly /ˈmɑː.kɪd.li/ zřetelně
maroon /məˈruːn/ kaštanově
hnědý
mask /mɑːsk/ maska, maskovat
mass /mæs/ hmotnost, hmota,
objem, hromadění velké množství
massage /ˈmæs.ɑːʒ/ masáž,
masírovat
MAST, Military Anti-Shock
Trousers vojenské protišokové
pneumatické kalhoty viz také
PASG
mastoid /ˈmæs.tɔɪd/ mastoidní,
bradavkový
maternal /məˈtɜː.nəl/ těhotenský,
mateřský
matter /ˈmæt.ər/ hmota
mature /məˈtjʊər/ dospělý, zralý
maxillary /mækˈsɪl.ər.i/ čelist,
čelistní
maximal /ˈmæk.sɪ.məl/ maximální
mean /miːn/ znamenat
means /miːnz/ možnosti,
prostředky
measure /ˈmeʒ.ər/ měřit, opatření
measurement /ˈmeʒ.ə.mənt/
měření, míra, velikost
mechanic /mɪˈkænɪk/
mechanismus
mechanics /məˈkæn.ɪks/
mechanika
meconium /mɪˈkəʊ.nɪ.əm/
mekonium, smolka, první stolice
novorozeněte
medial /ˈmiː.di.əl/ středový

mediastinal /ˌmiː.di.əsˈtaɪ.nəl/
mediastinální, mezihrudní
medical /ˈmed.ɪ.kəl/ léčebný,
léčivý, lékařský
medication /ˌmed.ɪˈkeɪ.ʃən/
medikace, léky
medium /ˈmiː.di.əm/ -sized /saɪzd/
středně velký
medium /ˈmiː.di.əm/ středně velký,
průměrný, medium, přenašeč,
střed, prostřední
melaena /məˈliː.n.ə/ melena, černě
zabarvená stolice natrávenou krví
membrane /ˈmem.breɪn/
membrána, blána, blána kryjící
tělesnou část, orgán ap.
meningitis /ˌmen.ɪnˈdʒaɪ.tɪs/
meningitida, zánět mozkových
blan, aseptic m. virová
meningitida
mental /ˈmen.təl/ duševní
mental /ˈmen.təl/ status /ˈsteɪtəs/
duševní stav
mentally /ˈmen.təl.i/ psychicky
mentation /menˈteɪ.ʃən/ duševní
pochody
mercury /ˈmɜː.kjʊ.ri/ rtuť
messy /ˈmes.i/ nepořádný,
neuspořádaný, špinavý
metabolize /mɪˈtæbə.laɪz/
metabolizovat, přeměňovat, trávit
metallic /məˈtæl.ɪk/ kovový
metastatic /ˌmet.əˈstæt.ɪk/ metastatický, týkající se
metastázy
methamphetamine /ˌmeθ.æmˈfet.ə.miːn/ metamfetamin, též
pervitin, syntetické stimulancium z
řad amfetaminů

method /'meθ.əd/ metoda, způsob
meticulous /mə'tɪk.jʊ.ləs/
úzkostlivě pečlivý
METTAG, Medical /'med.ɪ.kəl/
Emergency /ɪ'mɜː.dʒənt.si/ Triage
/'traɪ.ɪdʒ/ Tag /tæg/ označování
pacientů dle závažnosti
zdravotního stavu
MI, Myocardial /maɪ.ə‚kɑː.di.əl/
Infarction /ɪn'fɑːk.ʃən/ infarkt
myokardu
mid /mɪd/ střední
midaxillary /mɪd.æk'sɪl.ər.i/ střed
podpaží
midclavicular /mɪd.klə'vɪk.jʊ.lər/
týkající se střední části klíční kosti
middle /'mɪd.l/ age /eɪdʒ/ střední
věk, 40 – 65 let
middle /'mɪd.l/ prostřední
midline /'mɪd.laɪn/ střednice
migrate /maɪ'greɪt/ migrovat,
stěhovat se
mild /maɪld/ mírný, klidný, slabý,
lehký
military /'mɪl.ɪ.tər.i/ armáda,
vojenský
mimic /'mɪm.ɪk/ napodobovat
mind /maɪnd/ mysl, paměť
minimise / 'mɪn.ɪ.maɪz/
minimalizovat
minor / 'maɪ.nə/ menší, drobný,
malý, nezletilý
miosis /maɪ'əʊ.sɪs/ mióza,
abnormální kontrakce zornice
miscarriage /'mɪs‚kær.ɪdʒ/ potrat
(samovolný)
misinterpret /‚mɪs.ɪn'tɜː.prɪt/
nesprávně interpretovat, mylně
vyložit

misleading /‚mɪs'liː.dɪŋ/ zavádějící,
klamný, mylný
misperception /‚mɪs.pə'sep.ʃən/
klamné vnímání
mist /mɪst/ mlha, aerosol
mistaken /mɪ'steɪ.kən/ mylný,
nesprávný, chybný
misunderstanding /‚mɪs.
ʌn.də'stæn.dɪŋ/ nedorozumění,
špatné pochopení
mitral valve /'maɪ.trəl‚vælv/
mitrální, dvojcípá chlopeň
mittelschmerz /mɪtl.ʃmərθ/ bolest
v oblasti vaječníků uprostřed
ovulačního cyklu
mnemonic /nɪ'mɒn.ɪk/
mnemotechnická pomůcka
MO, Medical /'med.ɪ.kəl/ Officer /
'ɒf.ɪ.sər/ zdravotnický důstojník
modality /məʊ'dæl.ə.ti/ modalita,
možný způsob
mode /məʊd/ způsob, styl, režim
moderate /'mɒd.ər.ət/ mírný,
nevelký, střední, umírněný,
přiměřený
moderately /'mɒd.ər.ət.li/ mírně,
přiměřeně
modify /'mɒdɪ‚faɪ/ modifikovat,
pozměnit
modulation /‚mɒd.jʊ'leɪ.ʃən/
modulace, změna, úprava
moist /mɔɪst/ mokrý, vlhký
(vzduch)
moisten /'mɔɪsən/ navlhčit,
zvlhnout
molecule /'mɒl.ɪ.kjuː.l/ molekula
mood /muːd/ disorder /dɪ'sɔː.dər/
porucha nálady, nejčastější je
deprese a bipolární porucha

mood /muːd/ nálada

mood /muːd/ **swing** /swɪŋ/ výkyv nálady (prudký)

moral /ˈmɒrəl/ morálka, mravy

morbidly /ˌmɔːˈbɪd.ɪ.ti/ chorobně, patologicky

morgue /mɔːg/ márnice

morphine /ˈmɔː.fiːn/ morfium, morfin

morphine /ˈmɔː.fiːn/ **sulphate** /ˈsʌl.feɪt/ morfin sulfát

mortality /mɔːˈtæl.ə.ti/ mortalita, úmrtnost

motion /ˈməʊʃən/ pohyb, pokynout

motionless /ˈməʊ.ʃən.ləs/ nehybný, bez hnutí

motor /ˈməʊ.tər/ motorický, pohybový

mottled /ˈmɒt.|d/ skvrnitý, flekatý, žilkovaný

mouth /maʊθ/ ústa, hrdlo, otvor

move /muːv/ pohnout, hnout

movement /ˈmuːv.mənt/ pohyb

moving /ˈmuːvɪŋ/ pohyblivý

MPH, **Miles** /maɪlz/ **Per** /pə/ **Hour** /aʊə/ mil za hodinu (1 pozemní míle 1609 m)

mucosa /mjuːˈkəʊ.sə/ mukóza, sliznice

mucous membrane /ˌmjuː.kəsˈmem.breɪn/ sliznice

mucus /ˈmjuː.kəs/ mukus, hlen, sliz

muffle /ˈmʌf.ˌl/ utlumit, ztlumit, ztišit

mulch /mʌltʃ/ mulč

multi /mʌl.ti-/ více, mnoha

multifocal /mʌl.tiˈfəʊ.kəl/ víceohniskový

multigravida /mʌl.tiˈgræv.ɪ.də/ vícekrát těhotná

multipara /mʌl.tiˈpær.ə/ vícerodička, žena, která vícekrát rodila

multiparity /mʌl.tiˈpær.ɪt.ɪ/ vícečetný porod

multiple /ˈmʌl.tɪ.p|/ násobek, mnohonásobný, mnohočený

multiplex /ˈmʌl.tɪ.pleks/ mnohonásobný

multiplexing /ˈmʌltiˌpleksɪŋ/ multiplexování, více analogových signálů nebo digitálních datových toků je kombinováno do jednoho signálu, cílem je nejefektivnější využití daného přenosového média

multiply /ˈmʌl.tɪplaɪ/ násobit, rozmnožit

multisystem /ˈmʌl.tɪˈsɪs.təm/ vícesystémový

murmur /ˈmɜː.mər/ šelest, šeptat

Murphy's /ˈmɜː.fiz/ **sign** /saɪn/ Murphyho příznak, pacient je vyzván k nádechu při hluboké palpaci pod pravým žeberním okrajem, při choleocystitidě ucítí bolest

muscle /ˈmʌsəl/ sval

muscle /ˈmʌsəl/ **tone** /təʊn/ tonus svalové napětí

muscular /ˈmʌs.kjʊ.lər/ svalová, svalnatý

mustard /ˈmʌs.təd/ hořčice

MVC, **Motor** /ˈməʊtə/ **Vehicle** /ˈviː.ɪ.kl/ **Collision** /kəˈlɪʒ.ən/ srážka motorového vozidla

mydriasis /maɪˈdraɪ.ə.sɪs/ mydriáza, rozšíření zornice

myocardial /maɪ.əˌkɑː.di.əl/
myokardiální, týkající se srdeční
svaloviny
myocardium /ˌmaɪ.əˈkɑː.di.əm/
myokard, srdeční svalovina

N
NaCl, sodium /ˈsəʊ.di.əm/
chloride /ˈklɔːraɪd/ chlorid sodný,
kuchyňská sůl
nail /neɪl/ bed /bed/ nehtové lůžko
nail /neɪl/ polish /ˈpɒl.ɪʃ/ lak na
nehty
Naloxone /nəˈlɒksəʊn/ naloxon,
antidotum narkotik
narcotic /nɑːˈkɒt.ɪk/ narkotikum,
omamná látka
narrative /ˈnærətɪv/ vyprávění,
příběh
narrow /ˈnær.əʊ/ úzký, těsný,
omezený, zúžit
nasal /ˈneɪ.zəl/ flaring / fleər.
ɪŋ/ zvětšení nosních dírek
při dýchání, klasický příznak
závažného astmatu
nasal /ˈneɪ.zəl/ nosní
nasopharyngeal /ˌneɪ.zə.fəˈrɪn.dʒi.
əl/ nazofaryngeální, nosohltatový
nasopharynx /ˌneɪ.zəˈfær.ɪŋks/
nosohltan
nasotracheal /ˌneɪ.zə.trəˈkiː.əl/
nazotracheální, týkající se nosu a
průdušnice
nature /ˈneɪ.tʃər/ povaha, podstata,
charakter
nausea /ˈnɔː.zi.ə/ nevolnost,
nutkání k zvracení
near /nɪər/ téměř, blízko

nebulized /ˈneb.jə.laɪzd/
nebulizovaný, ve spreji
nebulizer /ˈneb.jə.laɪz.ər/
nebulizér, rozprašovač
necessitate /nəˈses.ɪ.teɪt/
vyžadovat, vynutit si
necrosis /neˈkrəʊsɪs/ nekróza,
odumření, místní odumírání tkáně
need /niːd/ potřeba, nutnost
needle /ˈniː.dl̩/ jehla, střelka
needle /ˈniː.dl̩/ stick /stɪk/ píchnutí
jehlou
negative /ˈneg.ə.tɪv/ bez nálezu,
onemocnění
neglect /nɪˈglekt/ zanedbání,
zanedbávat
negligence /ˈneglɪdʒəns/ nedbalost
negligent /ˈneg.lɪ.dʒənt/ nedbalý
neonate /ˌniː.əʊˈneɪ.t/ neonatus,
novorozenec
neoplasm /ˌniː.əʊˈplæz.əm/
zhoubný nádor
nerve /nɜːv/ nerv
nest /nest/ hnízdo, uhnízdit se
neural /ˈnjʊə.rəl/ neurální, nervový
neurogenic /ˌnjʊə.rəˈdʒen.ɪk/
neurogenní, nervového původu,
vznikající v nervovém systému
neurological /ˌnjʊə.rəˈlɒdʒ.ɪ.kəl/
neurologický
neuropathy /ˌnjʊəˈrɒp.ə.θi/
neuropatie, onemocnění nervů
neurosis /njʊəˈrəʊ.sɪs/ neuróza
neurotoxicity/ˌnjʊər.ə.tɒkˈsɪs.ɪ.ti/
neurotoxicita, schopnost ničit
nervovou tkáň
neutral /ˈnjuː.trəl/ neutrální,
nestranný
newborn /ˈnjuː.bɔːn/ novorozenec

nightmare /ˈnaɪt.meər/ noční
můra, zlý sen
niple /ˈnɪp‚l/ prsní bradavka
nitrogen /ˈnaɪ.trə.dʒən/ dusík,
dusíkatý
nitroglycerin /ˌnaɪ.trəʊˈglɪs.ər.i:n/
nitroglycerin, lék pro zklidnění
srdečních arytmií a snižování
krevního tlaku
Nitronox /ˌnaɪ.trə.nɒks/ nitronox
nitrous oxide /ˌnaɪ.trəsˈɒk.saɪd/
oxid dusný
no matter /ˈmætə/ nehledě na co
nocturnal /nɒkˈtɜ:.nəl/ noční
noise /nɔɪz/ hluk, rámus
non-judgemental /ˌnɒn.dʒʌdʒˈmen.
təl/ neodsuzující
non-productive /ˌnɒn.prəˈdʌk.tɪv/
neproduktivní, suchý (kašel)
nonadherent /ˌnɒn.ədˈhɪə.rənt/
nepřilnavý
noncompliance /ˌnɒn.kəmˈplaɪəns/
nedodržování, nesoulad
nondeliverable /ˌnɒn.dɪˈlɪv.ər.ə.b‚l/
neporoditelný
nondiscernible /ˌnɒn.dɪˈsɜ:.nɪ.b‚l/
nerozeznatelný, neviditelný
nonintact /ˌnɒn.ɪnˈtækt/ neintaktní,
nikoli nedotčený
nonketotic /ˌnɒn.ke.tɒt.ɪk/
neketotický
nonperfusing /ˌnɒn.pər.fju:z.ɪŋ/
neprosakující, nepronikající
nonrebreather /ˌnɒn.rəbrə.
ðər/ **mask** / mɑ:sk/ dýchací
maska jednocestnou klapkou,
vydechnutý oxid uhličitý je
vyloučen a není znovu vdechován

nonsalvageable /ˌnɒn ˈsæl.vɪdʒə.b‚l/
nezachranitelný
norepinephrine /nɔrˌep.əˈnef.
rɪn/ norepinefrin, noradrenalin,
hormon a neurotransmiter
normal /ˈnɔ:.məl/ normální,
obvyklý
note /nəʊt/ zaznamenat, zapsat,
poznámka, vzkaz, zpráva
notice /ˈnəʊtɪs/ zpozorovat,
povšimnout si
noticeable /ˈnəʊ.tɪ.sə.b‚l/ patrný,
zjevný, nápadný
noticeably /ˈnəʊ.tɪ.sə.bli/ zjevně,
znatelně
notify /ˈnəʊtɪ‚faɪ/ oznámit,
uvědomit, informovat
nucha /nju:kə/ šíje, vaz
nuchal /nu:.kəl/ šíjový
nullipara /nʌˈlɪp.ər.ə/ žena, která
dosud nerodila
numbness /ˈnʌm.nəs/ necitlivost,
znecitlivění, ochromení, pocit
necitlivosti
numerous /ˈnju:.mə.rəs/ početný
nurse /nɜ:s/ zdravotní sestra,
ošetřovat
nursing /ˈnɜ:.sɪŋ/ ošetřování, péče,
kojení, krmení
nutrient /ˈnju:.tri.ənt/ výživná
látka, živina

O

obesity /əʊ ˈbi:.sɪ.ti/ obezita
object /ˈɒb.dʒɪkt/ objekt, věc
obscenity /əbˈsen.ɪ.ti/ obscénnost,
sprosté slovo
observable /əbˈzɜ:vəbəl/
pozorovatelný, znatelný

observation /ˌɒb.zəˈveɪ.ʃən/ pozorování, postřehy

observe /əbˈzɜːv/ pozorovat, sledovat, dodržovat

obstetrics /ɒbˈstetrɪks/ porodnictví

obstruct /əbˈstrʌkt/ zablokovat, ucpat

obstruction /əbˈstrʌk.ʃən/ překážka, ucpání

obstructive /əbˈstrʌk.tɪv/ obstrukční, bránící čemu, obstruktivní, ucpávající

obtain /əbˈteɪn/ získat, dosáhnout

obtrude /əbˈtruːd/ narušovat, rušit

obvious /ˈɒb.vi.əs/ zjevný, jasný, zřejmý, očividný, samozřejmý, nápadný

occasion /əˈkeɪ.ʒən/ příležitost, událost

occasional /əˈkeɪʒənəl/ příležitostný, občasný

occasionally /əˈkeɪ.ʒən/ příležitostně, občas

occipital /ɒkˈsɪp.ɪ.təl/ okcipitální, týlní, zátylní

occlusion /əˈkluː.ʒən/ okluze, uzavření

occlusive /ɒˈkluː.sɪv/ **dressing** /ˈdres.ɪŋ/ okluzní obvaz, uzavřený obvaz

occlusive /ɒˈkluː.sɪv/ uzavřený

occupational /ˌɒk.jʊˈpeɪ.ʃən.əl/ pracovní, zaměstnanecký, profesní

occur /əˈkɜːr/ objevit se, nastat, přihodit se, vyskytovat se, nacházet se, existovat

occurrence /əˈkʌr.ənt s/ případ výskytu

odour /ˈəʊ.dər/ odér, pach, zápach

oedema /ɪˈdiː.mə/ edém, otok

oedematous /ɪˈdiː.mə.təs/ edémový, oteklý

oesophageal /iːˌsɒfəˈdʒiːəl/ ezofageální, týkající se jícnu

oesophagus /ɪˈsɒf.ə.gəs/ ezofagus, jícen

officer /ˈɒf.ɪ.sər/ referent, důstojník

official /əˈfɪʃəl/ úředník, představitel, funkcionář

ominous /ˈɒmɪnəs/ zlověstný, hrozivý

oncoming /ˈɒŋˌkʌmɪŋ/ blížící se, protijedoucí

oncotic /ɒŋ.kɒ.tɪk/ **pressure** /ˈpreʃ.ər/ onkotický tlak, osmotický tlak koloidu na membráně pro koloid nepropustné. O. t. nitrobuněčných bílkovin zajišťuje objem intracelulární tekutiny. O. t. plasmatických bílkovin přispívá k udržení dostatečného cirkulujícího objemu krve

ongoing /ˈɒŋˌɡəʊ.ɪŋ/ trvající, pokračující, přetrvávající, dále probíhající

onion /ˈʌn.jən/ cibule (zelenina)

online /ˈɒn.laɪn/ online, přímo spojený

onlooker /ˈɒnˌlʊk.ər/ přihlížející, divák

onset /ˈɒnˌset/ propuknutí, začátek

OPA, Oropharyngeal /ˌɔː.rəˈfərɪn.dʒi.əl/ **Airway** /ˈeə.weɪ/ zařízení používané k udržení otevřených horních dýchacích cest

IRENA BAUMRUKOVÁ

opening / ˈəʊ.pən.ɪŋ/ otevření, otvor

operation /ˌɒp.ərˈeɪ.ʃən/ operace, zásah, akce

ophthalmologist /ˌɒf.θælˈmɒl.ə.dʒɪst/ oftalmolog, oční lékař

opiate /ˈəʊ.pi.ət/ opiát, lék obsahující opium nebo jeho alkaloidy

opinion /əˈpɪn.jən/ názor, mínění

opponent /əˈpəʊ.nənt/ oponent, soupeř, protihráč

opportunistic /ˌɒp.ə.tjuːˈnɪs.tɪk/ oportunistický

opposite /ˈɒp.ə.zɪt/ proti, protilehlý, protějšek

OPQRST, Onset, Provocation, Quality, Radiation, Severity, Time cílená anamnéza, kdy bolest začala, co ji zhoršuje, jak je pociťována, zda se přemisťuje, jak je vážná, jak dlouho trvá

opt /ɒpt/ vybrat si, zvolit

option /ˈɒpʃən/ možnost, volba

orally /ˈɔː.rə.li/ ústně

order /ˈɔː.dər/ pokyn, příkaz, nařízení, pořadí

order /ˈɔːdə/ příkaz

ordered /ˈɔː.dəd/ nařízený, předepsaný

organophosphates /ɔːˌgæn.əʊˈfɒs.feɪts/ organofostáty, organické sloučeniny fosforu

oriented /ˈɔːrɪəntɪd/ orientovaný

original /əˈrɪdʒ.ɪ.nəl/ originální, prvotní, původní

originate /əˈrɪdʒ.ɪ.neɪt/ vzniknout, vytvořit

oropharyngeal /ˈɔː.rə ˌfəˈrɪn.dʒi.əl/ orofaryngeální, týkající se úst a hltanu

oropharynx /ˈɔː.rə ˈfær.ɪŋks/ orofarynx, ústní část hltanu

orthostatic /ˌɔː.θəˈstæt.ɪk/ ortostatický, ve vzpřímené poloze

os /ɒs/ ossa kost

osmolarity /ɒz.məˈlær.ə.ti/ osmolarita, celkové množství osmoticky aktivních částic rozpuštěných v litru rozpouštědla, obv. vody

osmosis /ɒzˈməʊ.sɪs/ osmóza, samovolné pronikání molekul rozpouštědla z méně koncentrovaného roztoku do roztoku koncentrovanějšího

osmotic /ɒzˈmɒt.ɪk/ pressure /ˈpreʃ.ər/ osmotický tlak, tlak tekutiny rozpouštědla na biologické polopropustné membráně

osteomyelitis /ˌɒs.ti.əʊ.maɪ.əlˈaɪ.tɪs/ osteomyelitida, zánět kosti a kostní dřeně

osteoporosis /ˌɒs.ti.əʊ.pəˈrəʊ.sɪs/ osteoporóza, prořídnutí kostí, onem. kosti způsobující úbytek kostní tkáně

otherwise /ˈʌð.ə.waɪz/ jinak, v jiném případě

outcome /ˈaʊtˌkʌm/ výsledek, výsledek čeho, jak věc dopadne, závěr

outermost /ˈaʊ.tə.məʊst/ nejvzdálenější (od středu)

outpatient /ˈaʊt.peɪ.ʃənt/ ambulantní pacient

outpouching /ˈaʊt.paʊtʃ.ɪŋ/ posunutí části tkáně zevnitř navenek, vytvoření váčku
output /ˈaʊtˌpʊt/ výdej, objem, výkon
outset /ˈaʊt.set/ začátek, počátek
outside /ˌaʊtˈsaɪd/ vnější strana, venku
outstretched /ˌaʊtˈstretʃt/ roztažený, natažený, napřažený
outward /ˈaʊt.wəd/ zevní, směřující ven, zevnějšek
ovarian /əʊˈveə.ri.ən/ ovariální, týkající se vaječníků
ovary /ˈəʊ.vər.i/ vaječník
overactive /ˈəʊ.vərˈæk.tɪv/ nadměrně aktivní, čilý
overall /ˌəʊ.vəˈrɔːl/ celkový, celkově
overcooling /ˌəʊ.vəˈkuː.lɪŋ/ nadměrné zchlazení
overdose /ˈəʊ.və.dəʊs/ nadměrná dávka, předávkování
overhear /ˌəʊvəˈhɪə/ vyslechnout (náhodou)
overhydration /ˌəʊvə.haɪˈdreɪ.ʃən/ nadměrná hydratace, zavodnění
overinflation /ˌəʊvə.ɪnˈfleɪʃ.ən/ nadměrné naplnění vzduchem, nahuštění
overload /ˌəʊ.vəˈləʊd/ přetížit, přetížení
overly /ˈəʊ.vəl.i/ přespříliš, až moc
overpressure /ˌəʊ.vəˈpreʃ.ər/ nadměrný tlak
overuse /ˌəʊ.vəˈjuːz/ nadužívat, nadměrné používání
overweight /ˌəʊ.vəˈweɪt/ nadváha, mít nadváhu

overwhelm /ˌəʊ.vəˈwelm/ přemoci, zdolat
ovum /ˈəʊ.vəm/ **ova** vajíčko
oxygen /ˈɒk.sɪ.dʒən/ kyslík
oxygenate /ˈɒk.sɪ.dʒə.neɪt/ okysličovat
oxygenation /ˈɒk.sɪ.dʒə.neɪ.ʃən/ oxygenace, okysličení
oxytocin /ˌɒk.sɪˈtəʊ.sɪn/ hormon tvořený v hypothalamu a vylučovaný do krve v zadním laloku hypofýzy, má význam pro stahy dělohy při porodu

P
pace /peɪs/ tempo, rychlost, krok, chůze
pack /pæk/ zábal, obal
packing /ˈpæk.ɪŋ/ balení, balicí materiál
PaCO2, partial /ˈpɑːʃəl/ **pressure** /ˈpreʃ.ər/ **of carbon** /ˈkɑː.bən/ **dioxide** /daɪˈɒk.saɪd/ **in arterial** /ɑːˈtɪərɪəl/ **blood** /blʌd/ parciální tlak oxidu uhličitého v alveolu, ovlivňuje jej alveolární ventilace
padded /ˈpæd.ɪd/ vycpaný, s vycpávkou
padding /ˈpæd.ɪŋ/ vycpávka, vatování
paediatric /ˌpiː.diˈæt.rɪk/ pediatrický
paediatrics /ˌpiː.diːˈæt.rɪks/ pediatrie
pain /peɪn/ bolest, bolet, trápit
painful /ˈpeɪn.fəl/ bolestivý, působící bolest
painless /ˈpeɪn.ləs/ bezbolestný
pale /peɪl/ bledý

palliative /'pæl.i.ə.tɪv/ paliativní, utišující, bolest zmírňující

pallor /'pæl.ər/ bledost, sinalost

palm /pɑːm/ dlaň

palpable /'pæl.pə.bl̩/ hmatný, zřetelný

palpate /'pæl.peɪt/ provádět palpaci, vyšetřovat pohmatem

palpation /pæl'peɪ.ʃən/ palpace, pohmat, prohmatávání

palpitations /ˌpæl.pɪ'teɪ.ʃənz/ palpitace, zrychlené bušení srdce

palsy /'pɔːl.zi/ obrna, ochrnutí, paralýza

pancreas /'pæŋ.kri.əs/ pankreas, slinivka břišní

pancreatic /ˌpæŋ.krɪ'æ.tɪk/ pankreatický, týkající se slinivky břišní

pancreatitis /ˌpæŋ.kri.ə'taɪ.tɪs/ pankreatitida, zánět slinivky břišní

pant /pænt/ těžce oddechovat, supět, popadat dech

paradoxical /ˌpær.ə'dɒk.sɪ.kəl/ paradoxní

paradoxically /ˌpær.ə'dɒk.sɪ.kəl.i/ paradoxně

paradoxus /'pær.ə.dɒk.səs/ paradoxní

paralyse /'pær.əl.aɪz/ paralyzovat, ochromit

paralysis /pə'ræl.ə.sɪs/ paralýza, ochrnutí

paramedic /ˌpærə'medɪk/ zdravotnický záchranář, člen RZP

paramount /'pær.ə.maʊnt/ prvořadý, nejzásadnější

parasympathetic /'pær.əˌsɪm.pə'θet.ɪk/ parasympatický,

týkající se autonomího nervstva s opačným účinkem než sympatikus

parental /pə'ren.təl/ rodičovský

parenteral /pə'ren.tə.rəl/ mimostřevní

parietal /pə'raɪə.təl/ parietální, temenní

parity /'pærɪtɪ/ rovnost, rovnoprávnost

paroxysm /'pær.ɒk.sɪ.zəm/ paroxysmus, náhlý záchvat

paroxysmal /ˌpær.ɒk.'sɪz.məl/ paroxyzmální, záchvatový

part /pɑːt/ část, součást, role, spoluúčast, rozdělit

partial /'pɑː.ʃəl/ částečný, dílčí

partial /'pɑːʃəl/ pressure /'preʃ.ər/ parciální tlak

partially /'pɑː.ʃəl.i/ částečně, zčásti

particle /'pɑː.tɪ.kl̩/ částice, částečka

particularly /pə'tɪk.jʊ.lə.li/ hlavně, zejména, obzvlášť

particulate /pə'tɪ.kjuː.lət/ z drobných částic

PASG, Pneumatic /njʊ'mætɪk/ Antishock /'æn.tɪ.ʃɒk/ Garment / 'gɑːmənt/ nafukovací oblek, používaný k potlačení šoku, stabilizaci zlomenin, podporování hemostázy a zvýšení periferní cévní rezistence, viz také MAST

pass /pɑːs/ out /aʊt/ omdlít, ztratit vědomí

pass /pɑːs/ projít, minout

passage /'pæsɪdʒ/ průchod, trubice, kanálek

past /pɑːst/ minulý, dřívější

pasty /'pæs.ti/ bledý, bílý

patency /'peɪ.tənt.si/ průchodnost

patent /'peɪ.tənt/ průchodný

path /pɑ:θ/ cesta, dráha pohybu

pathogen /'pæθ.ə.dʒən/ patogen, původce, choroboplodný zárodek

pathogenic /ˌpæθ.ə'dʒen.ɪk/ patogenní, choroboplodný

pathology /pə'θɒl.ə.dʒi/ patologie

pathophysiology /ˌpæθ.ə.fɪz. i'ɒl.ə.dʒi/ patofyziologie, nauka o chorobných pochodech a změnách funkcí organizmu během nemoci

pathway /'pɑ:θ.weɪ/ cesta, dráha pohybu

pattern /'pæt.ən/ model, schéma, systém, obrazec, struktura, vzor

PCP, phencyclidine /fɛn'sɪklɪˌdi:n/ fencyklidin, disociativní anestetikum, zneužíván jako taneční droga, jako anestetikum se přestal používat kvůli psychickým nežádoucím účinkům

PEA, Pulseless /pʌls.ləs/ **Electrical** /ɪ'lek.trɪ.kəl/ **Activity** /æk'tɪv.ɪ.ti/ bezpulzní elektrická aktivita

peak /pi:k/ **flow** /fləʊ/ **meter** /m.ɪ.tər/ výdechoměr, pomůcka pro měření vrcholu výdechové průtokové rychlosti, což je největší možné vydechnutí plícemi po co největším možném vdechu

peak /pi:k/ **flow** /fləʊ/ vrcholový výdechový průtok

peak /pi:k/ špička, vrchol maximum, nejvyšší stupeň

pearly /'pɜ:.li/ perlový, růžový

pedal /'ped.əl/ nožní, nohou se týkající

pedestrian /pɪ'destrɪən/ chodec

peers /pɪərz/ vrstevníci

pelvic /'pel.vɪk/ **inflammatory** / ɪn'flæm.ə.tər.i/ **disease** /dɪ'zi:z/ zánětlivé onemocnění pánve

pelvis /'pel.vɪs/ pánev

pending /'pen.dɪŋ/ brzký, bezprostředně hrozící

penetrate /'pen.ɪ.treɪt/ proniknout, vniknout, prorazit

penetrating /'pen.ɪ.treɪ.tɪŋ/ pronikavý

percentage /pə'sen.tɪdʒ/ procento, procentní podíl

perception /pə'sep.ʃən/ vnímání, vjem, pohled

percuss /pə'kʌs/ proklepat, vyšetřit poklepem

percussion /pə'kʌʃ.ən/ poklep, perkuse

perfect /'pɜ:.fekt/ perfektní, dokonalý, bezvadný

perforate /'pɜ:.fər.eɪ.t/ propíchnout, proděravět

perforation /ˌpɜ:.fər'eɪ.ʃən/ perforace, proniknutí, propíchnutí

perform /pə'fɔ:m/ vykonat, provést, udělat, fungovat

perfuse /pə'fju:z/ perfundovat, promývat

perfusion /pə'fju:.ʒən/ perfuze, promývání, zásobování orgánů tekutinou

pericardial /ˌper.ɪ'ka:di. əl/ perikardiální, týkající se osrdečníku

pericardium /ˌper.ɪˈkaːdi.əm/ osrdečník, perikard

perineum /ˌper.ɪˈniː.əm/ hráz, u muže úsek mezi análním otvorem a odstupem šourku, u ženy mezi análním otvorem a spojením stydkých pysků

period /ˈpɪə.ri.əd/ doba, lhůta

periorbital /ˌper.ɪ.ˈɔːbɪtəl/ periorbitální

peripheral /pəˈrɪf.ər.əl/ periferní, okrajový, obvodový

peritoneal /ˌper.ɪ.təˈni.əl/ peritoneální, pobřišniční

peritonitis /ˌper.ɪ.təˈnaɪ.tɪs/ peritonitida, zánět pobřišnice

periumbilical /ˌper.ɪ.ʌmˈbɪl.ɪ.kəl/ periumbilikální, ležící kolem pupku

permissible /pəˈmɪs.ə.bl̩/ přípustný, dovolený

permission /pəˈmɪʃ.ən/ povolení, dovolení

permit /pəˈmɪt/ povolit, dovolit

persist /pəˈsɪst/ přetrvávat, pokračovat, vytrvat

persistent /pəˈsɪs.tənt/ perzistentní, trvalý, přetrvávající, úporný, nepolevující

personnel /ˌpɜːsəˈnel/ personál

persuade /pəˈsweɪd/ přesvědčit, přimět

pertinent /ˈpɜːtɪnənt/ týkající se, související, případný

pertussis /pəˈtʌ.sɪs/ černý kašel

petechia /piˈtiː.ki.ə/ pl petechiae petechie, tečkovité krvácení z kapilár

petechial /piˈtiː.ki.əl/ petechiální, týkající se petechie

petit mal /ˌpəˈtiːˈmæl/ malý epileptický záchvat

pH /ˌpiːˈeɪtʃ/ pH kyselost či zásaditost prostředí

phase /feɪz/ fáze, stádium, etapa

phenomenon /fəˈnɒm.ɪ.nən/

phenomena fenomén, jev, úkaz

phlegm /flem/ hlen

phobia /ˈfəʊ.bi.ə/ fobie, chorobný strach

physical /ˈfɪz.ɪ.kəl/ tělesný, lékařská prohlídka

physician /fɪˈzɪʃ.ən/ lékař, doktor

physiological /ˌfɪz.i.ˈɒl.ə.dʒi.kəl/ fyziologický

pickup /pɪkʌp/ vozidlo s valníkovým nákladním prostorem

Pickwickian /pɪkˈwɪk.i.ən/

syndrome /ˈsɪndrəʊm/ Pickwikův syndrom, břišní obezita, která omezuje možnost dýchacích pohybů bránice

PID, Pelvic /ˈpel.vɪk/ **Inflammatory** /ɪnˈflæm.ə.tər.i/ **Disease** /dɪˈziːz/ zánětlivé onemocnění pánve

pierce /pɪəs/ propíchnout, probodnout

pigmentation /ˌpɪg.mənˈteɪ.ʃən/ pigmentace

pile /paɪl/ hromada

pill /pɪl/ pilulka, prášek, tabletka

pill-rolling /ˈpɪlˌrəʊ.lɪŋ/ **tremor** /ˈtrem.ər/ klidový třes palce a prstů ruky u Parkinsonovy choroby

pin /pɪn/ špendlík, spona

pin-point, pinpoint /ˈpɪn.pɔɪnt/ velmi přesný, špička špendlíku

pinch /pɪntʃ/ štípnout, stisknout

pinna /pin.ə/ aurikula, ušní boltec

pipe /paɪp/ trubka, potrubí, trubice

pit /pɪt/ viper /ˈvaɪ.pər/ chřestýšovec, chřestýšovitý had

pitch /pɪtʃ/ výška, poloha (tónu)

pitting /pɪt.ɪŋ/ oedema /ɪˈdiː.mə/ jamkovitý otok

pituitary gland /pɪˈtjuː.ɪ.tər. iˌglænd/ hypofýza, podvěsek mozkový

place /pleɪs/ místo, umístit, položit

placement /ˈpleɪs.mənt/ umístění, rozmístění

placenta /pləˈsen.tə/ praevia / priː.vi.ə/ vcestné lůžko, překrývá děložní otvor a brání normálnímu průběhu porodu

plain /pleɪn/ prostý, jednoduchý

plant /plɑːnt/ továrna

plaque /plɑːk/, /plæk/ plát, destička

plasma /ˈplæz.mə/ plazma

platelet /ˈpleɪt.lət/ krevní destička

pledge /pledʒ/ závazek, slib

pleura /ˈplʊə.rə/ pleura, pohrudnice

pleural /ˈplʊə.rəl/ pleurální, pohrudniční

pleuric /ˈplʊə.rɪk/ disease /dɪˌziːz/ onemocnění pohrudnice

plug /plʌg/ čípek, zátka, zásuvka, ucpat, uzavřít

PND, Paroxysmal /ˌpær.ɒk.ˈsɪz. məl/ Nocturnal /nɒkˈtɜː.nəl/ Dyspnea /dɪs.pniː.ə/ záchvatovitá (paroxysmální) noční dušnost

pneumatic /njuˈmætɪk/ vzduchový, na stlačený vzduch

pneumonia /njuːˈməʊ.ni.ə/ zápal plic

pneumothorax /ˌnjuːməʊˈθɔːræks/ pneumotorax, hrudní plynatost, vzduch v pohrudniční dutině hrudní

poikilothermy /ˌpɔɪ.kɪl.əˈθɜːm.i/ poikilotermie, neschopnost udržet stálou tělesnou teplotu

point /pɔɪnt/ okamžik, bod, hrot, špička, pracovní konec nástroje

point /pɔɪnt/ to /tə/ ukázat, namířit, upozornit

poison /ˈpɔɪ.zən/ jed, otrávit

poisoning /ˈpɔɪ.zən.ɪŋ/ otrava

pole /pəʊl/ sloup, stožár, telefonní ap.

polite /pəˈlaɪt/ slušný, zdvořilý

polycythaemia /ˌpɒl.ɪ.saɪˈθiːm.ɪ.ə/ polycytemie, zmnožení všech krevních elementů v krvi

polydipsia /ˌpɒl.ɪˈdɪp.sɪ.ə/ polydipsie, chorobná žíznivost

polyphagia /ˌpɒl.ɪˈfeɪ.dʒə/ polyfagie, zvýšená chuť k jídlu, pojídání velkého množství jídla

polyuria /ˌpɒl.ɪˈjʊə.rɪ.ə/ polyurie, nadměrné močení

pool /puːl/ bazén, nahromadit se

pool /puːl/ hall /hɔːl/ biliárová herna

pool /puːl/ stick /stɪk/, pool cue / kjuː/ tágo

pooling /puːl.ɪŋ/ nahromadění krve nebo jiné tekutiny, nahromadění krve je následkem dilatace a zastavení oběhu v kapilárách a žilách v oblasti

poorly /ˈpɔː.li/ chabě, nevalně, nemocný

pop /pɒp/ prasknout

popliteal /ˌpɒp.lɪˈtiːəl/ podkolenní, zákolenní

portion /ˈpɔː.ʃən/ část, díl, rozdělit

position /pəˈzɪʃ.ən/ pozice, poloha, umístit

positive /ˈpɒz.ə.tɪv/ pozitivní, kladný

possession /pəˈzeʃ.ən/ majetek, vlastnictví

posterior /pɒsˈtɪə.ri.ər/ posteriorní, zadní

postictal /ˈpəʊstˈɪkt.əl/ následně po prodělaném záchvatu, po mrtvici, po epileptickém záchvatu

postpartum /ˌpəʊstˈpɑː.təm/ poporodní, následující po porodu

posttraumatic /ˌpəʊst.trɒˌmæt.ɪk/ posttraumatický, poúrazový

postural /ˈpɒst.ʃər.əl/ posturální, postojový, týkající se držení těla

posture /ˈpɒs.tʃər/ držení těla, postoj, postavení těla, dát do pozice

potassium /pəˈtæs.i.əm/ draslík

potent /ˈpəʊ.tənt/ silný, účinný

potential /pəˈten.ʃəl/ potenciál, možnost, schopnost

power /ˈpaʊə/ **line** /laɪn/ elektrické vedení

power /ˈpaʊə/ pravomoc, kompetence, elektřina, elektrický

power /paʊər/ **company** /ˈkʌm.pə.ni/ elektrická společnost

power /paʊər/ **of attorney** /əˈtɜː.ni/ plná moc, oprávnění advokáta

practice /ˈpræk.tɪs/ praxe, praktika, postup

pre-existing /ˌpriː.ɪgˈzɪs.tɪŋ/ dřívější, již existující

prearrival /ˌpriː.əˈraɪ.vəl/ před příjezdem

precaution /prɪˈkɔː.ʃən/ opatrnost, preventivní opatření, bezpečnostní opatření, předběžné opatření

precede /prɪˈsiːd/ předcházet časově

precipitous /prɪˈsɪp.ɪ.təs/ prudký, překotný

predispose /ˌpriː.dɪˈspəʊz/ predisponovat, učinit náchylný

preeclampsia /ˌpri.ɪˈklæmp.si.ə/ preeklampsie, těhotenské onemocnění s otoky, bílkovinou v moči a vysokým krevním tlakem

pregnancy /ˈpreg.nən.si/ těhotenství

pregnant /ˈpregnənt/ těhotná

prehospital /ˌpriːˈhɒs.pɪ.təl/ přednemocniční

preliminary /prɪˈlɪm.ɪ.nər.i/ předběžný, přípravný

preload /ˌpriːˈləʊd/ preload, předpětí, předtížení, náplň srdeční komory na konci diastoly, enddiastolický objem, zvyšování p. je jedním z kompenzačních mechanismů při srdečním selhání

premature /ˈprem.ə.tʃər/ předčasný, nedonošený, předčasně narozený

prerespiratory /ˌpriːˈres.pər.əˌtɔr.i/ předrespirační

prescribe /prɪ'skraɪb/ předepsat, naordinovat lék

presence / 'prez.ənt s/ účast, přítomnost (osoby, věci ap.), zevnějšek

present /'prez.ənt/ projevovat, naléhat (na pánev o plodu)

presentation /ˌprez.ən'teɪ.ʃən/ vzhled, projevení představení, prezentace

presenting /prɪ'zent.ɪŋ/ **part** /pɑ:t/ procházející část, při porodu

preserve /prɪ'zɜ:v/ zachovat, uchovat

press /pres/ tlačit, tisknout

pressure /'preʃ.ə/ **dressing** /'dres.ɪŋ/ tlakový obvaz

pressure /'preʃ.ə/ tlak, stisk, napětí

pressurized /'preʃ.ər.aɪzd/ přetlakový, s regulovaným tlakem

presume /prɪ'zju:m/ předpokládat, domnívat se

pretend /prɪ'tend/ předstírat, tvrdit

preventable /prɪ'ven.tə.b|/ jemuž lze předejít, ne nevyhnutelný

previous /'pri:.vi.əs/ předchozí, předešlý

primarily /praɪ'mer.ɪ.li/ především, hlavně

primary /'praɪ.mə.ri/ primární, prvořadý

prior /'praɪə/ **to** /tʊ/ před, přede

priority /praɪ'ɒr.ɪ.ti/ priorita, přednost

privacy /'praɪvəsɪ/ soukromí

procedure /prə'si:dʒə/ postup, procedura

proceed /prə'si:d/ pokračovat, postupovat

produce /prə'dju:s/ způsobit, vyvolat, zapříčinit

product /'prɒd.ʌkt/ produkt, výsledek

production /prə'dʌk.ʃən/ produkce, tvoření, tvorba

productive /prə'dʌk.tɪv/ produktivní, vlhký kašel

profound /prə'faʊnd/ hluboký, silný

profoundly /prə'faʊnd.li/ hluboce, nesmírně

profusely /prə'fju:s.li/ hojně, silně

profusion /prə'fju:.ʒən/ hojnost, spousta

prognostic /prɒg'nɒs.tɪk/ prognostický, předpovídající

progress /'prəʊ.gres/ postup, vývoj, probíhat

progressively /prə'gres.ɪv.li/ progresivně, postupně

projected /prə'dʒek.tɪd/ promítaný

projectile /prə'dʒek.taɪl/ projektil, střela, náboj

prolapsed /prəʊ'læpst/ vyhřezlý, snížený trubicový orgán

prolonged /prə'lɒŋd/ prodloužený, dlouhotrvající, vleklý

promote /prə'məʊt/ podporovat, prosazovat

prompt /prɒmp t/ promptní, okamžitý, pohotový, přimět, dohnat koho k čemu

promptly /'prɒmptlɪ/ ihned, okamžitě

pronation /prəʊ'neɪ.ʃən/ pronace, stočení ruky s vnitřní polohou palce, stočení končetiny dovnitř podle podélné osy

prone /prəʊn/ **to** /tə/ mající sklony, náchylný

prone /prəʊn/ na břiše ležící

pronounced /prəˈnaʊnst/ vyslovovaný, zřetelný, výrazný

propelled /prəˈpeld/ poháněný, hnaný

proper /ˈprɒpə/ vhodný, pořádný, náležitý, vlastní, samotný

properly /ˈprɒp.əl.i/ vhodně, náležitě, řádně

property /ˈprɒp.ə.ti/ majetek, vlastnictví, vlastnost, charakter materiálu

proportionally /prəˈpɔː.ʃən.əli/ úměrně, přiměřeně

protection /prəˈtekʃən/ ochrana, zabezpečení

protective /prəˈtek.tɪv/ ochranný, ochrana

protein /ˈprəʊ.tiːn/ protein, bílkovina

proteinuria /ˈprəʊ.tiːn.jʊəˈriː.ə/ proteinurie, vylučování bílkovin močí

protrude /prəˈtruːd/ vyčnívat

protrusion /prəˈtruː.ʒən/ výčnělek, výrůstek

prove /pruːv/ dokázat, prokázat

proven /ˈpruːvən/ prokázaný, ověřený

provide /prəˈvaɪd/ poskytnout, dodat, zajistit

provided /prəˈvaɪ.dɪd/ pokud, za předpokladu že

provider /prəˈvaɪ.dər/ poskytovatel, dodavatel

provocation /ˌprɒvəˈkeɪʃən/ vyprovokování

provoke /prəˈvəʊk/ vyprovokovat, vyvolat

proximal /ˈprɒk.sɪ.məl/ proximální, bližší trupu nebo hlavě

proximate /ˈprɒk.sɪ.mət/ nejbližší, bezprostřední

proxy /ˈprɒk.sɪ/ zástupce, zmocněnec

prudent /ˈpruː.dənt/ prozíravý, opatrný

pruritus /prʊəˈraɪ.təs/ svědění, projev alergie nebo způsobené emocionálním stresem

pseudoseizure /ˈsjuː.dəʊ.ˈsiː.ʒər/ falešný, nepravý záchvat

psychiatric /ˌsaɪ.kiˈæt.rɪk/ psychiatrický, psychický

psychogenic /ˌsaɪ.kəʊˈdʒɛ.nɪk/ psychogenní, mentálního původu

psychosis /saɪˈkəʊ.sɪs/ psychóza, porucha myšlení a jednání s následným rozpadem osobnosti

puffy /ˈpʌf.i/ opuchlý, oteklý

pull /pʊl/ táhnout, zatahat

pulmonary /ˈpʊl.mə.nə.ri/ **congestion** /kənˈdʒes.tʃən/ překrvení plic

pulmonary /ˈpʊl.mə.nə.ri/ pulmonální, plicní

pulsate /pʌlˈseɪ.t/ pulzovat, tepat, bušit

pulsatile /ˈpʌlsəˌtaɪl/ **mass** /mæs/ pulzatilní hmota

pulsation /pʌlˈseɪ.ʃən/ pulzace, tepot

pulse /pʌls/ **oximeter** /ˈɒk.sɪ.m.ɪ.tər/ pulzní oximetr

pulse /pʌls/ **oximetry** /ˈɒk.sɪ.m.ə.tri/

pulzní oxymetrie, neinvazivně měří saturaci hemoglobinu kyslíkem v arteriální části krevního řečiště (pulzatilní tok), místem umístění detektoru jsou prsty končetin nebo ušní lalůčky

pulse /pʌls/ pulz, rytmus, tepat

pulseless /pʌls.ləs/ bez pulzu

pulselessness /pʌls.ləs.nəs/ nepřítomnost pulzu

pulsus /pʌls.əs/ **paradoxus** / ˈpær.ə.dɒks.əs/ paradoxní puls, tep, jehož vlny jsou při nádechu menší než při výdechu, patologickým se stává např. při tamponádě srdce či perikarditidě

pump /pʌmp/ pumpovat, čerpat

puncture / ˈpʌŋk.tʃə/ punkce, vpich, otvor propíchnutí, propíchnout

pupil /ˈpjuːpəl/ zornička

pupillary /pjuː.pɪl.ər.i/ pupilární, zornicový

pure /pjʊər/ čistý, bez příměsí

purplish /ˈpɜː.pl.ɪʃ/ nafialovělý

purpose /ˈpɜː.pəs/ účel, záměr, mít v úmyslu

purse /pɜːs/ našpulit rty

pursed /pɜːsd/-**lip** /lɪp/ našpulené rty

push /pʊʃ/ tlačit, posunout, postrčit, strčit, prodrat se

put /pʊt/ **pressure** /ˈpreʃ.ər/ vyvinout tlak na

PVCs, Premature /ˈpreməˌtjʊə/ **Ventricular** /venˈtrɪk.jə.lər/ **Contractions** /kənˈtrækʃəns/ předčasné stahy srdečních komor

Q

quadrant /ˈkwɒd.rənt/ kvadrant, čtvrtina kruhu

quality /kwɒlɪtɪ/ povaha, vlastnost

quantity /ˈkwɒn.tɪ.ti/ kvantita, počet, množství

questionable /ˈkwes.tʃə.nə.bl̩/ pochybný, sporný

R

rabies /ˈreɪ.biːz/ vzteklina

raccoon /rəˈkuːn/ **eyes** /aɪz/ „mývalí oči", zhmožděniny kolem očí

radial /ˈreɪ.di.əl/ radiální, vřetenní

radiate /ˈreɪ.di.eɪt/ vyzařovat, rozbíhat se (paprskovitě)

radiation /ˌreɪ.diˈeɪ.ʃən/ **sickness** / ˈsɪk.nəs/ nemoc z ozáření

radiation /ˌreɪ.diˈeɪ.ʃən/ vyzařování

radius /ˈreɪ.di.əs/ vřetenní kost

railing /ˈreɪ.lɪŋ/ zábradlí, ohrada

railroad /ˈreɪl.rəʊd/ železniční trať

raise /reɪz/ vytáhnout, zvýšit, zvýšení, zvednout, zřídit

rake /reɪk/ hrabat, hrábě

rale /raːl/ šelest, šelesty

rambling /ˈræm.blɪŋ/ nesouvislý, zmatený

range /reɪndʒ/ rozmezí, rozsah, pohybovat se, být v rozmezí

rape /reɪp/ znásilnit, znásilnění

rapid /ˈræp.ɪd/ rapidní, rychlý, překotný

rapport /ræˈpɔːr/ vzájemné porozumění, souznění

rarely /ˈreə.li/ vzácně, jen zřídka

rash /ræʃ/ vyrážka

rate /reɪt/ tempo, rychlost, frekvence, míra, ohodnotit, řadit

ratio /'reɪ.ʃi.əʊ/ podíl, vzájemný poměr, vztah

rattle /'ræt.l̩/ rachotit, drnčet

reach /riːtʃ/ dorazit, dosáhnout, dostat se

reactive /ri'æk.tɪv/ reaktivní (chemicky)

reading /'riː.dɪŋ/ odečet, údaj

rear-end /'rɪə.rend/ zadní část auta, nabourat zezadu

reasonable /'riː.zən.ə.b|/ přijatelný, rozumný

reassess /ˌriː.ə'ses/ přehodnotit, znovu posoudit

reassessment /ˌriː.ə'ses.mənt/ přehodnocení, nové zhodnocení

reassure /ˌriː.ə'ʃɔːr/ uklidnit, utěšit

rebound /ˌriː'baʊnd/ odražení, odskok

rebound /ˌriː'baʊnd/ **tenderness** /'ten.dər.nəs/ zvýšená bolestivost při náhlém uvolnění tlaku

receive /rɪ'siːv/ přijmout

recent /'riː.sənt/ nedávný, poslední

recheck /ˌriː.tʃek/ znovu zkontrolovat

recirculate /riː'sɜː.kjʊ.leɪt/ recirkulovat

recliner /rɪ'klaɪ.nər/ polohovací, sklápěcí křeslo

recognition /ˌrek.əg'nɪʃ.ən/ rozpoznání, zjištění, uznání, pochopení

recognize /'rek.əgˌnaɪz/ rozpoznat, uznat, ocenit, poznat

recoil /rɪ'kɔɪl/ zarazit se, ucuknout

recommended /ˌrekə'mendɪd/ doporučený

recompression /ˌriː.kəm'preʃ.ən/ **chamber** /'tʃeɪm.bər/ rekompresní komora

record /'rekɔːd/ záznam, nahrát, zapsat

recording /rɪ'kɔː.dɪŋ/ záznam, nahrávka

recover /rɪ'kʌv.ər/ zotavit se, uzdravit se

recumbent /rɪ'kʌm.bənt/ ležící

recurrence /rɪ'kʌr.əns/ recidiva, opakování, opětovný výskyt

red /red/ **blood** /blʌd/ **cell** /sel/ červená krvinka

redden /'red.ən/ zčervenat, zrudnout

reduce /rɪ'djuːs/ snížit, omezit, zmenšit

reevaluate /ˌriː.ɪ'væljueɪt/ znovu zhodnotit, přehodnotit

reexperience /ˌriː.ɪk'spɪə.ri.əns/ znovu prožít, prodělat

refer /rɪ'fɜːr/ mluvit o kom/čem, odkázat se, odvolávat se na co, svěřit, odkázat, poslat ke specialistovi

reference /'ref.ər.ənt s/ doporučení

referral /rɪ'fɜː.rəl/ doporučení kam, odkázání ke specialistovi, předání do péče

referred /rɪ'fɜːd/ **pain** /peɪn/ přenesená bolest, bolest pociťovaná v jiném místě než kde je její příčina

refill /'riː.fɪl/ plnění, doplnění, doplnit, dolít, znovu se naplnit

reflect /rɪ'flekt/ odrážet

reflux /ˈriːˌflʌks/ zpětný tok, zpětné proudění

refreeze /ˌriːˈfriːz/ znovu zmrznout

refusal /rɪˈfjuːzəl/ odmítnutí

refuse /rɪˈfjuːz/ odmítnout, nepřijmout

regain /rɪˈgeɪn/ znovu získat, vrátit

regarding /rɪˈgɑː.dɪŋ/ ohledně, pokud jde o

regardless /rɪˈgɑːd.ləs/ bez ohledu na co

regimen /ˈredʒ.ɪ.mən/ režim, životospráva

region /ˈriː.dʒən/ oblast, krajina

regional /ˈriː.dʒən.əl/ regionální, týkající se dané oblasti

regular /ˈreg.jʊ.lər/ pravidelný, častý, obvyklý

regularity /ˌreg.jʊˈlær.ə.ti/ pravidelnost, pravidelný jev

regulate /ˈregjʊˌleɪt/ regulovat, usměrňovat, řídit

regulation /ˌreg.jʊˈleɪ.ʃən/ regulace, řízení, usměrňování

reinflate /ˌriː.ɪnˈfleɪt/ znovu nafouknout

reinsert /ˌriː.ɪnˈsɜːt/ znovu vložit, vsunout

relate /rɪˈleɪt/ týkat se, vztahovat se, souviset

relation /rɪˈleɪ.ʃən/ vztah, souvislost

relationship /rɪˈleɪ.ʃən.ʃɪp/ vztah, příbuznost

relaxation /ˌriː.lækˈseɪ.ʃən/ relaxace, odpočinek, zmírnění

relaxed /rɪˈlækst/ uvolněný

relay /ˈriːleɪ/ přenos, vysílání

release /rɪˈliːs/ propustit, povolit, vypouštět, uvolňovat

relief /rɪˈliːf/ úleva, pomoc

relieve /rɪˈliːv/ utišit, zmírnit, pomoci

rely /rɪˈlaɪ/ **upon** /əˌpɒn/ spoléhat, být odkázán na koho, co

remain /rɪˈmeɪn/ vytrvat, zbývat, zůstat

remove /rɪˈmuːv/ odstranit, vyjmout, svléknout si

renal /ˈriː.nəl/ **calculi** /ˈkæl.kjʊ.laɪ/ ledvinové kameny

renal /ˈriː.nəl/ renální, ledvinový

reorient /ˌriːˈɔː.ri.ənt/ přeorientovat se

repeatedly /rɪˈpiː.tɪd.li/ opakovaně, opětovně

replacement /rɪˈpleɪs.mənt/ navrácení, náhrada, nahrazení, nové umístění, vrácení

report /rɪˈpɔːt/ hlášení, oznámit, podat zprávu, informovat

reportable /rɪˈpɔːt'ebəl/ podléhající hlášení

reposition /ˌriːpəˈzɪʃən/ přemístit, přesunout, posunout

reproducible /ˌriː.prə.djuːsɪ.bl̩/ opakující se

require /rɪˈkwaɪər/ nutně potřebovat, požadovat

requirement /rɪˈkwaɪə.mənt/ požadavek, podmínka

Res ipsa loquitur lat. věc mluví sama za sebe (za vše)

rescue /ˈreskjuː/ zachránit, pomoc, vysvobodit

rescuer /ˈres.kjuː.ər/ zachránce

reserve /rɪˈzɜːv/ rezerva, vyhradit si, zamluvit

reservoir /ˈrez.ə.vwɑːr/ ložisko, rezervoár, nádrž

residence /ˈrez.ɪ.dəns/ rezidence, obydlí

residual /rɪˈzɪd.ju.əl/ residuální, zbylý, zbytkový

residue /ˈrez.ɪ.djuː/ reziduum, zbytek

resistance /rɪˈzɪs.tənt s/ rezistence, odpor, odolnost

resolve /rɪˈzɒlv/ vyřešit, vstřebat se

resource /rɪˈzɔːs/ zdroje, možnosti, prostředky

respiratory /rɪˈspɪr.ə.tər.i/ **pattern** /ˈpæt.ən/ dechový vzorec

respond /rɪˈspɒnd/ reakce, odpověď, reagovat, odpovědět

responder /rɪˈspɒnd.ər/ reagující osoba

response /rɪˈspɒns/ odpověď, reakce

responsibility /rɪˌspɒn.səˈbɪ.lɪ.tɪ/ zodpovědnost, povinnosti, závazky pracovní

responsible /rɪˈspɒnt.sɪ.bļ/ odpovědný, zodpovídat se

responsive /rɪˈspɒnt.sɪv/ vnímavý, reagující, citlivý na co

responsiveness /rɪˈspɒn.sɪv.nəs/ schopnost reagovat, reakce

rest /rest/ spočívat, záviset, ležet

restate /ˌriːˈsteɪt/ jinak formulovat, přeformulovat

restless /ˈrest .ləs/ neklidný, nepokojný

restlessness /ˈrest.ləs.nəs/ neklid, nepokoj

restore /rɪˈstɔːr/ obnovit, znovu zavést, vrátit

restrain /rɪˈstreɪn/ zadržet, potlačovat

restraint /rɪˈstreɪnt/ restrikce, zamezování, omezení, překážka, zabezpečení v autě

restricted /rɪˈstrɪk.tɪd/ omezený, nepřístupný

result /rɪˈzʌlt/ výsledek, mít za následek

resume /rɪˈzjuːm/ pokračovat, zvovu začít

resuscitate /rɪˈsʌs.ɪ.teɪt/ oživovat

retain /rɪˈteɪn/ udržet si, ponechat, zachovat, uchovat, zadržet, uvíznout

retinal /ˈret.ɪ.nəl/ retinální, sítnicový

retraction /rɪˈtræk.ʃən/ retrakce, stažení, odtažení, zatažení

retroperitoneal /ˌret.rəʊˌper.ɪ.təʊ.ˈniː.əl/ ležící za pobřišnicí

reveal /rɪˈviːl/ odhalit, prozradit, objevit

reverse /rɪˈvɜːs/ zvrátit, změnit, otočit, opačně, pozpátku

revise /rɪˈvaɪz/ revidovat, opravit, přehodnotit

revision /rɪˈvɪʒ.ən/ revize, pozměnění, přepracování

revolve /rɪˈvɒlv/ rotovat, otáčet se, točit se

rewarm /ˌriːˌwɔːm/ znovu zahřát

rhonchus /rongˈkəs/ pl. -chi chrapot

rib /rɪb/ **cage** /keɪdʒ/ hrudní koš

rib /rɪb/ žebro

rider /'raɪ.dər/ jezdec, cyklista, řidič motocyklu

rifle /'raɪ.fl̩/ puška, kulovnice

right /raɪt/ právo

rigid /'rɪdʒ.ɪd/ rigidní, tvrdý, pevný, přísný, neohebný, tuhý, strnulý

rigidity /rɪ'dʒɪd.ɪ.ti/ rigidita, tuhost, ztuhlost, pevnost, tvrdost

rigor mortis /ˌrɪg.ə'mɔː.tɪs/ posmrtná ztuhlost

ring /rɪŋ/ kruh, kroužek, prstenec, kruhový otvor

Ringer's lactate /læk'teɪt/ Ringerův roztok, infuzní roztok, podobně jako fyziologický roztok je izotonický a obsahuje ionty sodíku a chloru, navíc pak obsahuje ionty draslíku a vápníku, čímž je bližší složení krevní plasmy

ringing /'rɪŋ.ɪŋ/ zvonění

rip /rɪp/ trhat, rvát

rise /raɪz/ zvednout, stoupat

rock /rɒk/ kámen, skála, zatřást, otřást

roll /rəʊl/ **over** /'əʊ.vər/ překulit se

roll /rəʊl/ stočit, svinout, rulička

roller /'rəʊ.lər/ **bandage** /'bæn.dɪdʒ/ obinadlo

rollover /'rəʊl.əʊ.vər/ převrácení (se na střechu)

rooftop /'ruːf.tɒp/ střecha, vršek střechy

room /ruːm/ prostor, místo, pokoj

roommate /'rʊm.meɪt/ spolubydlící

rotate /rəʊ'teɪt/ točit se, obíhat, střídat se

rotation /rəʊ'teɪ.ʃən/ rotace, otáčení, obíhání

rotator /rəʊ'teɪt.ər/ **cuff** /kʌf/ rotátorová manžeta, pouzdro ramenního svalu je zesíleno kloubními vazy a šlachami kolemjdoucích svalů (m. subscapularis, m. supraspinatus, m. infraspinatus, m. teres minor)

rotator /rəʊ'teɪt.ər/ rotátor, sval, který provádí rotaci

rotor /'rəʊtə/ rotor, pohyblivá část motoru

rough /rʌf/ drsný, hrubý

round /raʊnd/ kolem, kulatý, obchůzka

route /ruːt/ cesta, trasa

routine /ruː'tiːn/ rutina, běžná praxe

RSV, Human /hjuːmən/ **Respiratory** /rɪ'spɪr.ə.tər.i/ **Syncytial** /sɪn'sɪ.ʃɪ.əl/ **Virus** /'vaɪrəs/ lidský respirační syncyciální virus, je častým původcem těžkých respiračních infekcí v pediatrii

rub /rʌb/ mnout, masírovat, potřít, namazat, drhnout, otřít

rubivirus /ruːbɪ'vaɪ.rəs/ rubivirus, virus způsobující rubeolu (zarděnky)

rule /ruːl/ **out** /aʊt/ vyloučit

rule/ ruːl/ **of nines** /naɪnz/ pravidlo devíti, pravidlo pro přibližné posouzení rozsahu popálenin, povrch těla je rozdělen na zóny představující 9 % tělesného povrchu (BSA)

runny /'rʌn.i/ slzící oči z rýmy

rupture /'rʌp.tʃər/ ruptura, natržení, protržení, zlomení, kýla, výhřez

rush /rʌʃ/ in unáhlit se, vřítit se dovnitř
rush /rʌʃ/ spěchat, udělat ve spěchu, příval, nával

S
sac /sæk/ váček, vak
sacral /'seɪ.krəl/ sakrální, křížový
safety /'seɪftɪ/ bezpečnost, ochranný
Salicylates /sə'lɪs.ɪˌleɪts/ salicitáty (aspirin, anopirin, superpirin)
saline /'seɪ.laɪn/ slaný, solný roztok, fyziologický roztok
salivation /'sæl.ɪ.veɪ.ʃən/ salivace, slinění
salvageable /'sæl.vɪdʒə.bl̩/ zachranitelný
sample /sɑː.mpl̩/ vzorek, ukázka
SAMPLE, Signs and **Symptoms, Allergies, Medications, Past medical history, Last oral intake** mnemotechnická pomůcka (příznaky a symptomy, alergie, léky, minulá zdravotní anamnéza, poslední příjem ústy, události vedoucí k poranění či nemoci) pro klíčové otázky při posuzování stavu pacienta, užívá se spolu s hodnocením životních znaků, viz také OPQRST
sarcoma /sɑː'kəʊ.mə/ sarkom, zhoubný nádor pojivové tkáně
saturate /'sæt.jʊ.reɪt/ saturovat, nasytit, nasáknout
saturation /ˌsæt.jʊ'reɪ.ʃən/ saturace, nasycení
saw /sɔː/ pila, řezat
scale /skeɪl/ škála, rozsah

scalp /skælp/ vlasová pokožka, kůže pokrývající lebeční kosti, kůže na temeni hlavy
scalpel /'skæl.pəl/ skalpel
scapula /'skæp.jʊ.lə/ pl -ae lopatka
scar /skɑːr/ jizva, zjizvit
scenario /sɪ'nɑː.ri.əʊ/ scénář, možný vývoj
schizophrenic /ˌskɪt.sə'fren.ɪk/ schizofrenický, schizofrenik
scissors /'sɪz.əz/ nůžky, sevření
sclera /'sklɪə.rə/ skléra, oční bělmo
scold /skəʊld/ vynadat
scope /skəʊp/ prostor, příležitost, rozsah
score /skɔː/ docílit, skóre, dosažený výsledek
scream /skriːm/ křičet, ječet, křik, výkřik, jekot
scuba diving /'skuː.bəˌdaɪ.vɪŋ/ potápění s dýchacím přístrojem, sportovní potápění
seal /siːl/ tuleň, lachtan
seal /siːl/ utěsnit, zalepit, neprodyšně uzavřít
search /sɜːtʃ/ for /fɔː/ hledat
seat /'siː.t/ uložit do pozice, usadit, sedadlo
seat /siːt/ belt /belt/ bezpečnostní pás
seated /'siː.tɪd/ posazený, uložený
secondary /'sek.ən.dri/ sekundární, druhotný, vedlejší
secretion /sɪ'kriː.ʃən/ sekrece, vylučování, výměšky
section /'sek.ʃən/ část, úsek, průřez, odříznutí, pitva
secure /sɪ'kjʊə/ zajistit, zabezpečit, upevnit

security /sɪˈkjʊə.rɪ.ti/ bezpečnost, ostraha, zajištění, zabezpečení

sedation /sɪˈdeɪ.ʃən/ uklidňující lék

sedative /ˈsed.ə.tɪv/ sedativum, utišující lék

seek /siːk/ (sought, sought) hledat, usilovat, požadovat

segment /ˈseg.mənt/ segment, úsek, část, díl, článek orgánu

seize /siːz/ chytit, ovládnout, mít záchvat

seizure /ˈsiː.ʒə/ **disorder** /dɪˌsɔː.dər/ epilepsie

seizure /ˈsiː.ʒə/ křečový stav, záchvat (nemoci), záchvatový

seldom /ˈsel.dəm/ zřídka, málokdy

self-induced /ˌself.ɪnˈdjuːst/ způsobený sám sebou

semi /ˌsem.i/ -**seated** /ˈsiː.tɪd/ zpola posazený, v polosedě

semiconscious /ˌsem.iˈkɒn.ʃəs/ zpola při vědomí

sender /ˈsen.dər/ odesilatel

senile /ˈsiː.naɪl/ senilní

sensation /senˈseɪ.ʃən/ pocit, cit, čití, dojem, vjem, vnímání, smyslové vnímání

sense /sens/ smysl, pocit, vjem, rozum, chápat, mít smysl

sensory /ˈsent.sər.i/ smyslový

sentence /ˈsen.təns/ věta

separate /ˈsep.ər.ət/ oddělený, samostatný

separation /ˌsepəˈreɪʃən/ separace, oddělení, odloučení, rozdělení

sepsis /ˈsep.sɪs/ sepse, otrava krve, zaplavení organismu bakteriemi

septic /ˈsep.tɪk/ septický, zanícený, zhnisaný

septum /ˈsep.təm/ přepážka

serious /ˈsɪə.ri.əs/ opravdový, vážný, závažný, těžký

seriously /ˈsɪə.ri.əs.li/ vážně, těžce

setting /ˈset.ɪŋ/ prostředí

sever /ˈsev.ər/ oddělit, přerušit, urvat, odseknout

severe /sɪˈvɪə/ závažný

severity /sɪˈver.ɪ.ti/ krutost, vážnost, útrapy

sexual /ˈsek.sjuəl/ **intercourse** /ˈɪn.tə.kɔːs/ pohlavní styk

shaft /ʃɑːft/ diafýza, střední část dlouhé kosti

shake /ʃeɪk/ (shook, shaken) třást, otřást, chvět

shaken /ˈʃeɪkən/ **baby** /ˈbeɪ.bi/ **syndrome** /ˈsɪn.drəʊm/ syndrom třeseného dítěte, zdravotní poškození malého dítěte nešetrným třesením a cloumáním (zejména hlavičky a krku)

shallow /ˈʃæl.əʊ/ mělký

shaped /ʃeɪpt/ tvarovaný, ve tvaru, formovaný

sharp /ʃɑːp/ ostrý předmět, prudký, náhlý

shear /ˈʃɪə.r/ nůžky, stříhat, utrhnout se

sheet /ʃiːt/ prostěradlo, útržek, plátek, list, vrstva

shellfish /ˈʃel.fɪʃ/ měkkýši, korýši

shelter /ˈʃel.tər/ přístřeší, úkryt

shield /ʃiːld/ ochrana, štít, zastínit

shift /ʃɪft/ posunovat, přemístit, přesun, směna

shine /ʃaɪn/ svítit, zářit, lesk

shiver /ˈʃɪv.ər/ chvění, třes, třást se, chvět se

shock /ʃɒk/ šok, otřes, náraz

shockable /ˈʃɒk.ə.bļ/ umožňující úder (defibrilátor)

shopping /ˈʃɒp.ɪŋ/ **mall** /mɔːl/ nákupní středisko

short /ʃɔːt/ **of st** nedostávat se, chybět

shorten /ˈʃɔː.tən/ zkrátit

shortness /ˈʃɔːt.nəs/ nedostatečnost

shortness /ˈʃɔːt.nəs/ **of breath** / breθ/ dyspnoe, dušnost

shoulder /ˈʃəʊl.dər/ **blade** /bleɪd/ ramenní lopatka

shoulder /ˈʃəʊl.dər/ rameno

shouting /ˈʃaʊ.tɪŋ/ pokřikování, křičení

show /ˈʃəʊ/ ukázat, zachycovat, jevit, projev

showing /ˈʃəʊ.ɪŋ/ výsledek, vykázaná hodnota

shuffle /ˈʃʌf.ļ/ šourat, vléci se

shunt /ʃʌnt/ posunout, přesunout, zkrat, posunutí, odklonit se od směru, umělá cesta pro odklonění tekutiny

shut /ʃʌt/ **off** /ɒf/ vypnout, zastavit, odtáhnout

sick-looking /sɪkˈlʊk.ɪŋ/ vypadající jako nemocný

side /saɪd/ **effect** /ɪˈfekt/ vedlejší účinek

side /saɪd/ strana, bok, vedlejší

sigh /saɪ/ povzdech, vzdechnutí, zavzdychat

sign /saɪn/ znak, známka, znamení, podepsat

signal /ˈsɪg.nəl/ signál, znamení, signalizovat, indikovat

significance /sɪgˈnɪf.ɪ.kəns/ význam, důležitost, hodnota

significant /sɪgˈnɪf.ɪ.kənt/ důležitý, význačný, významný

silence /ˈsaɪ.ləns/ ticho, mlčení

silo /ˈsaɪ.ləʊ/ silo, nádoba na skladování obilí

similar /ˈsɪm.ɪ.lər/ podobný

simple /ˈsɪm.pļ/ prostý, jednoduchý

simplex /ˈsɪm.pleks/ jednosměrný přenos (tech.)

simultaneous /ˌsɪm.əlˈteɪ.ni.əs/ souběžný, současně probíhající

singe /sɪndʒ/ ožehnutí, lehká popálenina

single /ˈsɪŋɡəl/ jeden, jediný, jednoduchý

sinus /ˈsaɪ.nəs/ sinus, dutina (nosní)

siren /ˈsaɪərən/ siréna

site /saɪt/ místo, poloha, plocha, oblast, umístění, být umístěn

size /saɪz/ **up** /ʌp/ hodnotit, zhodnotit, posoudit, ujasnit

size /saɪz/ velikost, rozměry

skate /ˈskeɪ.t/ bruslit

skeletal /ˈskel.ɪ.təl/ skeletální, kosterní

skid /skɪd/ skluz, smyk

skill /skɪl/ dovednost, schopnost, zkušenost

skull /skʌl/ lebka

slander /ˈslɑːndə/ pomluva, hanobení

slang /slæŋ/ slang, hantýrka, nadávat

slap /slæp/ poklepat, fackovat, pohlavkovat, rána

slight /slaɪt/ nepatrný, mírný, drobný

slightly /ˈslaɪt.li/ trochu, nepatrně

slip /slɪp/ sklouznout, protáhnout, vsunout

slipper /ˈslɪp.ər/ bačkora, trepka

slippery /ˈslɪp.ər.i/ kluzký, klouzavý

slope /sləʊp/ sklon, svah

slowdown /ˈsləʊ.daʊn/ zpomalení

sludge /slʌdʒ/ kal, usazenina

SLUDGE, Salivation, Lacrimation, Urination, Diarrhoea, Gastrointestinal distress, Emesis příznaky otravy, slinění, slzení, močení, průjem, zažívací potíže, zvracení

slump /slʌmp/ prudce poklesnout, propadnout se, krize

slur /slɜːr/ mumlat opile, ospale apod.

slurred /ˈslɜːd/ nejasný

small /smɔːl/ bowel /ˈbaʊ.əl/ tenké střevo

smell /smel/ čich, cítit (čichem), být cítit

smooth /smuːð/ hladký, klidný

snake /sneɪk/ had

snap /snæp/ zapadnout, prasknout

sneeze /sniːz/ kýchnout, kýchnutí

sniffing /snɪf.ɪŋ/ čichání

snore /snɔːr/ chrápat, zachrápání

soaked /səʊkt/ nasáklý, promáčený

sob /sɒb/ vzlykat, vzlyk

soccer /ˈsɒk.ər/ fotbal

sodium /ˈsəʊ.di.əm/ chloride / ˈklɔːraɪd/ chlorid sodný, kuchyňská sůl

sodium /ˈsəʊ.di.əm/ sodík

sodium bicarbonate /ˌsəʊ.di.əm. baɪˈkɑː.bən.ət/ hydrouhličitan sodný, soda

soft /sɒft/ měkký, jemný

softly /ˈsɒft.li/ jemně, tlumeně

sole /səʊl/ chodidlo, ploska

solid /ˈsɒl.ɪd/ pevný, tvrdý, jednolitý

solution /səˈluː.ʃən/ řešení, roztok, rozpuštění

solvent /ˈsɒl.vənt/ ředidlo, rozpouštědlo

somatic /səˈmæt.ɪk/ somatický, tělesný, tělový

somewhat /ˈsʌm.wɒt/ trochu, poněkud

sore /sɔː/ throat /θrəʊt/ bolest v krku

sore /sɔːr/ bolavý, bolestivý

sorting /sɔːt.ɪŋ/ třídění, roztřídění, řazení

sound /saʊnd/ zvuk, znít

source /sɔːrs/ zdroj, příčina

space /speɪs/ prostor, mezera, vzdálenost

spasm /ˈspæz.əm/ křeč, záchvat

spasmodic /spæzˈmɒd.ɪk/ spazmický, křečovitý

specific /spəˈsɪf.ɪk/ specifický, konkrétní, přesný

specify /ˈspes.ɪ.faɪ/ specifikovat, vymezit, určit

speck /spek/ skvrnka

speech /spiːtʃ/ řeč, mluvení

speed /spiːd/ rychlost, řítit se

speed up /ˈspiːd.ʌp/ zrychlit, zvýšit rychlost

spell /spel/ doba, (krátké) období

sphincter /ˈsfɪŋk.tər/ svěrač

spider /ˈspaɪ.dər/ pavouk

spiderweb /ˈspaɪ.dəz.web/ pavoučí síť

spill /spɪl/ rozlít, rozsypat, vysypat

spinal /ˈspaɪ.nəl/ **cord** /kɔːd/ mícha

spinal /ˈspaɪ.nəl/ páteřní, míšní

spine /spaɪn/ **board** /bɔːd/ páteřní deska

splash /splæʃ/ postříkat, šplíchnutí

spleen /spliːn/ slezina

splenic /spliːn.ɪk/ splenický, slezinný

splint /splɪnt/ dlaha, zpevnit dlahou

sponge /spʌndʒ/ mycí houba, omývat

spontaneous /spɒnˈteɪ.ni.əs/ spontánní, samovolný

spot /spɒt/ skvrna, zpozorovat, všimnout si

spotting /spɒt.ɪŋ/ krvavý výtok z dělohy mezi menstruačními obdobími

spousal /ˈspaʊzəl/ manželský

spouse /spaʊs/ choť, manžel/ka

sprain /spreɪn/ podvrtnout, vymknout, vyvrtnutí, výron

spray /spreɪ/ rozprašovač, postříkat

spurt /spɜːt/ prýštit, tryskat, vystříknutí, proud

sputum /ˈspjuː.təm/ sputum, hlen při vykašlávání

squad /skwɒd/ oddíl, tým

squeeze /skwiːz/ zmáčknout, stisknutí

stab /stæb/ bodnout

stabilization /ˌsteɪ.bɪ.laɪˈzeɪ.ʃən/ stabilizace, ustálení

stable /ˈsteɪ.bl̩/ stabilní, stabilizovaný, stálý

stage /steɪdʒ/ stádium, etapa

stagnate /stægˈneɪt/ stagnovat, váznout

stain /steɪn/ skvrna, zašpinit

stand /stænd/ **for** /fə/ znamenat, značit

stand /stænd/ **in** zastoupit, zaskočit

standard /ˈstæn.dəd/ standard, zásada, obvyklý, běžný

standing /stænd.ɪŋ/ **order** /ˈɔːdə/ trvalý příkaz

state /steɪt/ stav, uvádět, prohlašovat

statement /ˈsteɪt.mənt/ prohlášení, výpověď

station /ˈsteɪ.ʃən/ být umístěný, pozice, stanoviště

status /ˈsteɪ.təs/ **asthmaticus** /æsθˈmæt.ɪk.əs/ status asthmaticus, těžký a prolongovaný záchvat bronchiálního astmatu se závažnou poruchou dýchání, změnami v parciálním tlaku krevních plynů a ve vnitřním prostředí

status /ˈsteɪ.təs/ status, stav

statute /ˈstætju:t/ zákon, předpis

steadily /ˈsted.ɪ.li/ stále, plynule

steady /ˈsted.i/ stálý

steering /'stɪər.ɪŋ/ wheel /wiːl/ volant

sternal /'stɔː.nəl/ sternální, týkající se hrudní kosti

sternum /'stɜː.nəm/ sternum, hrudní kost

stethoscope /'steθ.ə.skəʊp/ stetoskop, přístroj zesilující zvuky v tělních dutinách (na poslech hrudníku)

stick /stɪk/ (stuck, stuck) uvíznout, píchnout, bodnout

stick /stɪk/ hůl k chůzi

stiff /stɪf/ tvrdý, ztuhlý, neohebný

stiffness /'stɪf.nəs/ strnulost, ztuhlost, ztuhnutí

stimulant /'stɪm.jʊ.lənt/ stimulant, povzbuzující prostředek

stimulus /'stɪm.jʊ.ləs/ stimuli podnět, popud

sting /stɪŋ/ štípnutí, bodnutí, žihadlo, píchnout

stingray /'stɪŋ.reɪ/ trnucha, rejnok s jedovým bodcem na ocase

stoma /'stəʊ.mə/ ústa, malý otvor, pór, uměle vytvořený otvor mezi dutinami

stomach /'stʌm.ək/ žaludek, břicho

stonelike /'stəʊn.laɪk/ kameni podobný

stool /stuːl/ stolice, výkaly

storage /'stɔː.rɪdʒ/ ukládání, uchovávání, uschování

storm /stɔːm/ bouře

straight /streɪt/ přímo, přímý, rovný

strain /streɪn/ nápor, zátěž, namáhat, přetěžovat

streak /striːk/ stopa, proužek

stream /striːm/ proud, pramínek, téci

strenuous /'stren.ju.əs/ namáhavý, vysilující

stressor /'strɛs.ə/ stresor, prostředek, stav či podnět, který způsobí stres

stretch /stretʃ/ protáhnout, protažení

stretcher /'stretʃə/ nosítka pro zraněné

stridor /straɪd.ər/ stridor, pískavý zvuk při ztíženém dýchaní

strike /straɪk/ (struck, struck) zasáhnout, postihnout, udeřit

strike /straɪk/ úder

striking /'straɪ.kɪŋ/ nápadný, výrazný

stroke /strəʊk/ mozková mrtvice, úder, bití pulsu

stroke /strəʊk/ volume /'vɒl.juːm/ tepový objem, objem krve, který srdce vypudí při jednom srdečním stahu tepu, systole

structural /'strʌkt.ʃərəl/ konstrukční, stavební

structure /'strʌk.tʃər/ struktura, stavba

stupor /'stjuː.pər/ mrákoty, otupělost, bezvědomí

subarachnoid /ˌsʌb.ə'ræk.nɔɪd/ subarachnoideální, ležící pod pavučnicovou blánou

subclavian /sʌb'kleɪv.ɪ.ən/ podklíčkový, uložený pod klíční kostí

subconjunctival /ˌsʌb.kɒn.dʒaŋk.'tɪ.vəl/ subkonjunktivální, podspojivkový

subcutaneous /ˌsʌb.kjʊˈteɪ.ni.əs/ subkutánní, podkožní

subdiaphragmatic /ˌsʌbˌdaɪə.frægˈmæt.ɪk/ subdiafragmatický, ležící pod bránicí

subdural /sʌbˈdjʊ.ə.rəl/ subdurální, ležící pod tvrdou plenou mozkovou

subglottic /sʌbˈglɒt.ɪk/ subglotický, pod hlasivkami

sublingual /sʌbˈlɪŋ.gwəl/ sublingvální, podjazykový

subluxation /ˌsʌb.lʌkˈseɪ.ʃən/ subluxace, neúplné vykloubení, posuntí

subsequent /ˈsʌb.sɪ.kwənt/ pozdější, následující

subside /səbˈsaɪd/ polevit, zmírnit

substance /ˈsʌb.stənt s/ substance, látka, hmota

substantial /səbˈstæn.ʃəl/ podstatný, značný, velký

substernal /sʌbˈstɜ.nəl/ substernální, ležící pod hrudní kostí

successfully /səkˈses.fə.li/ úspěšně

succession /səkˈseʃ.ən/ řada, série

suck /sʌk/ sát, odsávat

suction /ˈsʌk.ʃən/ odsávání, odsávat

sudden /ˈsʌd.ən/ náhlý, nečekaný

suddenly /ˈsʌd.ən.li/ náhle, najednou

sue /sju:/ zažalovat, podat žalobu

suffer /ˈsʌf.ər/ trpět, utrpět, zhoršit se

suffering /ˈsʌf.ər.ɪŋ/ **from** /frəm/ trpící čím

suggestive /səˈdʒes.tɪv/ připomínající, nasvědčující

suicidal /ˌsu:ɪˈsaɪdəl/ sebevražedný, se sklony k sebevraždě

suit /sju:t/ oblek

suitable /ˈsju:.tə.bļ/ vhodný

sulphate /ˈsʌl.feɪt/ sulfát, síran

superheat /ˈsu:.pəˌhi:t/ přehřát, přehřívat páru ap.

superior /su:ˈpɪə.ri.ər/ horní, vyšší

supervise /ˈsu:pəˌvaɪz/ dohlížet, mít na starost

supervisor /ˈsu:.pə.vaɪ.zər/ dozor, nadřízený

supination /ˈsu:.pɪn.əɪ.ʃən/ supinace, lat. supinus, obrácený vzhůru, rotace předloktí, kterou se u končetiny visící podél těla otočí dlaň dopředu, tzn. malíkem k tělu

supine /ˈsu:.paɪn/ ležící naznak, ležící na zádech, tváří vzhůru, klidný

supplement /ˈsʌp.lɪ.mənt/ doplnit, dodatek

supplemental /ˌsʌp.lɪˈmen.təl/ doplňkový, dodatečný

supply /səˈplaɪ/ zásobovat, doplnit, potřeby, zásoby

support /səˌpɔ:t/ podpora, podporovat, podepřít

supportive /səˈpɔ:.tɪv/ nápomocný, podporující

suppress /səˈpres/ potlačit, zastavit

suppression /səˈpreʃ.ən/ potlačení, potlačování

suppressive /səˈpres.ɪv/ potlačující, zatajující

supraventricular /ˈsuːprə.venˈtrɪk.jə.lər/ supraventrikulární, ležící nad srdeční komorou

surface /ˈsɜː.fɪs/ povrch, hladina, zevnějšek, vynořit

surfactant /sər.fakˈtənt/ surfaktant, povrchově aktivní látka, pokrývající vnitřek plicních sklípků, nedostatečně vyvinut u předčasně narozených dětí, poškozován i v průběhu těžkých plicních chorob dospělých

surgery /ˈsɜː.dʒər.i/ chirurgie, chirurgický zákrok

surround /səˈraʊnd/ obklopovat

surroundings /səˈraʊn.dɪŋz/ prostředí, okolní podmínky

survey /ˈsɜː.veɪ/ průzkum, přehled, vyšetření, prohlídka, posoudit

survivability /səˈvaɪv.əˈbɪl.ə.ti/ schopnost přežít, přetrvat

survival /səˈvaɪ.vəl/ přežití

survive /səˈvaɪv/ žít, přečkat, přetrvat

survivor /səˈvaɪ.vər/ přeživší, pozůstalý

susceptible /səˈsep.tɪ.bļ/ náchylný, snadno podléhající

suspect /səˈspekt/ mít podezření, domnívat se

suspected /səˈspek.tɪd/ suspektní, domnělý podezřelý

suspicion /səˈspɪʃən/ podezření, podezírání

suspicious /səˈspɪʃ.əs/ nedůvěřivý, podezíravý

sustain /səˈsteɪn/ vydržet, snést, utrpět

swallow / ˈswɒl.əʊ/ polykat, spolknout, hlt

sweat /swet/ pot, potit se

sweep /swiːp/ (swept, swept) shrnout, stáhnout, smést

swelling /ˈswelɪŋ/ otok, opuchlina

swiftly /ˈswɪft.li/ rychle, pohotově

swing /swɪŋ/ prudká změna, obrat, kývat

switch /swɪtʃ/ prohodit, vyměnit, přepnout

swollen /ˈswəʊ.lən/ oteklý, zduřelý

sympathetic /ˌsɪm.pəˈθet.ɪk/ týkající se sympatického nervového systému

sympathomimetic /ˌsɪm.pə.θə.mɪˈmet.ɪk/ **syndrome** /ˈsɪn.drəʊm/ sympatomimetický syndrom, soubor příznaků způsobený otravou látkami se sympatomimetickými účinky např. kofein, theofylin, kokain, amfetamin, efedrin

symptom /ˈsɪmp.təm/ symptom, příznak

syncope /ˈsɪŋ.kə.pɪ/ synkopa, přechodné náhlé bezvědomí v důsledku omezení krevního přísunu do mozku

syncytial /sɪnˈsɪ.ʃɪ.əl/ **virus** /ˈvaɪrəs/ syncytiální virus, způsobuje záněty dýchacích cest, množení viru vede ke splývání sousedních buněk a vzniku syncytia

syndrome /ˈsɪn.drəʊm/ syndrom

syphilis /ˈsɪf.ɪ.lɪs/ syfilis

syringe /sɪˈrɪndʒ/ injekční stříkačka

systemic /sɪˈstem.ɪk/ systemický, týkající se těla jako celku

systolic /sɪsˈtɑl.ɪk/ systolický, týkající se systoly

T

tachycardia /ˌtæk.ɪˈkɑː.di.ə/ tachykardie

tachydysrhythmia /ˌtæk.ɪ.dɪsˈrɪθ.mɪə/ tachyarytmie, nepravidelná a urychlená srdeční akce

tachypnoea /ˌtæk.ɪp.ˈniː.ə/ tachypnoe, zrychlené dýchání

tackle /ˈtæk.l̩/ zákrok, napadat hráče, obrat o míč

tag /tæg/ cedulka, visačka, označit jmenovkou, cedulkou

tail /teɪl/ zadní část, ocas

take /teɪk/ **breath** /breθ/ vdechnout

take /teɪk/ **care** /keər/ pečovat, starat se

take /teɪk/ **time** /taɪm/ trvat, věnovat čas

tamponade /tæm.pəˈneɪd/ tamponáda, stlačení srdce tekutinou nahromaděnou v perikardu, tamponování

tan /tæn/ opálit se, opálení

tank /tæŋk/ cisterna, nádrž

tap /tæp/ poklepat, zaťukání

tape /teɪp/ lepicí páska, přilepit, zalepit

target /ˈtɑː.gɪt/ cíl, úkol

tarry /ˈtær.i/ térový, dehtový

task /tɑːsk/ úkol, úloha

teammate /ˈtiːm.meɪt/ spoluhráč

tear /teər/ protržení, trhlina, trhat, odtrhnout, roztrhnout se, protrhnout se

tearing /ˈteər.ɪŋ/ prudký

tearing /tɪer.ɪŋ/ pláč

teary /ˈtɪə.r.i/ uslzený

telephone /ˈtel.ɪ.fəʊn/ telefon, telefonní

temporal /ˈtem.pər.əl/ temporální, spánkový

temporary /ˈtempərərɪ/ dočasný, přechodný

tend /tend/ **to the needs of sb** zajišťovat potřeby někoho

tendency /ˈten.dən.si/ tendence, sklon

tender /ˈten.dər/ měkký, citlivý

tenderness /ˈten.də.nəs/ bolestivost, citlivost na dotek

tendon tendines /ˈten.dən/ šlacha

tension /ˈtent.ʃən/ **pneumothorax** /ˌnjuːməˈθɔː.ræks/ tenzní pneumotorax, vzduch v pohrudniční dutině

tension /ˈtent.ʃən/ tenze, napětí, tlak, tonus

tepid /ˈtep.ɪd/ vlažný, vlahý

teres /ˈtiː.riːz/ **teretes** sval nebo vazivo cylindrického tvaru

term /tɜːm/ termín, název

terminal /ˈtɜː.mɪ.nəl/ konečný, smrtelný, konečné stádium nemoci, umírající pacient

terminate /ˈtɜː.mɪ.neɪt/ ukončit, přerušit

termination /ˌtɜː.mɪˈneɪ.ʃən/ ukončení

tertiary /ˈtɜː.ʃər.i/ terciární, třetího stupně

therapy /ˈθer.ə.pi/ terapie, léčba

thereby /ˌðeəˈbaɪ/ tímto, a tím

therefore /ˈðeə.fɔːr/ proto, toho důvodu

thermal /ˈθɜː.məl/ tepelný

thiamine /ˈθaɪ.ə.miːn/ thiamin, vitamin B 1

thick /θɪk/ hustý

thicken /ˈθɪk.ən/ tloustnout, zhušťovat se

thickness /ˈθɪknɪs/ síla, tloušťka v průřezu

thigh /θaɪ/ stehno

thin /θɪn/ tenký, prořídnout

thoracic /θɔːˈræs.ɪk/ **cavity** /ˈkæv.ɪ.ti/ dutina hrudní

thorax /ˈθɔː.ræks/ hrudník

thorough /ˈθʌr.ə/ důkladný, podrobný

thought /θɔːt/ myšlenka, myšlenkový

thrash /θræʃ/ bít, tlouci

thready /ˈθred.i/ nitkovitý

threat /θret/ hrozba, ohrožení, výhrůžka

threaten /ˈθret.ən/ hrozit, vyhrožovat

threshold /ˈθreʃ.h əʊld/ práh, hranice

thrombolytic /θrɒm.bɒˈlit.ɪk/ **therapy** /ˈθer.ə.pi/ trombolytická léčba, rozpuštění trombu

thrombolytic /θrɒm.bəˈlɪt.ɪk/ trombolytický, rozpouštějící krevní sraženinu, trombus

thrombosis /θrɒmˈbəʊ.sɪs/ trombóza, srážení krve v cévách za živa

through /θruː/ přes, skrz, napříč, po celém

throughout /θruːˈaʊt/ po celém, ve všech částech, po celou dobu

throw /θrəʊ/ (threw, thrown) mrštit, hodit

thrust /θrʌst/ úder, vražení, tah

thumb / θʌm/ palec na ruce

thyroid /ˈθaɪə .rɔɪd/ **storm** /stɔːm/ život ohrožující komplikace zvýšené činnosti štítné žlázy

thyroid gland /ˈθaɪə .rɔɪd ˌglænd/ štítná žláza, štítný, týkající se štítné žlázy

thyrotoxicosis /ˌθaɪˈrəˌtɒksiˈkəʊ. sɪs/ tyreotoxikóza, otrava způsobená hyperfunkcí štítné žlázy

tibia /ˈtɪb.i.ə/ pl -ae holeň, kost holenní

tidal /ˈtaɪ.dəl/ přílivový, týkající se respiračního vzduchu

tidal /ˈtaɪdəl/ **volume** /ˈvɒljuːm/ objem vzduchu při nádechu, dechový objem, objem vzduchu nadechnutého či vydechnutého při jednom dechu

tiered /tɪəd/ víceúrovňový

tight /taɪt/ těsný, pevný

tightly /ˈtaɪt.li/ těsně

tightness /ˈtaɪt.nəs/ tíseň, těsnost, napětí

tilt /tɪlt/ sklon, naklonit, sklopit

time /taɪm/ čas, načasovat, naplánovat

times /taɪmz/ krát, opakovaně

timing /ˈtaɪ.mɪŋ/ načasování

tip /tɪp/ naklonit se, sklonit se, špička, hrot

tired /ˈtaɪəd/ unavený, vyčerpaný

tiring /ˈtaɪə.rɪŋ/ vyčerpávající

tissue /'tɪʃ.u:/, /'tɪs.ju:/ tkáň, papírový kapesník

titrate /'taɪ.treɪt/ titrovat, (titrace, metoda určení přesné dávky léku pomocí zkusmého dávkování od nižší k vyšší dávce s pečlivým sledování efektu)

TKO, **To Keep** (**venous** /'vi:.nəs/ **infusion** / ɪn'fju:.ʒən/ **line** /laɪn/) **Open** udržovat otevřený vstup pro žilní infuzi

toddler /'tɒd.lər/ batole, dítě učící se chodit

toe /təʊ/ prst na noze

tolerance /'tɒl.ər.əns/ tolerance, snášenlivost

tolerate /'tɒl.ər.eɪt/ tolerovat snášet

tone /təʊn/ napětí svalu nebo cévní stěny, nervové napětí

tongue /tʌŋ/ jazyk, špice

tool /tu:l/ nástroj, pomůcka, prostředek

top /tɒp/ navršit, navýšit, vrchol, vrchní část

topical /'tɒp.ɪ.kəl/ místní

total /'təʊ.təl/ celkem, úplný

touch /tʌtʃ/ dotknout se, dotek

touching /'tʌtʃ.ɪŋ/ dotknutí se

tourniquet /'tʊə.nɪ.keɪ/ škrtidlo, tlakový obvaz

toward /tə'wɔ:d/ směrem k, ve vztahu k

towel /taʊəl/ ručník

toxaemia /tɒk'si:.mi.ə/ toxemie, otrava krve

toxicity /tɒk'sɪs.ɪ.ti/ toxicita, jedovatost

toxin /'tɒk.sɪn/ toxin, jedovatá látka

trachea /trə'ki:.ə/ trachea, průdušnice

tracheal /trə'ki:.əl/ tracheální, průdušnicový

tracheobronchial /trə.ki:.ə'brɒŋ.ki.əl/ tracheobronchiální, týkající se průdušnice a průdušek

tracheostomy /ˌtræk.i'ɒst.ə.mi/ tracheostomie, chirurg. vytvoření otvoru do průdušnice k umožnění dýchání

track /træk/ dráha, cesta, sledovat

traction /'træk.ʃən/ trakce, tah

trained /treɪnd/ školený, kvalifikovaný

transection /ˌtræn'sek.ʃən/ příčný řez

transfer /træns'fɜ:r/ přemístit, přesunout, přesun

transient /'træn.zi.ənt/ přechodný, nestálý

transition /træn'zɪʃ.ən/ přechod, změna stavu

transmit /trænz'mɪt/ přenášet, rozšířit

transparent /træn'spær.ənt/ transparentní, průhledný

transport /'træn.spɔ:t/ transport, doprava

trap /træp/ past, nástraha, zachycovat

trauma /'trɔ:.mə/ trauma, zranění

traumatic /trɔ:'mæt.ɪk/ traumatický, úrazový

travel /'træv.əl/ cestovat, putovat, pohybovat se

treat /tri:t/ zacházet, jednat, léčit

treatable /triːt.ə.bḷ/ léčitelný
treatment /ˈtriːt.mənt/ léčení, ošetření
tremendous /trɪˈmen.dəs/ ohromný, obrovský
tremor /ˈtrem.ər/ třes, chvění
trench /trentʃ/ zákop
Trendelenburg /tren.del.ˈen. berg/ **position** /pəˈzɪʃ.ən/ Trendelenburgova poloha, při níž pacient leží na zádech a jeho pánev je uložena výše než hlava, užívá se při šoku k zlepšení prokrvení životně důležitých orgánů
triad /ˈtraɪ.æd/ triáda, trojice
triage /ˈtraɪ.ɪdʒ/ rychlé třídění raněných a nemocných, stanovení priorit dle naléhavosti
tricuspid valve /traɪˈkʌs.pɪdˌvælv/ trikuspidální (trojcípá) chlopeň
trigger /ˈtrɪg.ər/ spustit, vyvolat, vzbudit, spoušť zbraně
trim /trɪm/ oříznout, ostříhnout, zkrátit
trimester /trɪˈmes.tər/ trimestr
trip /trɪp/ zakopnout, klopýtnout
tripod /ˈtraɪ.pɒd/ trojnožka
troubleshoot /ˈtrʌb.ḷ.ʃuːt/ řešit problémy, odstraňovat závady
truck /trʌk/ nákladní auto, kamión
trunk /trʌŋk/ trup
trunking /ˈtrʌŋkɪŋ/ systém sdílených telefonních linek, umožňuje služby pro velký počet lidí současně
trust /trʌst/ důvěra, věřit
tube /tjuːb/ trubice, trubička
tug /tʌg/ trhnutí, cuknutí

tumour /ˈtjuː.mər/ tumor, nádor
turn /tɜːn/ **blue** /bluː/ zmodrat
turn /tɜːn/ **off** /ɒf/ odbočit, vypnout
turn out /ˈtɜːnˌaʊt/ zahnout ven, naruby, projevit se
twist/ˌtwɪst/ zkroutit, stočit, vyvrtnout si
twitch /twɪtʃ/ škubat, trhat, záškuby částí svalů
tympanic /ˈtɪm.pə.nik/ **membrane** /mem.breɪn/ ušní bubínek
tympanic /ˈtɪm.pə.nik/ tympanický, bubínkový
tyre /taɪər/ pneumatika

U
ulcer /ˈʌl.sər/ vřed
ultimate /ˈʌl.tɪ.mət/ konečný, závěrečný, poslední
umbilical /ʌmˈbɪl.ɪ.kəl/ pupeční
umbilical cord /ʌmˈbɪl.ɪ.kəlˌkɔːd/ pupeční šňůra
umbilicus /ʌmˈbɪl.ɪ.kəs/ pupek
unaffected /ˌʌn.əˈfek.tɪd/ nedotčený, nezasažený
unambiguous /ˌʌnæmˈbɪgjʊəs/ jednoznačný, zcela jasný
unattended /ˌʌn.əˈten.dɪd/ bez dozoru, nehlídaný
unaware /ˌʌn.əˈweər/ netušící, neuvědomující si
uncomfortable /ʌnˈkʌmp f.tə.bḷ/ nesvůj, necítící se dobře
uncompensated /ˌʌnˈkɒmpənseɪtɪd/ nekompenzovaný
unconscious /ʌnˈkɒnʃəs/ v bezvědomí
unconsciousness /ʌnˈkɒn.ʃəs.nəs/ bezvědomí

uncontrollably /ˌʌn.kənˈtrəʊ.lə.bli/ neovladatelně

uncontrolled /ˌʌn.kənˈtrəʊld/ nekontrolovatelný, neovladatelný, neřízený

under /ˈʌn.dər/ pod, podle, v souladu

underage /ˌʌn.dəˈreɪdʒ/ nezletilý, neplnoletý

underground /ˌʌn.dəˈgraʊnd/ podzemní

underlying /ˌʌndəˈlaɪ.ɪŋ/ skrytý, pod povrchem, základní, spodní

underneath /ˌʌn.dəˈniːθ/ hned pod čím, bezprostředně pod

undernourished /ˌʌn.dəˈnʌr.ɪʃt/ podvyživený, trpící podvýživou

undetected /ˌʌn.dɪˈtekt.əd/ nezjištěný, neobjevený

uneasiness /ʌnˈiː.zi.nəs/ neklid, znepokojení, nepříjemný pocit

unequal /ʌnˈiː.kwəl/ nerovný, nedostatečný, neschopný zvládnout

unevenly /ʌnˈiː.vən.li/ nestejně, nerovnoměrně

unfamiliar /ʌn.fəˈmɪl.i.ər/ cizí, neznámý

unilateral /ˌjuː.nɪˈlæt.ər.əl/ unilaterální, jednostranný

unilaterally /ˌjuː.nɪˈlæt.ər.əl.i/ unilaterálně, jednostranně

unintentional /ˌʌn.ɪnˈten.ʃən.əl/ neúmyslný, bezděčný

unlawful /ʌnˈlɔːfʊl/ nezákonný, protizákonný

unlike /ʌnˈlaɪk/ na rozdíl od, odlišný od

unlikely /ʌnˈlaɪ.kli/ nepravděpodobný

unnoticed /ʌnˈnəʊ.tɪst/ nepozorovaný, nepovšimnutý

unprovoked /ˌʌn.prəˈvəʊkt/ nevyprovokovaný, ničím nevyvolaný

unrecognized /ʌnˈrek.əg.naɪzd/ nerozpoznaný, bez povšimnutí

unrelated /ˌʌn.rɪˈleɪ.tɪd/ netýkající se, vzájemně nesouvisející

unremarkable /ˌʌn.rɪˈmɑː.kə.bl̩/ nezajímavý, obyčejný

unresponsive /ˌʌn.rɪˈspɒnt.sɪv/ bez reakce, nereagující, netečný

unrestrained /ˌʌn.rɪˈstreɪnd/ nespoutaný, nevázaný

unsafe /ʌnˈseɪf/ nebezpečný, zdravotně závadný

unsalvageable /ʌnˈsæl.vɪdʒ.ə.bl̩/ nezachránitelný, jemuž není pomoci

unseen /ʌnˈsiːn/ neviditelný, nevídaný

unstable /ʌnˈsteɪ.bl̩/ nestabilní, nestálý

unsure /ʌnˈʃɔːr/ nejistý, nesmělý

untreated /ʌnˈtriː.tɪd/ neléčený, neošetřený

unwanted /ʌnˈwɒn.tɪd/ nechtěný, nežádoucí

upgrade /ʌpˈgreɪd/ zlepšit, stoupnout, zvýšení

uphill /ˌʌpˈhɪl/ nahoru

upon /əˈpɒn/ na, za, ihned po

upper /ˈʌp.ər/ horní

upright /ˈʌp.raɪt/ vzpřímeně, vertikálně, svisle

upset /ʌp'set/ podráždění, rozrušený, znepokojený, narušit

upwind /,ʌp'wɪnd/ proti větru

uraemia /jʊə'riː.mɪ.ə/ uremie, chronické selhání činnosti ledvin

uraemic /jʊə'riː.mɪk/ uremický, týkající se uremie

urea /jʊə'riː.ə/ **frost** /frɒst/ klinický nález při chronickém renálním selhání, koncentrace močoviny je výrazně zvýšená v potu a způsobuje srážení krystalizované močoviny v pokožce

urethra /jʊə'riː.θrə/ močová trubice

urge /ɜːdʒ/ naléhat, nutkání, naléhavá potřeba

urgent /'ɜː.dʒənt/ urgentní, naléhavý, neodkladný

urinate /'jʊə.rɪ.neɪt/ močit

urination /,jʊə.rɪ'neɪ.ʃən/ močení

urticaria /,ɔː.tɪ'keə.ri.ə/ kopřivka

use /juːz/ užít, použít, použití

uterine /'juː.tər.aɪn/ **wall** /wɔːl/ uterinní, děložní stěna

uterus /'juː.tər.əs/ uterus, děloha

utility /juː'tɪl.ɪ.ti/ služby (veřejné), technická infrastruktura, dodávky vody, doprava

utilize /'juː.tɪ.laɪz/ použít, uplatnit

V

vagal /'veɪ gəl/ **tone** /təʊn/ úroveň aktivity v parasympatickém nervovém systému

vagal /'veɪ gəl/ vagální, vztahující se k nervus vagus

vague /veɪg/ vágní, nejasný, neurčitý

vagus /vəɪ.gəs/ pl -gi bloudivý nerv, X. hlavový nerv

valid /'vælɪd/ platný, oprávněný

Valium /'væl.i.əm/ diazepam (benzodiazepinové anxiolytikum, antiepileptikum, uvolňuje svalové napětí)

vallecula /və'lek.jʊl.ə/ valekula, jamka, žlábek

Valsalva /væl'sæl.və/ **manoeuvre** / mə'nuː.vər/ Valsalvův manévr, přetlakování uší ucpáním nosu a zatlačením vzduchu do uší

valuable /'væl.jʊ.bļ/ cenný, hodnotný

value /'væl.juː/ hodnota, význam, cena

valve /vælv/ chlopeň, klapka, ventil

varicella /,vær.ɪ'sel.ə/ varicela, plané neštovice

varicose vein /,vær.ɪ.kəʊs'veɪn/ křečová žíla

varied /'veə.rɪd/ rozmanitý, různorodý, pestrý

variety /və'raɪə.ti/ rozmanitost, různost, různorodost

varix /,veə.rɪks/ **varices** /'vær.ɪ.siːz/ varix, křečová žíla, krevní městka

vary /'veə.ri/ lišit se, měnit se, kolísat

vascular /'væs.kjʊ.lər/ vaskulární, cévní

vasculature /'væs.kjʊ.lə.tʃər/ vaskularita, cévnatost

vasoconstriction /,veɪ.zə.kən'strɪk.ʃən/ vazokonstrikce, zúžení cév

vasodilatation /,veɪ.zə.daɪ.lə'teɪ.ʃən/ vazodilatace, rozšíření cév

vasodilator /ˌveɪ.zə.daɪˈleɪ.tər/ vazodilátor, vyvolávající rozšíření cévy

vasospasm /ˌveɪ.zəʊˈspæzm/ vazospasmus, stažení svalové stěny cév se zúžením průsvitu

vasovagal /ˌveɪ.zəʊˈvæg.əl/ vazovagální, popisující působení n. vagus na krevní oběh

vault /vɔːlt/ klenba

vein /veɪn/ žíla

velocity /vɪˈlɒsɪtɪ/ rychlost

vena cava /ˌviː.nəˈkeɪ.və/ dutá žíla

venipuncture /ˌve.niˈpʌŋk.tʃər/ nabodnutí žíly, puštění žilou

venom /ˈvenəm/ jed hadí ap.

venous /ˈviː.nəs/ **return** /rɪˈtɜːn/ žilní návrat

venous /ˈviː.nəs/ **capacitance** /kəˈpæs.ɪ.tənts/ žilní kapacitance (rozdíl objemu prázdné a krví naplněné žíly po nafouknutí tlakové manžety)

vent /vent/ ventilovat, otvor, průduch, ventil

ventilate /ˈven.tɪ.leɪt/ ventilovat, větrat

ventilation /ˌven.tɪˈleɪ.ʃən/ ventilace, dýchání, výměna plynů

ventilatory /ˈventɪˌleɪtə.rɪ/ ventilační, dechový

ventricle /ˈven.trɪ.kl̩/ ventrikl, komora, srdeční, mozková, tělní dutina, žaludek

ventricular /venˈtrɪk.jə.lər/ **fibrillation** /ˌfaɪ.brɪˈleɪ.ʃən/, /ˌfɪb. rɪˈleɪ.ʃən/ fibrilace srdečních komor

ventricular /venˈtrɪk.jə.lər/ ventrikulární, komorový

verification /ˌver.ɪ.fɪˈkeɪ.ʃən/ verifikace, ověření, potvrzení

verify /ˈver.ɪ.faɪ/ verifikovat, ověřit si, potvrdit

vertebral /ˈvɜː.tɪ.brəl/ vertebrální, obratlový, páteřní

vessel /ˈves.əl/ céva

vestibular /vesˈtɪb.jə.lər/ vestibulární, předsíňový

via /ˈvaɪə/ přes, prostřednictvím

viable /ˈvaɪ.ə.bl̩/ životaschopný, funkční

victim /ˈvɪk.tɪm/ oběť

violate /ˈvaɪəˌleɪt/ narušit, porušit, přestoupit

violence /ˈvaɪə.ləns/ násilí, násilný čin

violent /ˈvaɪələnt/ agresivní, prudký, silný, násilný

violently /ˈvaɪə.lənt.li/ násilně, agresivně

visceral /ˈvɪs.ər.əl/ viscerální, útrobní, vnitřní

visibility /ˌvɪz.ɪˈbɪl.ɪ.ti/ viditelnost

visible /ˈvɪz.ɪ.bl̩/ viditelný, zřejmý

visibly /ˈvɪz.ɪ.bli/ viditelně, očividně

vision /ˈvɪʒ.ən/ vidění, zrak

visualization /ˌvɪʒ.u.əl.aɪˈzeɪ. ʃən/ vizualizace, zviditelnění, představa

visualize /ˈvɪʒ.u.əl.aɪz/ zviditelnit, vizualizovat

vital /ˈvaɪ.təl/ **signs** /saɪnz/ životní znaky

vitals /'vaɪ.təlz/ známky života, fyziologické funkce
vocal /'vəʊkəl/ **cords** /kɔ:dz/ hlasivky
voice /vɔɪs/ hlas, hlasový, vyslovit vyjádřit (názor, mínění)
volume /'vɒl.ju:m/ objem, množství, hlasitost
voluntary /'vɒləntərɪ/ dobrovolný, vůlí ovladatelný
vomit /'vɒm.ɪt/ zvracet, zvracení
vomitus /'vɒm.ɪ.təs/ vomitus, zvratky

W
waist /weɪst/ pas
wander /'wɒn.dər/ toulat se, bloudit
warmed /ˌwɔ:md/ zahřátý, teplý
warning /'wɔ:.nɪŋ/ **sign** /saɪn/ varovné znamení
warning /'wɔ:.nɪŋ/ varování, upozornění
warrant /'wɒr.ənt/ oprávnit, opravňovat, vyžádat si, zasluhovat
waste /weɪst/ chřadnout, ochabovat, vyčerpat se
waste /weɪst/ **product** /'prɒdʌkt/ odpadní produkt
watch /wɒtʃ/ sledovat, pozorovat, dávat pozor
wave /weɪv/ vlna, kývat, mávnout čím
weak /wi:k/ slabý, křehký, nedostatečný
weakly /wi:k.li/ slabě
weakness /'wi:k.nəs/ ochablost, chatrnost, slabost

wear /weər/ vzít si na sebe, nosit oblečení
weight /weɪt/ **loss** /lɒs/ úbytek váhy
weight /weɪt/ váha, hmotnost
well /wel/ studna, šachta výtahová, schodišťová ap.
welt /welt/ šrám, podlitina
wheal /wi:l/ napuchlina, šrám, podlitina
wheeze /wi:z/ sípat, těžce dýchat, sípání
whereas /weər'æz/ kdežto, zatímco
whimper /'wɪmpə/ naříkat, skuhrat
whisper /'wɪs.pər/ šeptat, šepot
whistle /'wɪs.l/ pískat, hvízdat, pískání
white /waɪt/ oční bělmo
widen /'waɪ.dən/ rozšířit (se)
will /wɪl/ vůle
windshield /'wɪnd.ʃi:ld/ čelní sklo
wipe /waɪp/ otřít, utřít, ubrousek
wiper /'waɪp.ər/ utěrka
wire /waɪər/ drát
wire /waɪər/ **ladder** /'læd.ər/ typ dlahy
wish /wɪʃ/ přát, přání
withdraw /wɪð'drɔ:/ stáhnout, ustoupit, odejít
withdrawal /wɪð'drɔ:.əl/ ukončení, odstranění
withdrawn /wɪð'drɔ:n/ uzavřený, odtažitý
withhold /wɪð'həʊld/ zadržet, odebrat
within /wɪ'ðɪn/ uvnitř, v rámci
witness /'wɪt.nəs/ svědek, svědčit, potvrdit podpisem

worker /'wɜː.kər/ pracovník, zaměstnanec
workout /'wɜːkˌaʊt/ cvičení, trénink
worsen /'wɜː.sən/ zhoršit (se)
wounded /'wuːn.dɪd/ raněný
wrap /ræp/ zabalit, obal
wreck /rek/ zcela zničit, obrátit v trosky
wrestler /'res.lər/ zápasník
wrinkle /'rɪŋkəl/ vráska, záhyb
wrist /rɪst/ zápěstí

X
X-ray /'eks.reɪ/ rentgen, vyšetřit rentgenem
xiphoid /zi.foid/ **process** /'proʊ.ses/ měčovitý výběžek

Y
yard /jɑːd/ dvůr, zahrada
yell /jel/ ječet, ječení, výkřik
yellow jacket /'jel.oʊˌdʒæk.ɪt/ vosa, včela
yellowish /'jel.əʊ.ɪʃ/ nažloutlý

Z
zone /zəʊn/ zóna, oblast
zoster /zɒ.stər/ pásový opar

BIBLIOGRAPHY

- ABZ.cz: slovník cizích slov – on-line hledání: slovník-cizích-slov.abz.cz/

- Anglicko český slovník online: anglickoceskyslovník.cz/

- Cambridge Advanced Learner's Dictionary: http: dictionary.cambridge.org/

- CAMBRIDGE English Pronouncing Dictionary. 17th ed. Cambridge, Cambridge University Press 2006, 599 p.

- Marchetta Mark: Barron's Paramedic Exam. Barron's Emt Paramedic Exam. Barron's Educational Series 2008, 2nd ed. 275 p. ISBN: 9780764195587 (0764195581)

- Medical dictionary: medical-dictionary.thefreedictionary.com/

- Paramedic Certification Exam. Learning Express. New York 2009, 4th ed. 210 p. ISBN: 9781576856895

- Topilová, Věra: Anglicko-český, česko-anglický lékařský slovník. 1. vyd. Praha, Grada Publishing 1999, 878 s,

- IPA phonetic symbols – online keyboard: ipa.typeit.org/

- Velký lékařský slovník On-line: lékařské.slovniky.cz/

www.ingramcontent.com/pod-product-compliance
Lightning Source LLC
Chambersburg PA
CBHW020719180526
45163CB00001B/39